Perspectives on Biologically Based Cancer Risk Assessment

NATO • Challenges of Modern Society

A series of volumes comprising multifaceted studies of contemporary problems facing our society, assembled in cooperation with NATO Committee on the Challenges of Modern Society.

Recent volumes in this series:

Volume 7 AIR POLLUTION MODELING AND ITS APPLICATION IV
Edited by C. De Wispelaere

Volume 8 CONTAMINATED LAND: Reclamation and Treatment
Edited by Michael A. Smith

Volume 9 INTERREGIONAL AIR POLLUTION MODELING: The State of the Art
Edited by S. Zwerver and J. van Ham

Volume 10 AIR POLLUTION MODELING AND ITS APPLICATION V
Edited by C. De Wispelaere, Francis A. Schiermeier, and Noor V. Gillani

Volume 11 AIR POLLUTION MODELING AND ITS APPLICATION VI
Edited by Han van Dop

Volume 12 RISK MANAGEMENT OF CHEMICALS IN THE ENVIRONMENT
Edited by Hans M. Seip and Anders B. Heiberg

Volume 13 AIR POLLUTION MODELING AND ITS APPLICATION VII
Edited by Han van Dop

Volume 14 HEALTH AND MEDICAL ASPECTS OF DISASTER PREPAREDNESS
Edited by John C. Duffy

Volume 15 AIR POLLUTION MODELING AND ITS APPLICATION VIII
Edited by Han van Dop and Douw G. Steyn

Volume 16 DIOXIN PERSPECTIVES: A Pilot Study on International Information Exchange on Dioxins and Related Compounds
Edited by Erich W. Bretthauer, Heinrich W. Kraus, and Alessandro di Domenico

Volume 17 AIR POLLUTION MODELING AND ITS APPLICATION IX
Edited by Han van Dop and George Kallos

Volume 18 AIR POLLUTION MODELING AND ITS APPLICATION X
Edited by Sven-Eric Gryning and Millán M. Millán

Volume 19 METHODS OF PESTICIDE EXPOSURE ASSESSMENT
Edited by Patricia B. Curry, Sesh Iyengar, Pamela A. Maloney, and Marco Maroni

Volume 20 PLANNING ESTUARIES
Cees-Jan van Westen and Reinier Jan Scheele

Volume 21 AIR POLLUTION MODELING AND ITS APPLICATION XI
Edited by Sven-Eric Gryning and Francis A. Schiermeier

Volume 22 AIR POLLUTION MODELING AND ITS APPLICATION XII
Edited by Sven-Eric Gryning and Nadine Chaumerliac

Volume 23 PERSPECTIVES ON BIOLOGICALLY BASED CANCER RISK ASSESSMENT
Edited by Vincent James Cogliano, E. Georg Luebeck, and Giovanni A. Zapponi

Perspectives on Biologically Based Cancer Risk Assessment

Edited by

Vincent James Cogliano
United States Environmental Protection Agency
Washington, DC

E. Georg Luebeck
Fred Hutchinson Cancer Research Center
Seattle, Washington

and

Giovanni A. Zapponi
National Institute of Health
Rome, Italy

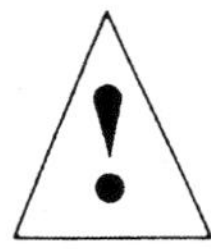

Published in cooperation with
NATO Committee on the Challenges of Modern Society

Kluwer Academic / Plenum Publishers
New York Boston Dordrecht London Moscow

Library of Congress Cataloging-in-Publication Data

Perspectives on biologically based cancer risk assessment / edited by
Vincent James Cogliano, E. Georg Luebeck, and Giovanni A. Zapponi.
p. cm. -- (NATO challenges of modern society ; v. 23)
"Published in cooperation with NATO Committee on the Challenges of
Modern Society."
Includes bibliographical references and index.
ISBN 0-306-46108-0. -- ISBN 0-306-46108-0
1. Carcinogens--Dose-response relationship. 2. Cancer--Risk
factors. 3. Health risk assessment. 4. Tumor markers.
I. Cogliano, Vincent James. II. Luebeck, E. Georg. III. Zapponi,
Giovanni A. IV. Series.
[DNLM: 1. Neoplasms--etiology. 2. Risk Assessment. QZ 202 P467
1999]
RC268.65.P47 1997
616.99'4071--dc21
DNLM/DLC
for Library of Congress 99-30081
CIP

Proceedings of the Final Report of the NATO CCMS Pilot Study on Dose Response Analysis and Biologically-Based Risk Assessment of Initiator and Promoter Carcinogens

ISBN: 0-306-46108-0

233 Spring Street, New York, N.Y. 10013

10 9 8 7 6 5 4 3 2 1

A C.I.P. record for this book is available from the Library of Congress

Printed in the United States of America

Preface

The first meeting of the NATO/CCMS Pilot Study "Dose-Response Analysis and Biologically-Based Risk assessment for Initiator and Promoter Carcinogens" was held in Rome, Italy, in the spring of 1991, and was followed by annual or bi-annual meetings held in Germany, Greece, Netherlands, Portugal, USA, up to the end of 1995; in large part supported by NATO/CCMS grants or fellowships, and organized by Pilot Study participants. The Pilot Study activity has been characterized by a higly collaborative atmosphere, which was essential for a deep and detailed analysis of a problem on which different points of view, methodological approaches and regulations exist in the various member countries.

The Pilot Study was aimed at proposing a carcinogenic risk assessment procedure which is based on a detailed analysis of the relevant biological processes, and may also consent the verification of hypotheses. The specific form of theoretical and mathematical models is identified by considering and using the whole set of objective data available. The multidisciplinary approach of the pilot study is reflected by the structure of this book. Each chapter is the result of the cooperation of several authors from different countries; its objective was to produce a comprehensive manual that includes both theoretical and practical information.

The main topics treated are:

- Basic Assumptions in Carcinogenic Risk Assessment
- The Biological Basis
- Data Sources
- The Use of Biomarkers in Risk Assessment
- Multistage Models
- Biologically-Based Modelling
- Statistical Considerations
- Case Studies and Practical Applications

The theoretical, mathematical and statistical basis of advanced carcinogenic risk assessment, together with its biological basis, are discussed in detail, keeping in mind the possible interests of readers specialized in this field as well as readers simply interested in the general aspects of carcinogenic risk assessment.

We are greatly indebted to the NATO/CCMS programme direction in Bruxelles and to our National CCMS Coordinators for the fundamental help they have provided to our work, as well as to all the institutes which have hosted and given support to the meetings.

The authors wish to express their appreciation to Ms. Lynn Schoolfield of the U.S. Environmental Protection Agency for her extra efforts to host three Pilot Study meetings in Washington and her devoted support of NATO-CCMS.

Contents

4. USE OF BIOCHEMICAL AND MOLECULAR BIOMARKERS FOR CANCER RISK ASSESSMENT IN HUMANS 81

J.J. Amaral-Mendes and E. Pluygers

Chapter 1

INTRODUCTION

V.J. Cogliano[1], E.D. Kroese[2], G.A. Zapponi[3], L. Attias[3] and I. Marcello[3]

[1]U.S. Environmental Protection Agency, Washington DC, USA
[2]Rijksinstituut voor Volksgezondheid en Milieuhygiene, Bilthoven, The Netherlands
[3]National Institute of Health, Rome, Italy

1.1. DOSE-RESPONSE ASSESSMENT IN NATO COUNTRIES

1.1.1. European Community

Chemical carcinogens represent a variety of (classes of) substances that are present in different media and compartments, which are determined by their sources, applications and use. With respect to dose-response assessment, within the context of quantitative risk assessment (QRA), these carcinogens are evaluated by various bodies, either on a national or international basis or both. For those chemicals present in air and water, an international harmonization of this risk evaluation is strived for by the Quality Guidelines of the World Health Organization (WHO, 1987, 1993). The same holds for food additives, contaminants, and pesticides, allowable levels of which are based on ADIs (allowable daily intakes) determined by the FAO/WHO committees JECFA and JMPR, respectively.

Most of the substances not considered by these international bodies, however, have to be dealt with on a national or continental level. On this level, there are substantial differences in the way the various countries or states approach this matter. Even within countries or states, different agencies or regulatory bodies may have different approaches to this subject. The basis for this is the different views held by experts in the field, the differences in legislation and regulatory history, public involvement, and government

[1]The views expressed in this chapter are those of the authors and do not necessarily reflect the views or policies of the U.S. Environmental Protection Agency.

Perspectives on Biologically Based Cancer Risk Assessment, edited by Cogliano *et al.*
Kluwer Academic/Plenum Publishers, New York, 1999.

structure between these countries or states. Also, the risk assessment approach used is influenced by the intended application of the results.

Within the European Union (EU) and its member states, dose-response assessment is commonly regarded as only one part of the broader process of risk assessment, generally agreed upon as consisting of the elements hazard identification, dose-response (effect) assessment and exposure assessment, and risk characterization (EU, 1993). Dose-response assessment and hazard identification are sometimes closely linked, however, as will be shown below.

1.1.1.1. European Union Within the EU carcinogens are classified depending on the weight of the evidence that the substance is a human carcinogen (EU, 1991). Dose-response analysis is not performed within the EU context, but on a member state level. This is due to the fact that in the hazard identification part of the risk assessment within the EU, the genotoxicity of the substance is also assessed. The outcome of this has consequences for the handling of these carcinogens and influences the procedures used for determining low-dose risks (EU, 1993). Carcinogens shown to be nongenotoxic are handled in the EU in the same way as noncarcinogenic substances, i.e., by identifying a no observed adverse effect level (NOAEL) and then using safety factors to arrive at an acceptable daily intake (ADI). The quantification of risks of genotoxic carcinogens (i.e., the dose-response analysis), is performed on a national basis within the EU member states. It is not expected that the EU itself will perform dose-response modeling or develop guidelines for it in the very near future. Considerations on carcinogenic potency may, on the other hand, be incorporated into the guidelines for setting specific concentration limits for carcinogens in substances or preparations (EU, 1995).

In most of the member states, genotoxic carcinogens are considered for a ban or an attempt is made to find a noncarcinogenic substitute. If these options are not possible, an exposure level associated with an acceptable risk level is determined by dose-response methodology, recognizing the absence of a safe dose, i.e., there is no threshold for the effect. The QRA methodology used here differs among countries; the evaluation of carcinogenicity and its underlying mechanisms is done by national expert committees on a case-by-case basis. Some of the national approaches in Europe will be shortly reviewed here.

1.1.1.2. The Netherlands In 1978 The National Health Council (NHC) proposed an approach to quantitative risk assessment of carcinogenic substances (NHC, 1978). Briefly, in this method a distinction is made between substances that induce DNA damage and may or may not stimulate precursor cell proliferation (now generally called genotoxic substances), and those that do not cause DNA damage but stimulate precursor cell proliferation only or have other effects relevant to carcinogenicity (now generally called nongenotoxic substances) (Kramers et al., 1991). In the quantitative risk evaluation, in deriving health-based recommended exposure limits for human exposure (to environmental carcinogenic substances), and for setting occupational standards, these differences in carcinogenic mechanism are accounted for. Mutagenesis is recognized as a stochastic process, i.e., the smallest dose is considered capable of inducing mutations, consequently this assumption implies the absence of a threshold. Nonmutagenic substances, on the other hand, are considered to act via a nonstochastic mechanism, since their effects are reversible, at least in an early stage, and the substance must bind to a large number of receptor sites or other molecules to induce its effects.

With respect to dose-response modeling, the following view was adopted and has recently been reestablished (NHC, 1994). The concept of the multistep nature of the process of carcinogenesis is well recognized. However, at very low dose levels the tumor induction will be a linear function of the dose, because it is assumed that the carcinogen will affect only a single hit (step), due to the abundance of endogenous and exogenous background hits (NHC, 1994; references cited herein). Even if a given agent acts purely by inducing mutations, without having promoting activity, or only having promoting activity, it may contribute to an increase in cancer risk if one assumes the existence of endogenous and ubiquitous exogenous factors that result in a background of initiated cells or promoting effects in every organism or tissue. Therefore, for genotoxic carcinogens or those carcinogens whose mechanism could not be resolved, a linear nonthreshold quantitative risk assessment method is used. Only a single (daily lifetime) dose-response data point is used, i.e., the lowest dose inducing an increased tumor-incidence relative to control incidence. From this dose a straight line through the origin is taken to estimate the exposure associated with an acceptable risk level or to arrive at the risk associated with actual human exposure. Thus, no further use is made of the dose-response curve or its data. In general, this method is regarded as conservative (i.e., overestimating risks), though it is recognized that in certain exceptional cases it may underestimate actual risks. This method is sometimes referred to as a "model-free" approach (Krewski et al., 1990).

For nongenotoxic carcinogens, an ADI is set by determining the NOAEL and appropriate safety factors.

The position towards mathematical or biologically based models in use for dose-response modeling elsewhere is that these rely on assumptions that cannot be verified, due to the absence of knowledge of the actual form of the dose-response curve in the low-dose range. The advantage of the Dutch method is its transparency and the fact that it is based only on the assumption of one-hit kinetics at low dose.

1.1.1.3. United Kingdom In the United Kingdom, also, a distinction is made on the basis of the mechanism by which chemicals induce cancer, i.e., between carcinogens that are genotoxic and those that are nongenotoxic (UK, 1991).

For carcinogens acting by a well understood nongenotoxic mechanism, it is considered that a safe level of exposure can be identified. Usually, a no observed effect level (NOEL) is determined from animal studies, and divided by a safety factor to arrive at an ADI. This safety factor should compensate for the uncertainty of extrapolating from findings in animals to humans and of interindividual variation. These ADIs are also used to calculate maximum residue levels for pesticides on food.

For carcinogens acting by a genotoxic mechanism, or for which the mechanism is unclear, no threshold is assumed (i.e., no "safe" dose can be identified) and exposure-related risks are evaluated by expert judgment and on a weight-of-the-evidence approach. All available evidence (e.g. human and animal data, mutagenicity data, and structure-activity relationships) is considered. Recommended are actions to reduce exposure levels to as low as is reasonably practical or to eliminate exposure entirely.

The mathematical models in use in other countries to quantify risks for humans at low exposure levels from data of highly dosed animals are not considered adequate because these models have not been validated, and are (on occasions) biologically implausible and, therefore, subject to a high degree of uncertainty. The animal data used are incomplete and inappropriate, the models are based more on mathematical assumptions than on established biochemical mechanisms, and risk estimates for low exposure levels vary orders of magnitude, depending on the model used. Moreover, these models and their estimates suggest a precision, which cannot be justified from the approximations and assumptions on which they are based (UK, 1991).

1.1.1.4. Germany Because environmental laws in Germany demanded the elimination of dangers to public health, any form of risk assessment to humans, e.g. the quantification of risks from exposure to carcinogens, was resisted until recently. Regulatory authorities, however, had to accept a form of quantitative risk assessment, as the need for it necessitated such. Although strongly influenced by United States Environmental Protection Agency methodology (U.S. EPA, 1986), German committees believe in a more flexible approach of selecting compounds for risk assessment and the choice of modeling, i.e., preferably on a case-by-case basis (FRG, 1993).

An intense debate and discussion regarding the ideas and methodology surrounding dose-response modeling is still ongoing, which has resulted in little QRA being completed to date. Although the existence of several modes of action of carcinogens has been recognized, a major point of discussion is that in many instances the existence of a threshold is not discernable (FRG, 1993). Only in two of these cases, i.e., with direct-acting genotoxic carcinogens and with nongenotoxic chemicals having carcinogenic effects found in close association with cytotoxicity in the target organ, the absence and presence of a threshold, respectively, is considered justified. In the latter case the NOAEL and safety factor approach is taken, though it is recognized that the NOAEL for cancer-inducing cytotoxicity may not be adequately determined. In case a nonthreshold approach is applicable, mostly the linearized multistage model, or unit risk values generated by U.S. EPA, is applied to arrive at an acceptable exposure level or estimate risks.

1.1.1.5. Denmark In Denmark also a distinction is made between genotoxic and nongenotoxic carcinogens. It is clearly stated that the preferable dose-response model for arriving at acceptable exposure levels for both genotoxic as well nongenotoxic carcinogens is a biologically based model, such as the one developed by Moolgavkar, Venzon, and Knudson (Moolgavkar and Venzon, 1979; Moolgavkar and Knudson, 1981). However, in practice these models cannot be used due to the absence of the "extra" experimental data needed, and more primitive models have to be relied on, preferably simplified versions of these biologically-based models. However, for genotoxic chemicals the one-hit or two-hit model may be used as an approximation instead, depending on whether the dose-response data are obtained from the lower or higher dose range, respectively. For nongenotoxic carcinogens, preferably referred to as promoters, in the absence of this "extra" data the Mantel-Bryan model may be used instead of a biologically based model, because this model is a conservative variant of the logit model, which has been shown to provide a good means of describing receptor-mediated processes in biology (Mantel and Bryan, 1961; DK, 1991). The maximum likelihood estimate (MLE) obtained by this latter procedure is, as stated, considered to be conservative. Even then, the 99-percent lower bound of this MLE value is taken for the determination of the virtually safe dose. It is well recognized that the available models are primitive and the extrapolations made introduce considerable uncertainty. Therefore, the purpose of quantitative risk analyses should be carefully evaluated.

In deriving at occupational exposure standards, Denmark also considers estimates generated elsewhere, e.g., U.S. threshold limit values and German MAK values.

1.1.1.6. Norway Norway has adopted a quite different approach for quantifying risks from exposure to carcinogenic agents in following Nordic recommendations (SFT, 1986). Carcinogens are divided into three subclasses based on their carcinogenic potency, instead of performing an extrapolation to risks at low human exposure levels. This approach is followed mainly because regulatory administrations were already practicing a system that had carcinogens grouped into three classes (though with a marginal role for potency only) for the purpose of labeling, and because the low dose extrapolation procedures in use elsewhere are based on calculations and models that are complicated and based on several assumptions that cannot be verified. The risk estimates that result from these calculations are, therefore, quite uncertain. The allocation to potency classes, on the other hand, does allow regulatory authorities in their cancer prevention programs to rank carcinogens with respect to their relative hazards.

The main element that determines the ranking of a carcinogen with respect to its potency is the lowest daily dose that has induced an increased frequency of tumors in a long-term animal carcinogenicity study. Also other elements bearing on dose-response relationships, information on mechanisms including genotoxicity, and toxicokinetics are considered hereby. Thus, basically only one point of the dose-response curve is used for the quantitative evaluation of carcinogens. Also, the clear distinction between genotoxic and nongenotoxic carcinogens made in EU member states that trigger different extrapolation procedures is basically not made here (FIKS, 1994).

1.1.1.7. Other countries Other countries do not have clearly developed and published quantitative cancer risk assessment procedures. Mostly these countries consider risk assessment-related information and exposure standards promulgated at the international level by organizations such as WHO, Codex Alimentarius Commission, International Labor Organization (ILO), International Program on Chemical Safety (IPCS),

Organization for Economic Cooperation and Development (OECD), European Community (EC), International Agency for Research on Cancer (IARC), the U.S. Food and Drug Administration (FDA), and the U.S. EPA.

1.1.1.8. Concluding remarks Although this overview on dose-response modeling is not complete, which is merely due to the absence of available literature and documentation on this subject, it does give a clear indication of the different procedures used and opinions held by the various countries. It should be remarked here, however, that the differences between countries or states with respect to QRA not only resides in dose-response analysis but also in differences in applying toxicokinetic data and in the use of various interspecies conversion factors for dose scales.

Before performing dose-response analysis, many of the countries in Europe first try to identify the mechanism of carcinogenesis for the substance under evaluation. Generally there are two possible outcomes, i.e., the carcinogen is recognized as being genotoxic or not. This outcome has consequences for the handling of these carcinogens and influences the procedures used for determining low-dose risks. In the majority of countries, nongenotoxic carcinogens are dealt with by the determination of a NOAEL and safety factors. Once identified as a genotoxic carcinogen, on the other hand, and recognizing that a ban or restricted use is not an option, all countries agree on a linear, nonthreshold, dose-response relationship. The dose-response methodology applied here, however, differs among countries. The basis for this is the different views held by experts in the field (who participate on the national expert committees), the differences in legislation and regulatory history, the intended application of the results of QRA, public involvement, and government structure between these countries or states.

Countries that do not make use of mathematical models for extrapolation to low-dose risks (e.g. The Netherlands, United Kingdom, and Norway), rely upon the validity of the available animal data solely, whereas those countries applying these mathematical tools additionally trust the validity of these models.

1.1.2. United States

1.1.2.1. Use of Dose-Response Assessment In the United States, dose-response assessment is commonly regarded as one phase of the broader process of risk assessment, used by both the public and private sectors as a tool for analyzing problems affecting public health and safety. Risk assessment is usually regarded as distinct from risk management, the process of using risk assessment and other information and constraints to come to a decision about what to do for a potential risk. Risk management involves more than risk assessment and scientific information; other considerations include applicable laws and regulations, cost, economic impacts, technical feasibility, equitable treatment of all, and public opinion.

The risk assessment process was characterized by four components by the National Research Council (NRC, 1983).

- Hazard identification, which involves evaluating epidemiologic studies, animal experiments, short-term tests, toxicokinetic studies, and other pertinent information to make a determination about whether a substance has the potential to induce cancer in humans.

- Dose-response assessment, which involves using quantitative information to estimate the human cancer response associated with different levels of exposure.

- Exposure assessment, which seeks to determine the potential routes of exposure to a substance and the amounts of exposure.

- Risk characterization, which integrates the results of the hazard identification, dose-response assessment, and exposure assessment. It includes a discussion of the strengths and limitations of the assessment.

In the United States, federal and state agencies have promoted the use of risk assessment as a way of analyzing public health issues and helping to guide subsequent action. These agencies include:

- Food and Drug Administration, responsible for ensuring the safety of foods, drugs, and cosmetics.

- Occupational Safety and Health Administration, responsible for ensuring worker safety.

- Consumer Product Safety Commission, responsible for ensuring the safety of consumer products.

- Environmental Protection Agency, responsible for protecting public health and the environment from the effects of pollution.

These and other agencies have sought to protect public health from exposure to carcinogens. All have used risk assessment to evaluate potential carcinogens that humans might be exposed to. With some small differences, these agencies have used a similar framework for dose-response assessment.

For most chemical carcinogens, default methods are used to estimate risks that may arise from exposure to a potential carcinogen, because either the mechanism of action is unknown or the information required by a mechanistic model is unavailable. NRC (1983) defined a default as "the option chosen on the basis of risk assessment policy that appears to be the best choice in the absence of data to the contrary." In the succeeding years, many risk assessments made use of default options for dose-response modeling. More than a decade later, the NRC (1994) reaffirmed the use of default options, recommending that one agency "should continue to regard the use of default options as a reasonable way to cope with uncertainty about the choice of appropriate models or theory."

It is instructive to describe default options as statements of science policy. That is, they have both a policy component and a science component. The policy objectives include:

- Protecting public health
- Promoting clarity and consistency across risk assessments

This first objective is achieved by methods that, using available information and making assumptions when information is lacking, are not likely to underestimate the risk to the public. The second objective is achieved by methods that can be applied in large numbers of cases.

The science component also plays a prominent role when developing and applying default options. The science objectives include ensuring that default methods are:

- Applicable to the generally available data set
- Consistent with prevailing views of carcinogenesis

These science objectives encourage default methods to keep pace with the kinds of information being generated in the laboratory and with current scientific thought. They are fundamental to maintaining the credibility of the default methods.

1.1.2.2. Evolution of Dose-Response Assessment The science objectives described above provide the impetus for evolution of default methods. This is because an agency's policy objectives might remain constant over a period of many years, while its science objectives must be able to incorporate new kinds of laboratory information and reflect emerging scientific understanding. The evolution of default dose-response methods can be seen as reflecting changes in the generally available data set as well as changes in the prevailing views of carcinogenesis.

Default methods for low-dose extrapolation have, indeed, evolved over the years. In the 1970's low-dose extrapolation was commonly performed using the log-probit model or the one-hit model. The log-probit model is often used for estimating the incidence of a general dose-related toxic effect, such as estimating LD50's from an acute toxicity study. This model has a fixed shape that assumes a highly nonlinear dose-response relationship at low doses. In contrast, the one-hit model has a fixed shape that assumes a linear dose-response relationship at low doses. It was generally fit through the single data point from a lifetime cancer study with one dosed group. In 1980 these models were generally replaced by the linearized multistage model (U.S. EPA, 1980), which is more flexible in shape and, thus, can fit a wider variety of dose-response relationships. It can be used to fit lifetime cancer studies with several dosed groups.

This evolution has reflected changes in the generally available data set. The log-probit model and the one-hit model reflect a time when many carcinogenicity studies were screening studies, often conducted at a single high dose. A special case of the log-probit model, known as the Mantel-Bryan model, was developed that could be fit to cancer studies using only one dose level. Because the shape of the dose-response curve is rigidly prescribed in these models, they are limited in their ability to fit the multiple-dose lifetime cancer studies of recent years. Thus, the linearized multistage model was adopted, in part because of its ability to reflect the steep high-dose curvature observed in many multiple-dose lifetime cancer studies that follow a "S"-shaped dose-response curve (U.S. EPA, 1980). Extensions of the multistage model have allowed it to be used with studies of time-dependent dosing patterns (Crump and Howe, 1984).

In recent years, other study designs that are not amenable to modeling by the linearized multistage model have become more common. These include initiation-promotion studies, mechanistic studies, and toxicokinetic studies. In order to be able to conduct dose-response assessments for the growing number of chemicals where these studies, but not lifetime cancer studies, are available, new default methods will have to be developed.

Similarly, the evolution of default dose-response methods has reflected changes in the prevailing views of carcinogenesis. The log-probit model, which has its roots in modeling noncancer effects such as acute lethality (LD50's), reflects an earlier view that cancer can be described by models of general toxicity. Later, the view of cancer as a nonthreshold process that can be linear at low levels of exposure came into prominence. This view led to the use of the low-dose linear one-hit model in preference to the highly nonlinear log-probit model. The one-hit model was, in turn, inconsistent with the accumulation of knowledge that cancer is a multistage process, which led to the replacement of the one-hit model by the multistage model.

The multistage model does not, however, explicitly describe several processes that have been shown to play an important role in carcinogenesis. These include the role of cell proliferation and death and the role of indirect mechanisms in carcinogenesis. In order to be able to conduct dose-response assessments for the chemicals where cell dynamics and indirect mechanisms play an important role in carcinogenesis, new default methods will have to be developed.

Thus, the evolution from the log-probit model to the one-hit model to the linearized multistage model can be understood as a response to changes in the generally available data set and changes in the prevailing views of carcinogenesis. The shift in the prevailing view of cancer as a linear, nonthreshold process led to a preference for the one-hit model over the log-probit model. The understanding of cancer as a multistage process, together with the availability of multiple-dose lifetime cancer studies that could not be fitted by the one-hit model, led to the replacement of the one-hit model by the linearized multistage model.

1.1.3. Differences between the United States and European Countries

From the above it is clear, that major differences exist between the U.S. and European countries in the way carcinogens are quantitatively evaluated (U.S. EPA, 1986). Whereas U.S. agencies have a default procedure for all carcinogens, most countries in Europe make a distinction in this respect between carcinogens identified as genotoxic and those identified as being nongenotoxic. Although both U.S. and European countries share a linear, nonthreshold extrapolation approach for genotoxic carcinogens, the dose-response methodology applied differs substantially from country to country. These different approaches may in the end lead to quite different allowable exposure standards

(Carnevale, 1987). Another deviation between these western unions, though not addressed here, also exist in the way some carcinogenic responses in animals are evaluated with respect to human relevance (Moolenaar, 1994).

1.2. FUTURE DIRECTIONS IN DOSE-RESPONSE ASSESSMENT

The Future of Default Methods To keep up with advances in the science, dose-response analysis will go through profound changes in the next few years. Methodology will attempt to reflect changes in the generally available data set, which will see fewer lifetime bioassays and more initiation-promotion studies, mechanistic information, and toxicokinetic studies. To accommodate contemporary changes in the available data and prevailing views of carcinogenesis, methodology may have to grow in several directions at once.

In the future, several different forms of quantitative risk characterization may be required. These include low-dose extrapolation, low-dose extrapolation for susceptible subgroups only, margin-of-exposure approaches when a threshold is indicated, benchmark (ED10) approaches, and comparison with noncancer estimates. This raises the question of whether there is a common framework for these applications.

One possible approach is to refine dose-response assessment into two steps: a modeling step and an extrapolation step. In the first step, the available dose-response data would be modeled in the range of observation. It would be reasonable to expect that the predictive ability of this model would be greatest in the range of observation, and that it would decline as the distance from the range of observation increases. A lowest reliable point could be determined, defined as the point below which the observed information no longer provides an estimate of risk of acceptable precision. This criterion may, perhaps, be expressed statistically; for example, the lowest reliable point might be defined as the point where the upper and lower bounds begin to differ by a factor of two or more.

The second step would be to extrapolate the dose-response relationship that was modeled in the range of observation to the lower exposure levels that are of interest. Because this extrapolation goes beyond the lowest reliable point of the modeled dose-response curve, the dose-response curve itself would not necessarily be the method of extrapolation. If supplemental data were available to indicate that the processes leading to cancer induction in the observed range are still operative below the lowest reliable point, and if the (lack of) precision below the lowest reliable point is acceptable, then the modeled dose- response curve could be used for extrapolation. On the other hand, if such supplemental data were not available, or if the imprecision below the lowest reliable point is unacceptably high, then other methods of extrapolation would be considered. One form of extrapolation would be a linear extrapolation from the lowest reliable point to zero. Besides giving a bound on the low-dose risk that would be consistent with low-dose linearity, such a linear extrapolation would explicitly recognize that the observed high-dose data provide uncertain projections of low-dose risk, and so the low-dose risk characterization would rely as much on policy (low-dose linearity when it is a plausible assumption in the absence of information to the contrary) as it would on the observed high-dose data.

This potential framework can be extended to incorporate more data or knowledge as it becomes available. Dose-response models in the range of observation can be guided by mechanism without invariably relying on the linearized multistage model to fit the observed data. Aside from tumor incidence data, these mechanistic models could also include information on premalignant lesions and their cell kinetics. In determining the lowest reliable point, supporting data on cellular responses and precancerous lesions could be used to extend the range of observation below the doses where tumors were observed. This framework has the potential to encourage experiments that allow better extrapolations and risk assessments based on more data.

1.3. BRIEF CONSIDERATIONS ON SOME COMMONLY USED PARAMETERS

1.3.1. Variation in Carcinogenic Potency and in Parameters Adopted for Carcinogen Regulation

As is well known, the dose estimated to induce tumors in 50 percent of exposed experimental animals (TD50) has been proposed as a suitable parameter for the quantitative characterization of carcinogenic potency (according to this definition, carcinogenic potency is inversely proportional to the TD50). Specific criteria have been proposed for the quantitative determination of the TD50, which is relatively independent of the mathematical model used for its estimation (IARC, 1986, Peto et al., 1984; Sawyer et al., 1984). Low-dose linear extrapolation from the TD50 has been used for estimating the doses corresponding to specific risk levels (Rulis, 1986). This procedure has been shown to lead to low-dose estimates generally similar to the ones based on the linearized multistage model (LMS) (Krewski et al., 1990), which is the model most frequently employed for low-dose risk assessment (Armitage, 1985; IARC, 1986; U.S. EPA IRIS files). The "Carcinogenic Potency Database", which includes data from approximately 3700 carcinogenicity experiments on rodents conducted by the U.S. National Cancer Institute/National Toxicology Program, as well as by other institutions, has been compiled and includes estimates of carcinogenic potencies (Gold et al., 1984; 1987; 1989).

Several authors have examined the main statistical characteristics of samples of carcinogenic potencies, using data from the "Carcinogenic Potency Database" (Rulis, 1986; Ashby and Tennant, 1988; Ashby et al., 1989; Gold et al., 1984, 1987, 1989; Krewski et al., 1990). The statistical distributions of the various subsets of carcinogenic potencies which have been examined appeared to be close to a lognormal statistical distribution; an analogous result was found for the doses corresponding to a specific low risk level (generally computed as a linear extrapolation from the TD50) (Rulis, 1986; Krewski et al., 1990). The analysis of these statistical distributions has indicated that the median of the approximately lognormally distributed carcinogenic potencies ranges between 10 and 45 mg/kg/day, while the median of the doses corresponding to a 10^{-6} risk level (calculated from the TD50 through linear extrapolation) was found to range between 20 and 90 ng/kg/day. The ratio between the 10th and the 90th percentiles of these distributions ranges up to three orders of magnitude.

In the specific case of food-contact articles, the reference to the parameters of this kind of statistical distribution and, in particular, to its ranges, percentiles, and extreme value distribution, has been proposed as a tool for extrapolating a "threshold for regulation policy", in the absence of specific complete data (Machuga et al., 1992; Rulis, 1986, 1989). More specifically, based on the ranges of toxicological and carcinogenic potencies, a concentration level for the dietary concentration of food-contact articles has been proposed ("threshold for regulation"), that would be "low enough to pose negligible safety concerns, even from potential carcinogens, but not so low to exclude almost all food-contact applications" (Machuga et al., 1992).

However, it may be interesting to notice that whenever the above-mentioned statistical distributions of carcinogenic potency include TCDD (2,3,7,8-tetrachlorodibenzo-p-dioxin), this latter chemical consistently exhibits the lowest TD50 and, therefore, the highest potency (Krewski et al., 1990), and appears in some sense as an "outlier". The occurrence of a carcinogenic potency such as that of TCDD is, in fact, scarcely predictable from the distribution of the potencies of the other chemicals, if reference is made to the lognormal distribution, its extreme range, and to the number of chemicals considered (Geigy Statistical Tables, 1982). If a similar analysis is effected on the chemicals included in the U.S. EPA Drinking Water Regulations and Health Advisories (1992), similar results arise (for 37 chemicals where both cancer and noncancer assessments are available). Also in this case, the statistical distribution of the doses estimated to induce a 10^{-4} risk level is not significantly different from a lognormal distribution (Kolmogorov-Smirnov test for one sample); the ratio between the 90th and 10th percentiles is consistent with the same parameter reported by Krewski et al. (1990) for a much more extended data set. The median of this distribution (1.2 g/kg/day) is in the same order of magnitude as the range reported by Krewski et al. (1990) for the same parameter (it is about 60 percent of the lower limit of that range).

The differences between the two methods adopted for the estimation of risk-specific doses (linearized multistage model and linear extrapolation from the TD50), as well as the small number of carcinogens evaluated by both methods, may account, at least in part, for the differences between the two estimates of the median value. Also in this case, the TCDD case appears as an "outlier". In particular, if the TCDD is excluded from the statistics, the lower tolerance limit (95 percent confidence) for the 97.5 percentile of the distribution of doses corresponding to a 10^{-4} risk level may be estimated to be 3 orders of magnitude higher than the TCDD dose which has been assessed to correspond to this risk level (Zapponi et al., 1994). These simple examples indicate that the adoption of criteria for a "threshold for regulation policy", based on the range and percentiles of carcinogenic potencies or of carcinogenic risk-specific doses, while possibly useful when dealing with specific and relatively homogeneous categories of risk factors, is questionable in cases like the ones above discussed, and that further research is needed on this topic.

The indication that some type of statistical distribution may be identified for the carcinogenic potencies of chemicals represents an important source of information. These distributions may reflect different classes of mechanisms of action involved in the carcinogenic processes (e.g., genotoxic, nongenotoxic, initiator, promoter, etc.), as well as structure-activity patterns and other parameters.

Lastly, it is useful to point out that TCDD is considered to be a nongenotoxic carcinogen, whose action is mediated by a specific cellular receptor (Okey et al., 1994). The extremely high carcinogenic potency in the experimental animals is indicated by the low dose levels that induced tumors in the experimental animals. This confirms the importance of devoting the same level of attention to both nongenotoxic and genotoxic carcinogens. It is also worthwhile to mention that in the case of a cellular receptor-mediated carcinogenic action, the carcinogenic process is considered to be generally effective even at very low doses, and the hypothesis of thresholds was questioned by Cohen and Ellwein (1990).

1.3.2. Toxicity Data and Carcinogenic Potencies: Correlation between Parameters Adopted for Risk Assessment

Various studies have been dedicated over the last years to the evaluation of the statistical relationships existing among various categories of toxicity data, including carcinogenic potencies. The correlation between carcinogenic potency, estimated by the dose that induces tumors in 50 percent of exposed animals (TD50) (IARC, 1986; Peto et al., 1984; Sawyer et al., 1984), and acute toxicity, estimated by the dose that kills 50 percent of exposed animals (LD50), was described by Zeise et al. (1984). Metzger et al. (1988) have analyzed the correlation between the TD50 and the LD50 for different data subsets (i.e., only data produced by the U.S. National Cancer Institute and the U.S. National Toxicology Program, only data by other sources, different categories of animal exposure and different species). The authors of this study conclude that carcinogenic potency and acute toxicity are proportional and that the TD50-LD50 correlations are robust with respect to differences in species and route of administration (Metzger et al., 1988). Correlations can also be found between carcinogenic potency and other toxicological parameters (e.g., mutations, reproductive toxicity, and acute, subchronic, and chronic toxicity); a battery of toxicological parameters was shown to account for 80 percent of the observed variability in carcinogenic potency in the most sensitive target organ in mice, this figure was 92 percent for variability in mouse liver tumor potency (Travis et al., 1990).

A possible explanation for these correlations is that toxic effects may induce tissue damage with subsequent cell proliferation. Through this process, the cancer risk may be increased; therefore, these correlations may account, in some sense, for some carcinogenic promotion activity induced by toxicity (Travis et al., 1990).

As is well known, toxicity has been shown to be involved in different mechanisms that lead to cell proliferation. They include reactions with specific cell receptors, cell regeneration/proliferation as a consequence of cytotoxicity, as well as stimuli to mitogenesis (Cohen and Ellwein, 1990; Butterworth and Goldsworthy, 1991; Travis and

Belefant, 1992). Moreover, cell proliferation may indirectly increase the mutation rate by converting the DNA adducts that have not yet been repaired into permanent mutations, and also as a result of errors in DNA replication (Bogen, 1989; Preston-Martin et al., 1990; Butterworth and Goldsworthy, 1991; Cohen and Ellwein, 1991; Portier and Kopp-Schneider, 1991; Monticello and Morgan, 1993).

However, along with this hypothesis, other processes have been indicated among the possible causes of the correlations found between carcinogenic potency and toxicity parameters. For example, the highest dose used in cancer bioassays is the "Maximum Tolerated Dose" (MTD), which is generally selected as a specific fraction of the LD50; as a consequence, the dose range adopted in carcinogenic experiments is dependent on the LD50 values. Owing to the very large variability of LD50s and carcinogenic potencies, this dependency may result in some correlation effect for the possible "tautologous nature of the correlation" (Bernstein et al., 1985; Crouch et al., 1987).

Zeise et al. (1986) propose the hypothesis that various processes, including absorption, transport, binding to molecules, metabolism, and others, may be common, at least in part, to mechanisms involved in both carcinogenicity and acute toxicity, thus contributing to the correlation between the two endpoints.

Even if much more research and data are necessary for an exhaustive explanation of the correlation between toxicity and carcinogenic potency, there is good ground for assuming that this correlation has a biological basis, and is not simply an experimental artifact.

These considerations may be extended to the main parameters adopted for cancer and noncancer assessment. As an example, a highly significant correlation ($r = 0.841, p < 0.001$) between the doses corresponding to a 10^{-4} carcinogenic risk level ($d(10^{-4})$) and the Reference Doses (RfDs) emerges for a subset of 37 drinking water contaminants where both cancer and noncancer assessments had been carried out for drinking water regulations and health advisories (U.S. EPA, 1992). This correlation appears to account for more than the 70 percent of the variability of the logarithms of the $d(10^{-4})$s. The slope and intercept of the linear regression are 0.80 (standard error = 0.09) and -2.48, respectively. If the TCDD doses, which are much lower than the others, are excluded from the analysis, the correlation remains highly significant (but lower) and the regression slope does not change significantly. The uncertainty level of the estimates that can be derived from this kind of regression spans up to two orders of magnitude, as indicated by the prediction interval (95 percent confidence) (Zapponi et al., 1994).

Moreover, for the same set of 37 chemicals, the statistical distribution of cancer risk levels computed at the reference dose does not differ significantly from a lognormal distribution (Kolmogorov-Smirnov test for one sample). These cancer risk levels (estimated through the linearized multistage model) range from 0.09×10^{-4} to 1200×10^{-4}, with a median value of around 4×10^{-4} (Zapponi et al., 1994). This suggests that, for carcinogens in this example, exposure at the level of the reference dose would often pose a cancer risk that has generally been regarded as unacceptable. However, for a significant fraction of these compounds, the exposure at the level of the reference dose may provide protection also for the risk of cancer. Lastly, these data suggest that the tolerance interval of the ratios of $d(10^{-4})$s to RfDs may provide a useful indicator in this kind of evaluation.

1.3.3. The Linearized Multistage Model and Benchmark Dose (BD) Approaches: Dose-Response Analysis May Provide a Unique Framework for Both the Carcinogenic and Noncarcinogenic Procedures

The benchmark dose (BD) is commonly defined as the lower confidence limit for the dose corresponding to a specified increase of health effects over background level. This increase would be near the lower limit of the experimental range (Crump, 1984). In practice, the lower confidence limits (usually 95 percent confidence level) of the doses expected to induce 1, 5, or 10 percent extra risk over the background (usually indicated as ED01, ED05, or ED10) are used (Crump, 1984; Auton, 1994). BDs are quantitatively defined through dose-response analysis using appropriate mathematical models. This definition is quite general, and applies to both carcinogenic and noncarcinogenic dose-response analysis. It is important to note that BDs are the result of a statistical-mathematical interpolation rather than extrapolation, or involve, at most, very limited extrapolation beyond the experimental dose range. As a consequence, the BD estimate is scarcely influenced by the selection of the model adopted for the dose-response mathematical description (this feature tends to overcome the well-known model dependency in low-dose extrapolation used for carcinogen risk assessment) (Crump, 1984). In noncancer assessment, BDs are proposed as an alternative to the No-Observed-Adverse-Effect-Level (NOAEL), which is an experimental dose rather than an interpolated dose. Similar to a NOAEL, BDs are divided by an appropriate Uncertainty Factor (UF) to derive Reference Doses (RfDs) or other similar parameters (e.g., Acceptable Daily Intakes - ADIs - etc.). It is useful to note that BDs are estimated by fitting a model to an entire set of dose-response data instead of choosing just one dose to be the NOAEL; therefore, BDs make more use of the information available from a dose-response data set (Crump, 1984; Gaylor, 1989). Moreover, the BD approach intrinsically takes into account experimental design and uncertainty, through use of lower confidence limits. Typically, the confidence interval will be narrower, and BDs larger, in the case of higher quality experimental data (well-designed bioassays using an larger number of experimental animals and experimental groups) than in the case of lower quality data. In the case of the NOAEL-based approach, the opposite is generally true; smaller experimental groups are less likely to detect an adverse effect, leading to NOAELs that are, in truth, false negatives. Therefore, the BD approach may encourage well designed studies, by allowing less conservative estimates of RfDs or equivalent parameters (Crump, 1984). Additionally, in the BD approach, the UF adopted in a specific assessment may sometimes be interpreted in terms of the risk under a worst-case hypothesis, at least if the dose-response is curving upward. For example, the response at the dose BD01/100 is expected to be lower than 10^{-4}, even under the pessimistic hypothesis of the absence of a low-dose threshold and of a linear low-dose trend for the specific effect (provided that the dose-response relationship is upward) (Gaylor, 1989). This interpretation assumes that the uncertainty factor (in this case, 100) is not used to adjust for differences between animals and humans or between experimental exposures and anticipated human exposures.

Lastly, the BD approach largely reduces the differences between carcinogen and noncarcinogen assessment procedures by making reference to dose-response analysis and modeling and by explicitly considering the confidence limits of the estimates. It provides a key to appropriately harmonizing the two methods. In fact, such methods have been proposed for carcinogen risk assessment (Van Ryzin, 1980; Gaylor and Kodell, 1980; Farmer et al., 1982; Krewski et al., 1990). The proposed procedures basically use a linear extrapolation from a measure or estimate of a dose corresponding to a specific risk level (generally, 1 percent).

As an example, for a subset of 22 chemicals assessed for drinking water regulation and health advisories (U.S. EPA, 1992), the BD approach is comparable to estimates from the linearized multistage procedure reported in U.S. EPA IRIS files. In particular, the correlation between the logarithms of the doses corresponding to a 10^{-4} carcinogenic risk level and the logarithms of the BD01s (for the same dose-response data set) was high (Zapponi et al., 1994). The BD01s used in this analysis were computed as the geometric mean of the BD01 values obtained by using the Weibull, lognormal, and multistage models (Crump, 1984). The slope of the regression (equal to 0.92, standard error = 0.24) was not significantly different from unity, and the intercept the regression line (equal to -4.5 log-unit) was not significantly different from the logarithm of 1/100. As expected, the regression parameters indicate that the $d(10^{-4})$s are substantially linearly proportional to the BD01s computed on the same data, and, on average, are about 1/100 of them. The uncertainty of the regression estimates was less than one order of magnitude.

Thus, the linearized multistage model (used for cancer assessment) and the BD approach (being considered for noncancer assessment) provide similar results, assuming comparability between 10^{-4} risk levels and BD01/100. Low-dose risk estimates obtained from the linearized multistage model or from a number of different linear models (including linear extrapolation from a parameter such as the BD01) have been shown to be substantially equivalent in various studies (Krewski et al., 1990). This finding suggests that the above conclusion may be quite general.

For example, for many years the U.S. EPA has used the ED10 benchmark dose to develop potency rankings of potential carcinogens in its emergency response program (U.S. EPA, 1988) and its Clean Air Act hazard ranking program (U.S. EPA, 1994). To develop these rankings, ED10s were used rather than low-dose extrapolation, because ED10s are mostly independent of choice of model and are statistically stable without use of upper bounds that can distort relative rankings (Cogliano, 1986; U.S. EPA, 1988). A comparison of ED10 benchmark doses to low-dose slopes from the linearized multistage procedure found a high correlation between these two measures in a database containing 86 potential carcinogens (Cogliano, 1986). This finding led the National Research Council (NRC, 1993) to remark that the ED10 can serve as a common measure for both potency ranking and a starting point for low-dose extrapolation.

1.4. STRUCTURE OF THIS REPORT

This volume follows a progression from cancer biology to related data sources to models to applications. Chapter 2 discusses the biological basis of cancer. Chapter 3 describes several sources of experimental data used in risk assessment; this discussion is extended to biochemical and molecular markers in Chapter 4. Chapter 5 describes the multistage models that have been used in risk assessment, and Chapter 6 presents biologically based models of carcinogenesis that are increasing in use. Chapter 7 discusses some statistical considerations involved in the use of these models. Chapter 8 applies these models in a series of case studies. Finally, Chapter 9 discusses some conclusions and recommendations.

1.5. REFERENCES

Armitage P. (1985): Multistage Models of Carcinogenesis, Environmental Health perspectives, 63, 195-201.

Ashby J. and Tennant R.W. (1988): Chemical structure, Salmonella mutagenicity, extent of carcinogenicity as indicators of genotoxic carcinogens among 222 chemicals tested in rodents by the U.S. NCI/NTP, Mutation Research, 204, 17-115.

Ashby J., Tenant R.W., Zeiger E., and Stasiewicz S. (1989): Classification according to chemical structure, mutagenicity to Salmonella and level of carcinogenicity of a further 42 chemicals tested for carcinogenicity by the U.S. National Toxicology Program, Mutation Research, 223, 73-103.

Auton T.R. (1994): Calculation of benchmark doses from teratology data, Regul. Toxicol. Pharmacol., 19, 152-167.

Bernstein L., Gold L.S., Ames B.N., Pike M.C. and Hoel D.G. (1985): Some tautologous aspects of the comparison of carcinogenic potency in rats and mice, Fundamentals of Applied Toxicology, 5, 79-86.

Bogen K.T. (1989): Cell proliferation kinetics and Multistage cancer risk models, Journal of the national Cancer Institute, 81, 4, 267-277.

Butterworth B.E., and Goldsworthy T.L. (1991): The role of cell proliferation in multistage carcinogenesis, Proceedings of the Soc. of Experimental Biology and Medicine, 198, 683-687.

Carnevale F., Montesano R., Partensky C. and Tomatis L. (1987): Comparison of regulations on occupational carcinogens in several industrialized countries. Am. J. Industr. Medicine, 12, 453-473.

Cogliano V.J. (1986): The U.S. EPA's methodology for adjusting the reportable quantities of potential carcinogens. Proceedings of the 7th National Conference on Management of Uncontrolled Hazardous Wastes (Superfund '86). Washington: Hazardous Materials Control Research Institute, 182-185.

Cohen S.M. and Ellwein L.B. (1990): Cell proliferation ion carcinogenesis, Science, 249, 1007-1011.

Cohen S.M., and Ellwein L.B. (1991): Genetic errors, cell proliferation, and carcinogenesis, Cancer Research, 51, 6493-6505.

Crump K.S. (1984): A new method for determining allowable daily intakes, Fundamental and applied toxicology, 4, 854-871.

Crump K.S. and Howe R.B. (1984): The multistage model with a time-dependent dose pattern: applications to carcinogenic risk assessment. Risk Analysis 4(3), 163-176.

DK (1991): Quantitative Risk Analysis for Carcinogens, National Food Agency of Denmark, Institute of Toxicology, Kopenhagen.

EU (1991): Classification on the basis of specific effects to human health. Official Journal of the European Communities, No.L 180 (8-7-91).

EU (1993): Commission Directive 93/67/EEC: Laying Down the Principles for the Assessment of Risks to Man and the Environment of Substances Notified in Accordance with Council Directive 67/548/EEC, July 20.

EU (1995): Guidelines for setting specific concentrations limits for carcinogens in Annex I of Directive 67/548/EEC, Inclusion of potency considerations. Commission Working Group on the Classification and Labeling of Dangerous Substances, Draft.

FRG (1993): Basisdaten Toxikologie für umweltrelevante Stoffe zur Gefahrenbeurteilung bei Altlasten, Berichte 4/93 (Eds. M.Hassauer, F.Kalberlah, J.Oltmanns and K.Schneider). Umweltforschungsplan des Bundesministers für Umwelt, Naturschutz und Reaktorsicherheit, Erich Schmidt Verlag, Berlin.

FIKS (1994): Guidelines for the Scientific evaluation of carcinogens (Eds. T.Sanner and E.Dybing), State Pollution Control Authority & Directorate of Labour Inspection's scientific group for identification of carcinogens, Norway.

Gaylor D.W. and Kodell R.L. (1980): Linear interpolation algorithm for low-dose risk assessment of toxic substances, Journal of Environmental Pathology and Toxicology, 4, 305-312.

Gaylor D.W. (1993): Quantitative risk assessment for quantal reproductive and developmental effects, Environmental Health Perspectives, 79, 243-246.

Gold L.S., Sawyer C.B., Magaw R., Backman G.M., de Veciana M., Levinson R., Hooper N.K., Havender W.R., Bernstein L., Peto R., Pike M.C. and Ames B.N. (1984): A carcinogenic potency database of the standardized results of animal bioassays, Environmental Health Perspectives, 58, 9-322.

Gold L.S., Slone T.H., Backman G.M., Magaw R., Lopipero P., Blumenthal M., and Ames B.N. (1987): Second chronological supplement to the Carcinogenic Potency Database: Standardized results of animal bioassays published through December 1984 and by the National Toxicological Program through May, 1986, Environmental Health Perspectives, 74, 237-329.

Gold L.S., Slone T.H., and Bernstein L. (1989): Summary of carcinogenic potency and positivity for 492 rodent carcinogens in the carcinogenic potency database, Environmental Health Perspectives, 79, 259-272.

IARC - International Agency for Research on Cancer (WHO) (1986): Statistical Methods in Cancer Research, Volume III: The design and analysis of long-term animal experiments, IARC, Lyon.

Kramers P.G.N., Knaap A.G.A.C., van der Heijden C.A., Taalman R.D.F.M. and Mohn G.R. (1991): Role of genotoxicity assays in the regulation of chemicals in The Netherlands. Mutagenesis, 6, 487-493.

Krewski D., Sziskowicz M., and Rosenkranz H. (1990): Quantitative factors in chemical carcinogenesis: Variation in carcinogenic potency, Regul. Toxicol. Pharmacol., 12, 13-29.

Luebeck E.G. and Moolgavkar, S.H. (1991): Stochastic description of initiation and promotion in experimental carcinogenesis, in Galli G., Rossi L., Vineis P., and Zapponi G.A. (eds): Risk assessment of chemical carcinogens, Annali Istituto Superiore di Sanità, 27, 4, 575-580.

Machuga E.J., Pauli G.H., and Rulis A.M. (1992): A threshold of regulation policy for food-contact articles, Food Control, Vol.3, 4, 180-182.

Mantel,N. and Bryan,W.R. (1961): Safety testing of carcinogenic agents. J.Natl. Cancer Inst., 27, 455-470.

Metger B., Crouch E., and Wilson R. (1989): On the relationship between carcinogenicity and acute toxicity, Risk Analysis, Vol.9, 2, 169-177.

Monticello T.M., and Morgan K.T. (1993): Cell proliferation and formaldehyde-induced respiratory carcinogenesis, Risk Analysis, 14, 3, 313-319.

Moolenaar, R.J. (1994): Carcinogen Risk assessment: International comparison. Regul. Toxicol.

Pharmacol., 20, 302-336.

Moolgavkar S.H. and Venzon D.J. (1979): Two-event models for carcinogenesis: incidence curves for childhood and adult tumors. Mathematical Biosciences, 47, 55-77.

Moolgavkar S.H. and Knudson A.G. Jr. (1981): Mutation and cancer: a model for human carcinogenesis. J. Natl. Cancer Inst., 55, 1032-1052.

NHC (1978): Health Council of The Netherlands (Gezondheidsraad), Commissie Beoordeling carcinogeniteit van chemische stoffen. Advies inzake de beoordeling van carcinogeniteit van chemische stoffen. No.1987/19, Rijswijk.

NHC (1994): Risk assessment of carcinogenic chemicals in The Netherlands. Health Council of The Netherlands (Gezondheidsraad), Committee on the Evaluation of the Carcinogenicity of Chemical Substances. Regul. Toxicol. Pharmacol., 19, 14-30.

NRC (National Research Council) (1983): Risk Assessment in the Federal Government: Managing the Process. Washington: National Academy Press.

NRC (National Research Council) (1993): Issues in risk assessment. Washington: National Academy Press.

NRC (National Research Council) (1994): Science and Judgment in Risk Assessment. Washington: National Academy Press.

Okey A.B, Riddick D.S., and Harper P.A. (1994): The Ah receptor: Mediator of the toxicity of 2,3,7,8-tetrachlorodibenzo-p-dioxin (TCDD) and related compounds, Toxicology Letters, 70, 1-22.

Parodi S., Taningher M., Baero P., and Santi L. (1982): Quantitative correlations amongst alkaline DNA fragmentation, DNA covalent binding, mutagenicity in the Ames test and carcinogenicity, for 21 compounds, Mutation Research, 93, 1-24.

Peto R., Pike M.C., Bernstein l., Gold L.S., and Ames B.N. (1984): The TD50: A proposed general convention for the numerical description of the carcinogenic potency of chemicals in chronic exposure animal experiments, Environmental Health Perspectives, 59, 1-8.

Portier C.J. and Kopp-Schneider A. (1991): A multistage model of carcinogenesis incorporating DNA damage and repair, Risk Analysis, 11,3, 535-543.

Preston-Martin S., Pike M.C., Ross R.K., Jones P.A., and Henderson B.E. (1990): Increased cell division as a cause of human cancer, Cancer Research, 50, 7415-7421.

Reichard E., Cranor C., Raucher R., and Zapponi G. (1990): Groundwater contamination risk assessment. A guide to understanding and managing uncertainties, International Association of the Hydrological Science (IAHS) Publications, Wallingford, Oxfordshire, U.K..

Rulis A.M. (1986): De minimis and the threshold of regulation, Food protection technology (C.W. Felix Ed.), 29-37, Lewis Publishers, Chelsea, MI.

Sawyer C., Peto R., Bernstein L., and Pike M.C. (1984): Calculation of carcinogenic potency from long-term animal carcinogenic experiments, Biometrics, 40, 27-40.

SFT (1986): Potency Ranking of Carcinogenic substances. Report from a Nordic Working Party. Nordisk Ministerrd. Miljorapport 1985: 4E, The State Pollution Control Authority, Oslo.

Travis C.C., Richter Pack S.A., Saulsbury A.W., and Yambert M.W. (1990): Prediction of carcinogenic potency from toxicological data, Mutation Research, 241, 21-36.

Travis C.C., and Belefant H. (1992): Promotion as a factor in carcinogenesis, Toxicology Letters, 60, 1-9.

UK (1991): Guidelines for the Evaluation of Chemicals for Carcinogenicity, Report on Health and Social Subjects No.42. Committee on Carcinogenicity of Chemicals in Food, Consumer Products and the Environment, Department of Health.

U.S. EPA (United States Environmental Protection Agency) (1980): Water quality criteria documents; availability. Federal Register 45(231), 79318-79379.

U.S. EPA (1986): Guidelines for carcinogen risk assessment. Federal Register, 33992-34003.

U.S. EPA (1988): Methodology for evaluating potential carcinogenicity in support of reportable quantity adjustments pursuant to CERCLA section 102. Washington: U.S. EPA, EPA/600/8-89/053.

U.S. EPA (1994): Technical background document to support rulemaking pursuant to the Clean Air Act section 112(g): ranking of pollutants with respect to hazard to human health. Research Triangle Park, NC: U.S. EPA, EPA 450/3 92 010.

U.S. EPA Integrated Risk Information Service - IRIS, EPA File on Line, 1995, U.S. EPA, Washington D.C..

U.S. EPA Office of Water (1992): Drinking water regulations and health advisories, U.S. EPA, Washington.

Van Ryzin J. (1980): Quantitative risk assessment, Journal of Occupational Medicine, 22, 321-326.

WHO (1987): Air Quality Guidelines for Europe. WHO Regional Office for Europe, Regional Publications, European Series No.23, Copenhagen.

WHO (1993): Guidelines for Drinking-water Quality, 2nd ed. Vol.1. Recommendations. Geneva.

Zapponi G.A., Attias L. and Marcello I. (1994): Dose-response analysis and low-dose risk assessment for carcinogenic and non-carcinogenic chemicals: some common criteria, ISS-IAHS International Symposium Assessing and managing health risks from drinking water contamination: approaches and applications, Rome, September 13-17, 1994, Abstract Book.

Zeise L., Wilson R., and Crouch E. (1984): Use of acute toxicity to estimate carcinogenic risk, Risk Analysis, 4, 187-199.

Zeise L., Crouch E.A.C., and Wilson, R. (1986): A possible relationship between toxicity and carcinogenicity, Journal of the American College of Toxicology, 137-151.

Chapter 2

THE BIOLOGICAL BASIS OF CANCER

V.J. Cogliano[1], A. Kappas[2], G. Voutsinas[2], and G.A. Zapponi[3]

[1]U.S. Environmental Protection Agency, Washington DC, USA
[2]National Centre for Scientific Research "Demokritus", Athens, Greece
[3]National Institute of Health, Rome, Italy

2.1. INTRODUCTION

Cancer is a multistage process, in which a series of events must transpire in the transformation of normal cells into a malignant tumor. Knowledge of the multistage nature of carcinogenesis comes from both epidemiologic and experimental data. Armitage and Doll (1954) observed how the incidence of cancer of several organs appeared to increase as a power function of age, and proposed a mathematical multistage model of cancer that was consistent with this relationship. Using this model, one could predict how the age-incidence curve would change in response to exposure to a carcinogen that affects a particular stage. Epidemiologic information was used to classify several human carcinogens as either early-stage or late-stage carcinogens.

Animal experiments, especially those conducted in mouse skin, have been used to distinguish between initiation and promotion. (It can be noted that the term "promotion" has been rather loosely used in describing a part of the process of carcinogenesis, while in multistage modeling the term refers to a specific cell population.) Several chemicals have been identified as initiators, and others as promoters. Application of an initiator followed by a promoter could induce high incidences of cancer, while either the initiator or the promoter alone was generally ineffective in inducing cancer. It was thus concluded that initiation and promotion were two distinct and necessary stages in the carcinogenesis process. Because application of a promoter followed by an initiator was also ineffective, the sequential nature of these two stages was demonstrated.

[1]The views expressed in this chapter are those of the authors and do not necessarily reflect the views or policies of the U.S. Environmental Protection Agency.

Perspectives on Biologically Based Cancer Risk Assessment, edited by Cogliano *et al.*
Kluwer Academic/Plenum Publishers, New York, 1999.

Other studies showed that a single dose of an initiator was sufficient to fulfill the initiation stage, while repeated doses of a promoter were often necessary. A long delay between application of initiator and promoter had little effect. From these results it was concluded that initiators caused irreversible changes, while promoters did not.

For a time, these two stages were adequate to explain a large body of experimental and epidemiologic observations. Initiation and promotion in animal experiments were considered analogous to early-stage and late-stage effects inferred from epidemiologic analyses. More recently, it has been shown that agents that affect the size of cell populations can also affect the incidence of cancer. An agent may, for example, dramatically increase the rate at which an initiated cell divides, causing clones of initiated cells to grow faster. As the number of initiated cells increases, there are more cells with the potential to progress to malignancy.

It is now convenient to talk of the carcinogenesis process as comprising initiation, promotion, and progression. Initiation is considered to be the event that transforms a normal cell into a pre-cancerous intermediate (or "initiated") cell. Promotion is often regarded as the proliferation of a single initiated cell into a clone of many initiated cells. Progression denotes the transformation of one of these initiated cells into a malignant cell, which then proliferates into a detectable malignant tumor.

Several types of events at the cellular level have been shown to affect initiation, promotion, or progression. Genetic changes, if not repaired, can cause irreversible changes in a cell. Mitogenesis, or the stimulation of cell division, can cause proliferation of cells. Cytotoxicity, or the killing of cells, can indirectly stimulate cell proliferation as surviving cells attempt to regenerate the tissue by increasing their rate of division.

At one time, it was considered that chemicals inducing genetic changes would act as initiators, while chemicals acting principally through cell proliferation would act as promoters. Current understanding shows that these distinctions are not so clear. Promotion of initiated cells is marked by an increase in these cells' rate of division, but such increase in rate can result from a genetic change. Similarly, initiated cells can result from either genetic damage or cell proliferation: when a cell divides, there is a small chance of a spontaneous mutation; thus, agents that stimulate cell division can increase the chance of a spontaneous mutation and, hence, initiation. In addition, although chemically induced mutations may be repairable, if the repair is not completed before the next cell division, the mutation becomes permanent; thus, agents that stimulate cell division decrease the time interval for repair and can enhance the effectiveness of mutations induced either spontaneously or by other chemicals.

The occurrence of spontaneous cancer in animals and humans has been taken as an indication that each of the stages of carcinogenesis can occur in the absence of external stimulation by a carcinogenic agent. Some initiated cells may be present at birth, and further formation of initiated cells is an expected consequence of spontaneous mutations occurring during the normal cycle of cell birth and cell death. Similarly, some promotion of initiated cells can be expected as cell populations grow. Thus, any agent that affects any of the stages of carcinogenesis has the capacity to increase the overall risk of cancer.

These considerations offer a view of carcinogenesis as a stochastic, nondeterministic process. Stochastic elements are present in the spontaneous occurrence of cancer.

For example, the normal cycle of cell birth and cell death can give rise to random spontaneous mutations. Alteration of cell dynamics by a carcinogen provides additional spontaneous elements. For example, increased cell replication, which shortens the time available for repair of genetic damage, can increase the probability of a mutation becoming permanent. By increasing the rate of one of these stochastic processes, a carcinogen can increase the overall probability of cancer.

As different kinds of information become available through new experimental protocols, the description of the carcinogenesis process can become more detailed and refined. For example, the rate of cell proliferation can be expressed using a single parameter to represent the rate of growth. With additional information, the rate of growth rate can be represented as the difference between two parameters, the rate of cell birth minus the rate of cell death. The same growth rate can result from a combination of birth and death rates that are either both high or both low. Newer protocols for initiation-promotion studies are collecting information that allow independent determination of the rates of cell birth and cell death. Such studies might reveal the presence of a small number of large initiated premalignant lesions, or alternatively, a large number of small initiated premalignant lesions. The presence of a small number of large lesions would suggest high birth and death rates, implying the extinction of many small lesions, while the presence of a large number of small lesions would suggest low birth and death rates, with little extinction of lesions.

2.2. CELL PROLIFERATION

Cell proliferation is presently recognized as a major factor in cancer induction. Both epidemiological evidence and experimental studies indicate that increased cell proliferation is involved in many carcinogenic processes (Monticello and Morgan, 1994; Cohen and Ellwein, 1990, 1991, 1993; Ellwein and Purtilo, 1992; Preston-Martin et al., 1990). Moreover, many studies underline that cancer risk assessment should consider that cell proliferation may increase the frequency of mutations as a consequence of errors in replication or of the conversion of endogenous or exogenous DNA adducts into stable mutations (Bogen, 1989; Butterworth and Goldsworthy, 1991). Ames and Gold (1990a, 1990b) have hypothesized that the relatively high doses used in bioassays (doses near the maximum tolerated dose, or MTD) may be responsible for overestimating cancer risk (both qualitatively and quantitatively), because these doses damage tissues and cause cell death, thereby stimulating an intense compensatory cell division process, whose consequence is an increase of tumor response ("mitogenesis increases mutagenesis").

It is, however, important to mention that Travis and Belefant (1992) report many data and evaluations supporting the hypothesis that the increased mutation rate attributable to this process is not a major factor in the induction of cancer in animal testing. In particular, they estimate that the pool of spontaneously initiated cells, already present in animal tissues at the beginning of bioassays, may be expected to be so large that the further addition of the cells that may be indirectly initiated through this process should not be significant. Further, they argue that most promoters exert their action at doses that are not cytotoxic, so that the biological effect connected with cytotoxicity may not be considered a necessary component of promotion (Travis and Belefant, 1992).

In relation to this subject, Weinstein (1991) argues that more than 90 percent of the carcinogenic effects observed at the highest doses in the experimental studies of the National Toxicology Program were also observed at lower doses, so that they cannot simply be assumed to be an indirect consequence of cytotoxic effects caused by excessive doses, as hypothesized by Ames and Gold (1990). Furthermore, Weinstein also underlines that often the observation of carcinogenic effects in rodents is not accompanied by the concomitant observation of obvious target organ toxicity. The same author observes that the estimated frequency of "spontaneous" or "background" DNA damage (up to 1 in 10,000 nucleotides) is much higher than the frequency of DNA-adducts (about 1/100,000 - 1/1,000,000) attributable to noncytotoxic doses of specific carcinogens known to be mutagenic and carcinogenic, while the effects attributable to the former do not appear to be as deleterious as those of the latter. Based on this consideration, Weinstein argues that the weight given by Ames and Gold to the role of endogenous DNA damage may be too high (Weinstein, 1991).

The classification scheme for carcinogens proposed by Cohen and Ellwein (1990), may offer a key for summarizing some main aspects of the above-discussed points. This classification considers genotoxic carcinogens (chemicals that react with DNA, for which a threshold is unlikely, though the dose-response may be affected by cell proliferation) and two subcategories of nongenotoxic carcinogens. The first of these includes nongenotoxic chemicals that induce cell proliferation through receptor-mediated processes, which are usually effective at very low doses and for which the threshold hypothesis is questionable. The second includes nongenotoxic chemicals that induce proliferation without specific reactions with cell receptors, usually as a consequence of toxicity and subsequent tissue regeneration, through mechanisms for which a threshold hypothesis is considered likely.

In the specific case of receptor-mediated processes, Cohen and Ellwein (1991) observe that a certain percentage of receptors in a cell must be occupied, and, therefore, more than a single molecule interacting with a cell's receptors is necessary for induction of the cellular response. Based on this observation, these authors argue that although chemicals acting through receptor-mediated mechanisms can be effective at very low doses, their action could likely have a threshold (Cohen and Ellwein, 1991). Accordingly, the number of molecules assumed to induce the effect represents a critical parameter from the point of view of the threshold hypothesis: genotoxic effects, for which a single molecule is theoretically sufficient, may be considered qualitatively different, in terms of low-dose threshold, from receptor-mediated proliferation effects, for which presumably a certain number of molecules, not only one, is necessary.

This point, however, needs to be discussed in more detail. A molecule of a genotoxic chemical that enters the cellular environment has to overcome a number of important obstacles before being able to exert its carcinogenic effect. These obstacles include the biological defense mechanisms of the cell, the possible presence of competing receptors, the difficulty of the molecule to reach the relatively scarce critical DNA targets, and the difficulty of the critical DNA adduct to survive DNA repair up to the time of cell division. These considerations indicate that the theoretical probability of a single genotoxic molecule to exert a carcinogenic effect can be expected to be low, even if it succeeds in entering one of the relatively rare susceptible (stem) cells.

Also to the point, in some cases a receptor can be occupied by different ligands (e.g., the aryl hydrocarbon receptor can be occupied by chlorinated dibenzo-p-dioxins and dibenzofurans, polychlorinated biphenyls, and polycyclic aromatic hydrocarbons). Each molecule contributes to the overall carcinogenic process; therefore, "one ligand-receptor molecule could theoretically produce a change (although undetectable) in gene expression" (IARC, 1992).

Based on these simple considerations, it can be assumed that for both genotoxic and receptor-mediated processes a certain number of molecules is necessary to reach a specific probability of inducing a response at cellular level. In other words, in the absence of a more precise analysis, based on specific data and probability evaluations, a distinction among these two processes only in terms of the number of molecules (e.g., "only one molecule", "more than one molecule", "a number of molecules", or "many molecules") may represent an oversimplification of the problem.

It would probably be better to consider a category of cellular processes that can be induced by relatively small numbers of molecules and for which single molecular events are meaningful. This category could include genotoxic effects as well as various types of receptor-mediated proliferation effects.

The example of the 2,3,7,8-tetrachlorodibenzo-p-dioxin (TCDD) (specifically treated elsewhere in this report) may be of interest in this discussion. As is well known, TCDD is one of the most potent rodent carcinogens, even if it is not considered genotoxic. TCDD induces an increased cell proliferation in the target organs and tissues, and its action has been indicated as being connected with a specific receptor (Okey et al., 1994; Cohen and Ellwein, 1991). The examination of data included in "Carcinogenic Potency Database" compiled by Gold et al. (1984, 1987, 1989) indicates that TCDD is characterized by the highest carcinogenic potency of the chemicals examined, and that the TCDD doses shown to be active in inducing cancer in rodents (effect doses) are lower than the doses that, for more than half of the other chemicals (genotoxic and nongenotoxic) included in the database, are estimated (through a linear low-dose extrapolation) to correspond to a 10-5 risk level (Krewski et al., 1990). These data seem to confirm the difficulty of a quantitative and qualitative distinction between genotoxic and nongenotoxic receptor-mediated processes, at least from the point of view of carcinogenic potency and risk-specific doses.

Therefore, for both genotoxic and receptor-mediated nongenotoxic effects, in the absence of specific objective data demonstrating the contrary (e.g., the demonstration of nonlinearities of the involved kinetics), it seems reasonable to assume, in the low-dose range of interest for risk assessment, that the likelihood of a carcinogenic response increases proportionally to the number of molecules present in the cellular environment, and, consequently, proportionally to the dose at the target. This is one of the arguments on which the low-dose linearity hypothesis has been based.

According to Lutz (1990), if the hypothesis of a specific nonlinearity is proposed for low-dose extrapolation purposes, its slope and range have to be appropriately investigated and evaluated for any relevant endpoint (e.g., DNA-adduct formation, activation of oncogenes, sustained hyperplasia) in the dose range of interest. In the absence of these data, low-dose linear extrapolation seems an appropriate hypothesis (Lutz, 1990).

2.3. CELL PROLIFERATION AND MUTATION

Specific consideration of the processes that can lead to mutations has been indicated as an important point in cancer risk modeling (Bogen, 1989; Portier and Kopp-Schneider, 1991; Butterworth and Goldsworthy, 1991; Ellwein and Purtilo, 1992; Lutz, 1990). This modeling approach examines the dynamics of DNA damage and its fixation by introducing a "damaged cell stage", which is potentially reversible, in the multistage models of carcinogenesis. According to these models, a specific cell, either normal or already initiated, is transformed into a "damaged cell" as a consequence of DNA adduct formation or other events (e.g., single strand breaks). The event inducing the damage is assumed to affect a single strand, so that the damage may be removed by the DNA repair system. The damage may be fixed into a stable mutation if the cell divides before the damage is repaired. In DNA damage and repair models, the processes of damage formation (leading to the transition from a previous stage to the damaged stage), back transition from the damaged stage to the previous stage (as a consequence of DNA repair), and damaged cell removal (as a consequence of death or differentiation) are quantitatively accounted for by their respective rates. These rates may be dependent on the dose of the specific carcinogen(s) under examination and on background conditions, as well as on time.

The incorporation of DNA damage and repair in cancer risk modeling may explicitly take into account events such as an increase of cell division rate or a reduction of DNA repair efficiency, which, even if not directly affecting DNA, may nevertheless enhance the mutation rate.

Moreover, a simple simulation analysis of mutation kinetics indicates that correlations between cell division events and the time series of DNA adduct formation and persistence may correspond to a significant increase in the expected mutation frequency without any change in the average rates of these two events. The synchronization of these two categories of cellular events may represent an important parameter by itself. The joint capacity of some carcinogenic agents for inducing both DNA adducts and some degree of cell proliferation may be regarded within this scheme.

These considerations indicate that, whenever necessary, the model parameter representing the transition rate between two consecutive stages should not only account for possible genotoxic action, but also for possible events secondary to cell proliferation, such as exogenous and endogenous DNA adduct fixation and DNA replication errors.

Lastly, it is worth noting that the dose-dependent increase in cell division rate, if it enhances the DNA damage fixation rate and, thereby, the mutation rate, should not be strictly considered within the "cancer promotion" framework. Rather, it must also be considered as part of the "initiation" framework. Further, it is worth noting that, whenever necessary, this process may be considered in cancer risk mathematical modeling by simply adopting, for the quantitative description of the transition probability from one stage to the successive one, a mathematical function that also accounts for "indirect" mutation events like the ones discussed above.

More generally, it is important to underline that the theory on which two-stage clonal expansion models are based explicitly considers the possibility that the same agent(s) may exert their impact on initiation, promotion, and conversion, without a priori distinguishing between "initiators", "promoters", or "completers". Rather, these models allow the estimate of the initiation, promotion, and conversion potential of carcinogenic agent(s) without restricting them to specific categories of action. This represents an important feature, which is of interest in both hypothesis identification and testing, and in practical risk assessment evaluations.

2.4. DIFFERENCES IN SUSCEPTIBILITY

As is well known, the factors modifying the toxicity of chemicals and the effects of exposure to infectious agents include species and strain, genetic differences, age, sex, diet, lifestyle, and health conditions (Carlson, 1987). In particular, differences among human individuals and subpopulations may involve absorption, distribution in the organism, tissue binding, half-life in body, metabolism, excretion rate, as well as mutagenicity and carcinogenicity. It is important to note that human heterogeneity in response to toxic agents can be expected to be much greater than that observed in inbred strains commonly used in toxicological experiments (intentionally selected for their homogeneity) (Calabrese, 1988). A factor 10 for human variability is commonly used in setting acceptable exposure standards for noncarcinogens; however, this aspect is generally not specifically considered in carcinogen risk assessment (Calabrese, 1988).

Many studies have pointed out the high variability of human populations with respect to most of biomarkers associated with the carcinogenic process, even when exposure levels are comparable or practically equivalent (Calabrese, 1988; Perera et al., 1991; Caporaso, 1991; Hattis, 1988). In particular, carcinogen binding to DNA has been shown to vary over a wide range up to more than a hundredfold, even in samples of cultured cells equally treated. This variability, which has been indicated to be not a simple consequence of intraindividual variability, which also exists (Thompson et al., 1989), may have important consequences on the definition of carcinogen risk. As an example, if carcinogen DNA binding levels are assumed as possible indicators of the "target active dose", not only the average levels of these parameters, but also their statistical distribution, may be important for risk assessment. Moreover, wide interindividual variation has been demonstrated in the metabolism of various carcinogens (Caporaso, 1991).

The individual sensitivities in human populations have been hypothesized to be lognormally distributed (Hattis, 1988). As is well known, the lognormal distribution is characterized by a long tail, which extends towards high values, and by particularly high upper extreme values (at least compared with a normal distribution). If the variability assessed for most biomarkers associated with carcinogenicity is assumed to be representative of the variability of the individual susceptibilities, and if these latter are lognormally distributed, it may be easily estimated that the "individual risk" for the "extreme" individuals in the population could be up to two orders of magnitude higher than the "average risk", and even more (depending on the number of individuals considered).

Moreover, the existence of different phenotypes and genotypes has been demonstrated, in relation to parameters that are recognized to be relevant for carcinogenic risk (Harris, 1991; Kawahjiri et al., 1990; Idle et al. 1981; Kaisary et al., 1987). For instance, based on a statistical sample of a typical Western population, a multimodal lognormal distribution has been shown to appropriately describe the distribution of individual metabolic ratios of the pharmacological drug debrisoquine (metabolic ratios being defined as molar ratios of debrisoquine to hydroxydebrisoquine, its main metabolite) (Caporaso, 1991). The three peaks of this distribution were associated with extensive metabolizers (homozygous), extensive metabolizers (heterozygous), and poor metabolizers (homozygous recessive). An association of the debrisoquine metabolic phenotype and lung cancer has been indicated by several epidemiological studies (Caporaso et al., 1989, 1990).

A detailed discussion of these topics is beyond the scope of this discussion. However, the above-reported data and evaluations indicate that a remarkably high interindividual variability, also due to the possible existence of different phenotypes and genotypes, may be encountered for parameters relevant to carcinogenic risk. This point may be particularly important in carcinogenic risk assessment, also from a ethical point of view. In other words, the "individual risk" may be something different from the "population risk": these data suggest that individuals and subpopulations might exist in the same population under examination, whose risk could be higher, even much higher, than the average risk. It seems reasonable that reference to relevant biomarkers, metabolic parameters, other relevant biological indicators of susceptibility, and, whenever necessary and possible, relevant phenotypic and genetic differences, may provide useful information for analyzing and considering these aspects. The importance and use in risk assessment of biomarkers and metabolic data and models will be examined in detail in other chapters of this report, so that it is not necessary to further discuss them here.

Lastly, it is worth noting that a well known set of mathematical models of common use in toxicology, the "tolerance distribution" mathematical models, of which the "probit" model is the classical example, assume, by definition, that different individuals are characterized by different tolerances and effect thresholds for the tested agent, and make explicit reference to the cumulative distribution of individual tolerances (Finney, 1987; IARC, 1986; Berkson, 1953). In other words, individual variability has long been a motivation for mathematical modeling in toxicology. This principle has also been discussed in relation to heterogeneous populations and to the "linearizing effect" in heterogeneous population dose-response relationships caused by the multifactorial variation of individual susceptibilities (Lutz, 1990).

2.5. MECHANISMS OF INHIBITION IN MUTAGENESIS AND CARCINOGENESIS

2.5.1. Introduction

Mutations in somatic and germ cells can be the cause of major health hazards. They can lead to various somatic and heritable diseases or have teratogenic effects. The relationship between somatic mutations and cancer is well established: cancer cannot be initiated without a mutation (Lawley, 1989; Hemminki, 1993). But, while mutations are required for initiation, a single mutation is not enough to cause cancer. Cancer is a multistage process that results from the occurrence of several independent accidents in one cell (Knudson Jr., 1986). The different operational stages thought to occur in carcinogenesis are initiation, promotion, and progression, but the course of events is not perfectly determined in the different forms of the disease. Initiation depends on mutation induction and is an irreversible process, while promotion is more complex, possibly influenced by one or more reversible steps (Ramel, 1990).

Genetic alterations acting or suspected to act during carcinogenesis include point mutations, insertions, deletions, translocations, inversions, sister chromatid exchanges, nondisjunction, recombination, disproportional replication of DNA, mitochondrial mutations, as well as events leading to the induction of indirect mutagenesis, such as imbalance of nucleotide pool, secondary formation of oxygen radicals, inactivation of defense mechanisms against free radicals, and endogenous formation of DNA adducts (Ramel, 1990).

Two classes of genes, the dominantly acting oncogenes and the recessive tumor suppressor genes were shown to play a leading role in the carcinogenic process. Oncogenes through activation by mutations, translocations, etc., and tumor suppressor genes through inactivation by mutations, deletions, etc. (Bishop, 1991; Weinberg, 1991).

Most cancers are initiated by genetic change, but heritable epigenetic events, such as changes in the methylation pattern of DNA, that affect gene expression without causing any changes in the DNA sequence are also thought to be involved in the carcinogenic process (Doerfler, 1983; Jones and Buckley, 1990).

Each step in the development of cancer is governed by multiple factors. Some depend on the genetic constitution of the individual, while others on the environment and lifestyle. Most cancers are the result of various environmental factors. This suggests that the identification of mutagenic agents in the environment and subsequent protection of humans from exposure to such agents might prevent certain human cancers (Henderson et al., 1991). In real life, hazardous chemicals are usually found in combination with other agents, which may enhance or inhibit their mutagenic or carcinogenic effects. Such interactions are important since induction of mutations might be preceded by a series of events involving biotransformation leading to formation of reactive metabolites, reaction of such metabolites with DNA, DNA repair, etc. (Ramel et al., 1986).

There are various chemical agents able to enhance or inhibit mutagenicity and carcinogenicity acting on the different steps of the process. Here we are dealing with

Classification
1. Extracellular inhibition
2. Intracellular inhibition
a) Inhibition of cancer initiation
b) Inhibition of tumor promotion and progression

Table 2.1: *Categories of inhibitors of mutagenesis and carcinogenesis*

the great variety of inhibitors of mutagenesis and carcinogenesis and their mechanisms of action.

2.5.2. Inhibition in Mutagenesis and Carcinogenesis

The multiple genetic alterations occurring along the different stages of carcinogenesis can be modulated through a variety of mechanisms by a broad range of inhibitors (Hartman and Shankel, 1990).

Inhibition of mutagenesis and carcinogenesis (also termed antimutagenesis and anticarcinogenesis) is effected at many levels, including prevention of mutagen formation, direct or enzymatic trapping of mutagens by compounds present in the cell or in the surrounding fluid, inhibition of metabolic activation of promutagens, modulation of DNA repair mechanisms, inhibition of oxidative DNA damage, etc.

Exact classification of all known inhibitors of mutagenesis and carcinogenesis is difficult since the precise mechanisms of action are not known for many compounds, while in several cases obtained results cannot be distinguished as being the cause or the consequence of inhibitory effects. In addition, many well-characterized compounds exhibit their inhibitory effect through a plethora of discrete mechanisms of action and thus belong to more than one class in classifications based on mechanistic principles. The different classification schemes proposed so far share the same main features (Wattenberg, 1985; Ramel et al., 1986; De Flora and Ramel, 1988).

According to the classification of De Flora and Ramel (1988), based on the mechanisms of action of the inhibitors of mutagenesis and carcinogenesis, antimutagenesis and anticarcinogenesis involve (1) inhibition in extracellular environments and (2) inhibition in the intracellular environment. The latter includes (a) agents inhibiting cancer initiation and (b) agents suppressing tumor promotion and progression (see Table 2.1).

2.5.3. Extracellular Inhibition

Events occurring in the extracellular environment such as different interactions and biotransformations may play a major role in mutation induction. Inhibition in the extracellular environment may be the result of inhibition of uptake of the mutagens or of their precursors, inhibition of endogenous formation of mutagens and inactivation of mutagens (De Flora and Ramel, 1988) (see Table 2.2).

There are several agents that can inhibit penetration of various mutagens into the cells. Short-chain fatty acids inhibit N-nitrosodimethylamine (NDMA) mutagenicity

Mechanism	Examples
Inhibition of uptake	Short-chain fatty acids, putrescine, vitamin C, dietary fibers
Inhibition of endogenous formation	Vitamin C, tocopherols, phenols (caffeic, ferulic, chlorogenic acids, etc.), aminobenzoic acid, p-aminosalicylic acid, butylated hydroxytoluene, thiols (glutathione, N-acetylcysteine), Lactobacillus acidophilus, Bifidobacterium longum
Inactivation of mutagens	Antioxidants (enzymes from cabbage, broccoli, etc., peroxidases of human saliva, uric acid, bilirubin), thiols, dietary fibers

Table 2.2: *Categories of extracellular inhibitors of mutagenesis and carcinogenesis*

in bacteria by interfering in the cellular uptake of NDMA metabolites (Hayatsu et al., 1988), putrescine prevents the cellular uptake of paraquat (Brooke-Taylor et al., 1983), while vitamin C blocks uptake of hexavalent chromium, thus inhibiting the clastogenic activity of lead chromate in Chinese hamster ovary cells (Wise et al., 1993).

Mutagens and carcinogens in the human organism are formed by transformation of promutagens in the acidic gastric environment and by biotransformation in the prokaryotic cells that constitute the microbial intestinal flora (Gichner and Veleminsky, 1988).

The most typical deleterious products formed through the nitrosation reaction in the acidic environment of the stomach are the N-nitroso compounds, which are well-known mutagens and carcinogens. The nitrosation reaction can be modulated by several catalysts or inhibitors (Gichner and Veleminsky, 1988). Vitamin C (ascorbic acid) was found to decrease nitrosamine production from secondary amines and nitrite in an acidic environment (Mirvish, 1981), while it was found to inhibit N-methyl-N'-nitro-N-nitrosoguanidine (MNNG) induced mutagenesis in vitro and in vivo (Jain et al., 1989; Kappas and Patrineli, 1992) and decrease the frequency of clastogenic and mitosis- disruptive events induced in mouse bone marrow cells by the pesticides endosulfan, phosphamidon, and mancozeb (Khan and Sinha, 1993). Vitamin E is a collective term comprising eight different phenolic compounds synthesized by plants of which the most common and biologically active is alpha-tocopherol. This compound was found to inhibit the formation of N-nitroso compounds by scavenging nitrite both in vitro and in vivo (Bartsch et al., 1988). Several naturally occurring phenolic acids were also shown to inhibit the formation of N-nitroso compounds (Stich et al., 1982). Caffeic, ferulic and chlorogenic acids were shown to block nitrosamine formation (Kuenzig et al., 1984; Pignatelli et al., 1982), gallic and tannic acids inhibited the N-nitroso compounds- induced mutagenicity in Salmonella (Gichner et al., 1987), while caffeic, ellagic, chlorogenic, and ferulic acids inhibited rat tongue carcinogenesis induced by 4-nitroquinoline-1-oxide (Tanaka et al., 1993).

An inhibitory action against N-nitroso compounds-induced mutagenicity and carcinogenicity is also exhibited by a variety of other natural or synthetic chemicals like aminobenzoic acid isomers (Gichner et al., 1994), p-aminosalicylic acid (Gichner et al., 1992), propyl gallate, butylated hydroxytoluene (Hirose et al., 1993), glutathione (Kako et al., 1992), N-acetylcysteine (Camoirano et al., 1988), catechins (Jain et al., 1989), etc., while enterobacteria of the human intestinal tract possessing appreciable amounts of glutathione exhibit a significant detoxifying activity (Owens and Hartman, 1986).

The conversion of promutagens into mutagens and carcinogens by the prokaryotic cells colonizing the human intestinal tract can be suppressed by Lactobacillus acidophilus through reduction of the activity of enzymes of bacterial source, such as beta-glucuronidase, nitroreductase, azoreductase (Goldin and Gorbach, 1977). Dietary supplementation of Bifidobacterium longum cultures was shown to inhibit colon and liver tumors induced by the food mutagen 2-amino-3-methylimidazo[4,5f]quinoline in rats (Reddy and Rivenson, 1993).

The anticarcinogenic effect of dietary fibers is attributed to their capacity in binding and irreversibly adsorbing carcinogenic chemicals. The decrease of transit time of the digestion products through the intestinal tract by dietary fibers prevents prolonged contact and subsequent absorption of the mutagens into the mucosal cells (Hayatsu et al., 1988). Insoluble polysaccharides from dietary fibers inhibit colon tumor development in laboratory animals through the binding of bile acids or bile salts (Reddy, 1975), while soluble fiber polysaccharides from unlignified cell walls lower the pH due to production of short-chain fatty acids, which are fiber degradation products (Bartram et al., 1993). The drop in pH decreases the potential tumor promoter activity of secondary bile acids due to diminished solubility of free bile acids and inhibition of colonic bacterial enzyme 7-alpha- dehydroxylase, which degrades primary to secondary bile acids (Rogers et al., 1993; Harris and Ferguson, 1993).

Several porphyrins like hemin, chlorophyll, and chlorophyllin inhibit the mutagenicity of various polycyclic chemicals through complex formation at the planar of their molecule (Arimoto et al., 1993; Hayatsu et al., 1993; Dashwood and Guo, 1993).

Mutagens and carcinogens can be inactivated in extracellular environments by physical, chemical, or enzymatic reactions. There are various detoxifying agents, basically possessing antioxidant activities, which modulate the concentration of electrophiles. Several enzymes from cabbage, radish, celery, broccoli, etc., possessing peroxidase and NADPH-oxidase activities exhibit antimutagenic activity through inactivation of certain pyrolysis products (Inoue et al., 1981). Some complex mixtures of human and animal origin like saliva, blood, urine and tissue homogenates, possess antioxidant activities (Gichner and Veleminsky, 1988). Inactivation of mutagens by human saliva is attributed to the action of peroxidases, while uric acid and bilirubin are effective antioxidants of the human blood plasma (Ames et al., 1981; Stocker et al., 1987).

2.5.4. Intracellular Inhibition

Cancer initiation involves an irreversible modification taking place in the intracellular environment most probably due to a mutation related to growth control and/or differentiation. The three steps hypothetically involved in the process of initiation are:

Mechanism	Examples
Inhibition of metabolic activation	Diallyl sulfide, catechins, ammonium metavanadate, oleic acid, wheat sprout, isothiocyanates, dithiocarbamates
Induction of a shift in monooxygenase isoenzymes	trans-stilbene oxide
Induction of cytochrome P-450	indole-3-carbinol, β-naphthoflavone
Induction of enzymatic conjugation of electrophiles	Phenols, indoles, isothiocyanates, coumarins, diterpenes, non polar flavones, dithiolthiones, thiols
Direct trapping of electrophiles	Ellagic acid, glutathione, N-acetylcysteine
Scavenging of free radicals	Antioxidants (tocopherols, β-carotene, vitamin C, etc.), antioxidant enzyme systems
Inhibition of oncogene expression	Protease inhibitors (antipain, leupeptine, etc.)
Modulation of DNA repair	Cinnamaldehyde, coumarin, umbelliferone, anisaldehyde, vanillin, tannic acid, cobaltous chloride, protease inhibitors
Modulation of DNA replication	Vitamin A, β-carotene, retinyl palmitate, anti-inflammatory steroids

Table 2.3: *Categories of intracellular inhibitors of mutagenesis and carcinogenesis blocking cancer initiation*

generation of electrophilic reactants formed spontaneously or after metabolic activation, binding of electrophilic reactants to cellular DNA and other macromolecules, and cell proliferation fixing the biochemical lesion (Rotstein and Slaga, 1988).

There are many agents acting intracellularly to block the initiation process. Intracellular inhibition may be due to modulation of cell metabolism, blocking of reactive chemical species, modulation of DNA replication, modulation of DNA repair, and modulation of cell replication (De Flora and Ramel, 1988) (see Table 2.3).

2.5.5. Inhibitors of Cancer Initiation

Except for direct-acting mutagens/carcinogens, genotoxic chemicals must be metabolically activated to reactive electrophilic species for to bind to cellular DNA and other macromolecules. Modulation of cell metabolism involves regulation of the rate of formation of electrophiles by monooxygenases versus the rate of disappearance of electrophiles due to enzymatic reactions, non- enzymatic breakdown and binding by cell components, in favor of the second. Modulation of the rate of disappearance of electrophiles mainly regards inhibition through interference with the enzymatic function of the microsomal monooxygenase system and may include inhibition of the biochemical mechanisms responsible for activation of promutagens to electrophilic metabolites, induction of a shift in the monooxygenase isoenzymes, induction of a competitive interaction for metabolic activation between structurally similar compounds and stimulation of enzymatic detoxification of chemicals (De Flora and Ramel, 1988).

There are various inhibitors of metabolic activation in the microsomal monooxygenase system. Diallyl sulfide, a natural ingredient of Allium vegetables, inhibits metabolic activation of nitrosamines (Hong et al., 1991); catechins contained in several tea extracts inhibit metabolic activation of benzo[]pyrenes (Sasaki et al., 1993); the vanadium compound, ammonium metavanadate, inhibits the activity of the cytochrome P-450-dependent monooxygenase system by acting at both the pre- and post-transcriptional levels (Del Carratore et al., 1993); oleic acid inhibits mutagenicity of food pyrolysate mutagens, polycyclic aromatic hydrocarbons, and nitrosamines by blocking metabolic activation of these agents (Hayatsu et al., 1988); wheat sprout extract inhibits mutagenicity induced by benzo[]pyrene, cyclophosphamide, and ethidium bromide by inhibiting the P-450-dependent monooxygenase system activity, due to the action of the flavonoids apigenin and shaftoside (Peryt et al., 1992); while nitropyrene-induced genotoxicity is modulated by apigenin, tannic acid, ellagic acid, and indole-3-carbinol (Kuo et al., 1992).

Other inhibitors of the microsomal monooxygenase system are several isothiocyanates (Wattenberg, 1981), dithiocarbamates (Gichner and Veleminsky, 1984), flavonoids (Edenharder et al., 1993), as well as ellagic acid (Wood et al., 1982), acetaminophen, methimazole (Gichner et al., 1993), arachidonic acid (Ho et al., 1992), etc.

The microsomal monooxygenase system can also be modulated through induction of a shift in monooxygenase isoenzymes, resulting in inhibition of formation of the ultimate mutagenic compound. For example, trans-stilbene oxide through induction of specific cytochrome P-450 isoenzymes synthesis shifts benzo[]pyrene metabolism from the highly mutagenic 7,8-dihydrodiol 9,10-epoxides to the less mutagenic 4,5-epoxide (Oesch, 1988).

Several inducers of cytochrome P-450, like indole-3-carbinol and beta-naphthoflavone, act as inhibitors of mutagenesis and carcinogenesis by increasing the production of activated metabolites in non-target tissues or by enhancing oxidative detoxification in all tissues. However, induction of cytochrome P-450 may lead to enhanced activation of a promutagen in a non-target tissue resulting in a shift in target organ (Morse and Stoner, 1993) (see Table 2.4).

Blocking of reactive chemical species refers to trapping of positively charged electrophilic metabolites and scavenging of oxygen radicals. It includes enzymatic conjugation of electrophiles by UDP glucuronyl transferases, sulfotransferases, acetyltransferases, glutathione S-transferase isoenzymes, DT diaphorase, etc., with the formation of inactive products (Wattenberg, 1985; De Flora and Ramel, 1988).

Glutathione S-transferase isoenzymes catalyze the nucleophilic addition of the thiol of glutathione to electrophilic acceptors including aryl and alkyl halides, olefins, organic peroxides, quinones and sulphate esters, while new substrates are continuously being reported in the literature. Glutathione S-transferase is induced by a variety of chemicals, such as phenols, indoles, aromatic isothiocyanates, coumarins, diterpenes, nonpolar flavones, dithiolthiones and thiols (Ketterer, 1988; Pickett and Lu, 1989).

Enzymatic detoxification of chemicals is also stimulated by the action of DT di-

Mechanism	Examples
Inhibition of cell proliferation, induction of cell differentiation	Retinoids, calcium, α-difluoromethylornithine
Modulation of the inflammatory response	Inhibitors of arachidonic acid metabolism (piroxicam, indomethacin, aspirin, ibuprofen, quercetin, curcumin)
Inhibition of oxidative DNA damage	Antioxidants (butylated hydroxytoluene and hydroxyanisole, vitamin C, vitamin E, disulfiram, etc.)
Inhibition of oncogene expression	Protease inhibitors
Modulation of signal transduction	Inhibitors of protein kinase C (tamoxifen, phentolamine, dibucaine, verapamil, staurosporine)

Table 2.4: *Categories of intracellular inhibitors of mutagenesis and carcinogenesis suppressing tumor promotion and progression*

aphorase inducers, including several natural or synthetic phenols, synthetic thiols, along with several flat planar aromatics (cytochrome P-450 inducers), such as polycyclic aromatic hydrocarbons, azo dyes, and beta-naphthoflavone (Hollander and Ernster, 1975; De Flora and Ramel, 1988; Morse and Stoner, 1993).

Cruciferous plants such as Brussels sprouts, cabbage, and broccoli, containing phenols, isothiocyanates, and indole derivatives, are capable of modifying the activities of enzymes involved in the metabolic transformation of chemicals (Benson and Barretto, 1985; Chung et al., 1993). Such an inducer of quinone reductase and glutathione S-transferases was recently isolated and characterized from Brassica oleracea italica (Zhang et al., 1992).

Besides enzymatic conjugation, trapping of electrophiles is also effected by direct reaction with nucleophilic inhibitors, such as ellagic acid, glutathione, N-acetylcysteine, etc. Ellagic acid is a naturally occurring plant phenol known to inhibit mutagenicity of epoxides of polycyclic aromatic hydrocarbons, aflatoxin B1 and N-nitroso compounds (Hayatsu et al., 1988). Glutathione, the tripeptide gamma-glutamyl-L-cysteinyl-glycine, is the most widely distributed thiol found in animals, plants, fungi, and many bacteria. It is present in high concentrations in the intracellular environment, but it is also found in extracellular environments. The mechanism of action of glutathione and related thiols involves attack on electrophilic carbons, nitrogens and oxygens (Ketterer, 1988). Vitamin A indirectly acts through formation of epoxides, which compete with carcinogenic epoxides in reaction with DNA or through enhancement of prostaglandin production, which inhibits binding of carcinogens to DNA (De Flora and Ramel, 1988).

Endogenous or exogenous free radicals can react with cellular macromolecules and lead to a variety of biological consequences such as mutation, transformation etc. The reduction of oxygen to superoxide anions in biological systems can lead to a rapid spontaneous and enzymatic formation of hydrogen peroxide, which undergoes a metal-catalyzed decomposition yielding reactive hydroxyl radicals that seem to be involved in the various stages of the carcinogenic process. Oxidant effects may be modulated through enzymatic activities or through direct reaction with several small scavenging molecules. Antioxidant enzyme systems include superoxide dismutases, catalases, selenium containing glutathione peroxidases, DT diaphorase, etc., while antioxidant scavenger molecules include tocopherols, beta-carotene, glutathione, uric acid, butylated hydroxyanisole, etc. (Hochstein and Atallah, 1988).

Alpha-tocopherol was found to trap unsaturated fatty-acid-derived chain-propagating peroxy radicals in lipid membranes and to scavenge superoxide anions (Simic, 1988); vitamin C and glutathione exhibited a protective action against oxidative damage caused by potassium bromate (Sai et al., 1992); two vitamin mixes, the first containing ascorbic acid, alpha-tocopherol, and lecithin and the second a rosemary extract, carnosic acid, and carnosol, were shown to strongly inhibit mutagenicity induced by the generation of oxygen radicals by tert-butyl-hydroperoxide and hydrogen peroxide (Minnunni et al., 1992); beta-carotene, tocopherols, butylated hydroxytoluene, dimethyl sulfoxide, and mannitol effectively inhibited nitric oxide-induced mutagenicity (Arroyo et al., 1992); while several protease inhibitors block the carcinogenic process mediated by active oxygen radicals (Hayatsu et al., 1988).

Activation of proto-oncogenes by a variety of mechanisms is involved in the different stages of the carcinogenic process (Bishop, 1983; Barbacid, 1987). Mutant Ha-ras genes were detected before tumor development in chemically-initiated mouse skin (Nelson et al., 1992). Several protease inhibitors have been found to inhibit oncogene expression, thus exhibiting anticarcinogenic properties. The protease inhibitor antipain suppressed c-myc expression in mammalian cells, while S-adenosyl-L-methionine inhibited c-Ha-ras and c-myc expression in rat liver (De Flora and Ramel, 1988).

Mutation induction is influenced by the DNA repair capacity of the cells (Walker, 1985). The efficiency of DNA repair depends on the nature of DNA lesion, the type of repair effected, the cell proliferation rate, etc. Slight DNA damage is repaired by the error-free excision or recombination repair systems, more severe DNA lesions are repaired by the SOS repair system, while alkylation damage is repaired by the induction of specific alkyl glycosylases and transferases of the adaptive response repair system (Kuroda and Inoue, 1988).

Several antimutagenic agents can act on the process of DNA repair and replication in affected cells. Cinnamaldehyde, coumarin, umbelliferone, anisaldehyde, vanillin, and tannic acid suppress the mutagenic effects of UV or chemicals in bacterial systems (Ohta et al., 1983a; Ohta et al., 1983b; Shimoi et al., 1985; Ohta et al., 1988). Cobaltous chloride decreases the proliferating activity of affected cells, prolonging cell cycles before DNA lesions are fixed; cinnamaldehyde and vanillin favor an error-free RecA-dependent recombinational repair; tannic acid stimulates DNA excision repair; while several protease inhibitors suppress error-prone DNA repair systems (Kuroda and Inoue, 1988). Conflicting are the results of experiments regarding the anticarcinogenic potential of several DNA repair inhibitors such as methylxanthines (e.g., caffeine), nicotinamide analogs (e.g., 3-aminobenzamide), etc. (Boothman et al., 1988).

Modulation of cell proliferation by antiproliferative agents can prolong the cell cycle providing time for efficient elimination of premutagenic lesions by DNA repair systems (Moon et al., 1983). Efficient inhibitors of cell proliferation are the retinoids vitamin A, beta-carotene, retinyl palmitate, retinyl acetate, etc., along with hydroxyurea, actinomycin D, and some anti-inflammatory steroids (Rotstein and Slaga, 1988).

2.5.6. Inhibitors of Tumor Promotion and Progression

Tumor promotion is operationally defined as an event leading to sustained hyperplasia and subsequent development of papillomas and is divided into two stages in the mouse skin model: a brief exposure to the potent tumor promoter 12-O-tetradecanoyl-13-phorbol acetate (TPA) in stage I is followed by a repeated treatment with a weaker promoter such as mezerein in stage II (Rotstein and Slaga, 1988).

Tumor progression, on the other hand, is a broadly defined stage in the carcinogenic process and each step involved may be the result of one or more new abnormalities within the initiated cell. Extended cell proliferation, invasion of adjacent tissue, and metastasis depend on the loss or gain of whole chromosomes, loss of chromosomal domains, increased rate of spontaneous and induced mutations, and enhanced gene amplification (Bishop, 1987; Bishop, 1991).

Inhibitors of tumor promotion and progression act on initiated or neoplastic cells to modulate the genetic or epigenetic events involved. Some of the mechanisms discussed in the previous sections can also apply to modulation of tumor promotion and progression, which may be the result of inhibition of cell proliferation and induction of cell differentiation, modulation of the inflammatory response, inhibition of oxidative DNA damage, inhibition of oncogene expression, modulation of signal transduction, etc. (Wattenberg, 1985; De Flora and Ramel, 1988; Morse and Stoner, 1993).

Polyamines are accumulated due to increased levels of ornithine decarboxylase, an enzyme catalyzing the conversion of ornithine to putrescine, and confer high proliferative ability to affected cells (Tabor and Tabor, 1984). Alpha-difluoromethylornithine, an ornithine decarboxylase inhibitor, prevents chemical carcinogenesis induced in various systems (Tanaka et al., 1993), while selenium salts alone (Ip, 1981) or in combination with alpha-difluoromethylornithine inhibit colon tumorigenesis in rats (McGarrity and Peiffer, 1993). Several retinoids and carotenoids inhibit cell proliferation and induce cell differentiation through regulation of gene expression (Sporn and Roberts, 1983) and modulation of gap junctional communication (Mehta et al., 1989; Bertram, 1993). Retinoids as well as calcium were found to stimulate cell differentiation and inhibit tumor promotion and progression in various experimental systems (Mawson et al., 1987; Chen et al., 1993).

Inflammation induced by promoters is a critical step in tumor promotion. Arachidonic acid seems to be a major contributor to the overall inflammatory response when metabolized through the cyclo-oxygenase or the lipoxygenase pathways leading to increased prostaglandin and 12-hydroxyarachidonic acid production (Rotstein and Slaga, 1988; Pegg, 1988). Inhibition of arachidonic acid metabolism by the cyclo-oxygenase and lipoxygenase pathways inhibitors piroxicam, indomethacin, aspirin, ibuprofen, 3,4,2',4'-tetrahydroxychalcone, quercetin, curcumin, etc., efficiently inhibits tumor promotion (Reddy et al., 1990; Narisawa et al., 1981; Reddy et al., 1993; Morse and Stoner, 1993).

Reactive oxygen forms such as superoxide, hydroxyl radical, and hydrogen peroxide can induce DNA lesions affecting gene expression in initiated cells during tumor promotion and progression. Characteristic DNA lesions produced are single and double strand breaks, apurinic and apyrimidinic sites, etc. Such DNA damaging agents are strong clastogens but weak mutagens preferentially inducing sequence rearrangements, while they can also participate in epigenetic mechanisms resulting in altered gene expression (Cerutti, 1985).

Several antioxidants exhibit an efficient antipromotional activity. Curcumin, butylated hydroxytoluene, and butylated hydroxyanisole were shown to inhibit tumor promotion induced by phorbol-12-myristate-13-acetate functioning as hydroxyl radical scavengers (Shih and Lin, 1993; Wattenberg and Lam, 1983). Several other antioxidants such as vitamins C and E, disulfiram, 4- parahydroxyanisole and copper(II) 3,5-diisopropylsalicylate are efficient inhibitors of tumor promotion induced by 12-O-tetradecanoyl-13-phorbol acetate (Rotstein and Slaga, 1988; Slaga et al., 1983; Egner and Kensler, 1985).

Other forms of inhibition of tumor promotion involve the action of specific protease inhibitors such as antipain, leupeptine, and Bowman-Birk soybean protease which were found to suppress tumor promotion in animal models (Nomura et al., 1980; Hozumi et al., 1972; Yavelow et al., 1983) or modulation of signal transduction through inhibition of protein kinase C and subsequent decrease in phosphorylation of regulatory proteins affecting cell proliferation (Castagna and Martelly, 1989). Agents known to exhibit an inhibitory effect towards protein kinase C activity are tamoxifen, phentolamine, dibucaine, verapamil, staurosporine, etc. (Morse and Stoner, 1993; Weinstein, 1988; Mori et al., 1980; Strickland et al., 1993).

2.5.7. Dual Effects of Inhibitors

There are some cases where the causative factor of cancer development is known and can be eliminated, as cigarette smoking. But in several other cases, even if the causes are known, they cannot be eliminated, as for example exposure to substances of natural or synthetic origin occurring in the environment or in the food or being produced as by-products of normal metabolism (Ames, 1983; Voutsinas et al., 1993; Ashby and Tennant, 1988; Sugimura, 1988; Ames and Gold, 1991).

The control of cancer by the administration of one or more chemical compounds, termed cancer chemoprevention, has received growing attention. As most of the human cancers are of unknown causes, a general strategy for cancer prevention could be an approach to reducing incidence of the disease (Wattenberg, 1985).

A major problem in the use of the various inhibitors of mutagenesis and carcinogenesis for cancer chemoprevention is that in many cases they exhibit toxic or even mutagenic and carcinogenic effects according to the conditions (De Flora and Ramel, 1988). For example, the variety of phenolic compounds contained in numerous plants are able to suppress the genotoxic activity of several carcinogenic compounds both in vitro and in vivo, but they also induce double strand breaks, DNA adducts, mutations, and chromosome aberrations in a variety of test systems (Stich, 1991). Ascorbic acid enhances SCEs induced by MNNG (Galloway and Painter, 1979), thiotepa, and L-ethionine (Lialiaris et al., 1987), while the frequencies of mutations induced by ethyl methanesulfonate are enhanced when Chinese hamster cells are pre- or post-treated with ascorbic acid (Kojima et al., 1992). o-Vanillin enhances chromosome aberrations induced by alkylating agents (Matsumura et al., 1993), vitamin E acts as a tumor promoter in 7,12-dimethylbenz[]anthracene-initiated mouse skin (Mitchel and McCann, 1993), and tamoxifen possess a strong hepatocarcinogenic effect in rats (Williams et al., 1993).

Moreover, interactions between different inhibitors or between inhibitors and xenobiotics can yield toxic chemical derivatives. For example, the conjugation product of glutathione and ethylene dibromide, S-(2-bromoethyl)-glutathione behaves as a sulphur mustard possessing mutagenic properties (Ketterer, 1988), while ascorbic acid in combination with the synthetic antioxidant butylated hydroxyanisole increases the incidences of squamous cell carcinomas and the multiplicity of forestomach tumors in rats (Shibata et al., 1993).

Additionally, there are inhibitors exhibiting anticancer activity in one tissue, while they are carcinogenic in other tissues. Alpha-tocopherol was found to increase the incidence of preneoplastic lesions in the stomach, while reducing the incidence and multiplicity of kidney atypical tubules; t-butylhydroquinone enhanced the frequency of esophagal papillomas, decreasing the multiplicity of colon adenocarcinomas; and butylated hydroxytoluene enhanced the development of thyroid hyperplasias, but reduced the incidence and multiplicity of colon adenocarcinomas in rats (Hirose et al., 1993).

This dual effect of inhibitors raises serious problems regarding their use in cancer chemoprevention. Further elucidation of the mechanisms of action of various modulators of mutagenesis and carcinogenesis may provide new ideas for a rational design of efficient chemopreventive measures.

2.6. REFERENCES

Alberts B., Bray D., Lewis J., Raff M., Roberts K. and Watson J.D. (1989): Molecular Biology of the Cell, Garland Publishing Inc., New York, pp. 1187-1218.

Ames B.N. (1983): Dietary carcinogens and anticarcinogens, Oxygen radicals and degenerative diseases, Science 221, 1256-1264.

Ames B.N., Cathcart R., Schwiers E. and Hochstein P. (1981): Uric acid provides an antioxidant defence in humans against oxidant- and radical-caused aging and cancer: A hypothesis, Proc. Natl. Acad. Sci. USA 78, 6858-6862.

Ames B.N. and Gold L.S. (1990a): Too many rodents carcinogens: mitogenesis increases mutagenesis, Science, 246, 970-971.

Ames B.N. and Gold L.S. (1990b): Chemical carcinogenesis: too many rodent carcinogens, Proc. Natl. Acad. Sci., 87, 7772-7776.

Ames B.N. and Gold L.S. (1991): Endogenous mutagens and the causes of aging and cancer, Mutation Res. 250, 3-16.

Arimoto S., Fukuoka S., Itome C., Nakano H., Rai H. and Hayatsu H. (1993): Binding of polycyclic planar mutagens to chlorophyllin resulting in inhibition of the mutagenic activity, Mutation Res. 287,

293-305.

Arroyo P.L., Hatch-Pigott V., Mower H.F. and Cooney R.V. (1992): Mutagenicity of nitric oxide and its inhibition by antioxidants, Mutation Res. 281, 193-202.

Ashby J. and Tennant R.W. (1988): Chemical structure, Salmonella mutagenicity and extent of carcinogenicity as indicators of genotoxic carcinogenesis among 222 chemicals tested in rodents by the U.S. NCI/NTP, Mutation Res. 204, 17-115.

Barbacid M. (1987): ras Genes, Annu. Rev. Biochem. 56, 779-827.

Bartram H.-P., Scheppach W., Schmid H., Hofmann A., Dusel G., Richter F., Richter A. and Kasper H. (1993): Proliferation of human colonic mucosa as an intermediate biomarker of carcinogenesis: effects of butyrate, deoxycholate, calcium, ammonia, and pH, Cancer Res. 53, 3283-3288.

Bartsch H., Ohshima H. and Pignatelli B. (1988): Inhibitors of endogenous nitrosation. Mechanisms and implications in human cancer prevention, Mutation Res. 202, 301-324.

Benson A.M. and Barretto P.B. (1985): Effects of disulfiram, diethylthiocarbamate, bisethylxanthogen and benzyl isothiocyanate on glutathione transferase activities in mouse organs, Cancer Res. 45, 4219-4223.

Berkson J. (1953): A statistically precise and relatively simple method of estimating the bioassay with quantal response based on the logit function, J. Am. Stat. Assoc. 48, 565-599.

Bertram J.S. (1993): Inhibition of chemically induced neoplastic transformation by carotenoids Ann. N.Y. Acad. Sci. 686, 161-176.

Bishop J.M. (1983): Cellular oncogenes and retroviruses, Annu. Rev. Biochem. 52, 301-354.

Bishop J.M. (1987): The molecular genetics of cancer, Science 235, 305-311.

Bishop J.M. (1991): Molecular themes in oncogenesis, Cell 64, 235-248.

Bogen K.T. (1989): Cell proliferation kinetics and Multistage cancer risk models, Journal of the National Cancer Institute, 81, 4, 267-277.

Boothman D.A., Schlegel R. and Pardee A.B. (1988): Anticarcinogenic potential of DNA-repair modulators, Mutation Res. 202, 393-411.

Brooke-Taylor S., Smith L.L. and Cohen G.M. (1983): The accumulation of polyamines and paraquat by human peripheral blood, Biochem. Pharmacol. 32, 717-720.

Butterworth B.E., and Goldsworthy T.L. (1991): The role of cell proliferation in multistage carcinogenesis, Proceedings of the Soc. of Experimental Biology and Medicine, 198, 683-687.

Calabrese E.J. (1988): Animal extrapolation and the challenge of human interindividual variation, in C.C. Travis (ed.): Carcinogen risk assessment, Plenum Press, N.Y., pp. 115-122.

Camoirano A., Badolati G.S., Zanacchi P., Bagnasco M. and De Flora S. (1988): Dual role of thiols in N-methyl-N'-nitro-N-nitrosoguanidine genotoxicity, Exp. Oncol. (Life Sci. Adv.) 7, 21-25.

Caporaso N., Hayes R., Dosemici M. et al. (1989): Lung cancer risk, occupational expopsure and the debrisoquine metabolic phenotype, cancer res., 49, 3675-3679.

Caporaso N., Tucker M.A., Hoover R.N., Hayes R.B. et al. (1990): Lung cancer and the debrisoquine metabolic phenotype, JNCI, 82, 1264-1272.

Caporaso N. (1991): Study design and genetic susceptibility in the risk assessment of chemical carcinogens, Ann. Ist. Super. Sanit, 27(4), 621-630.

Carlson G.P. (1987): Factors modifying toxicity, in R.G. Tardiff and J.V. Rodricks (eds): Toxic substances and human risk, Plenum Press, N.Y.

Castagna M. and Martelly I. (1989): Overview of promotion as a mechanism in carcinogenesis, in: C.C. Travis (ed.), Biologically Based Methods for Cancer Risk Assessment, Plenum Press, New York, pp. 141-153.

Cerutti P.A. (1985): Prooxidant states and tumor promotion, Science 227, 375-381.

Chen L.-C., Sly L., Jones C.S., Tarone R. and De Luca L.M. (1993): Differential effects of dietary β-carotene on papilloma and carcinoma formation induced by an initiation-promotion protocol in SENCAR mouse skin, Carcinogenesis 14, 713-717.

Chung F.-L., Morse M.A., Eklind K.I. and Xu Y. (1993): Inhibition of the tobacco-specific nitrosamine-induced lung tumorigenesis by compounds derived from cruciferous vegetables and green tea, Ann. N.Y. Acad. Sci. 686, 186-202.

Cohen S.M. and Ellwein L.B. (1990): Cell proliferation ion carcinogenesis, Science, 249, 1007-1011.

Cohen S.M., and Ellwein L.B. (1991): Genetic errors, cell proliferation, and carcinogenesis, Cancer Research, 51, 6493-6505.

Dashwood R. and Guo D. (1993): Antimutagenic potency of chlorophyllin in the Salmonella assay and its correlation with binding constants of mutagen-inhibitor complexes, Environ. Mol. Mutagen. 22, 164-171.

De Flora S. and Ramel C. (1988): Mechanisms of inhibitors of mutagenesis and carcinogenesis. Classification and overview, Mutation Res. 202, 285-306.

Del Carratore R., Morichetti E., Galli A., Galeotti C. and Bronzetti G. (1993): Inhibition of yeast cytochrome P-450 by ammonium metavanadate, Mutation Res. 301, 165-170.

Doerfler W. (1983): DNA methylation and gene activity, Ann. Rev. Biochem. 52, 93-124.

Edenharder R., von Petersdorff I. and Rauscher R. (1993): Antimutagenic effects of flavonoids, chalcones and structurally related compounds on the activity of 2-amino-3-methylimidazo-[4,5-f]quinoline (IQ) and other heterocyclic amine mutagens from cooked food, Mutation Res. 287, 261-274.

Egner P.A. and Kensler T.W. (1985): Effects of a biomimetic superoxide dismutase on complete and multistage carcinogenesis in mouse skin, Carcinogenesis 6, 1167-1172.

Ellwein L.B. and Purtilo D. (1992): Cellular proliferation and genetic events involved in the genesis of Burkitt lymphoma (BL) in immmune compromised patients, Cancer Genet. Cytogenet., 64, 42-48

Finney D.J. (1987): Statistical method in biological assay, Oxford University Press, Oxford.

Galloway S.M. and Painter R.B. (1979): Vitamin C is positive in the DNA synthesis inhibition and sister-chromatid exchange tests, Mutation Res. 60, 321-327.

Gichner T. and Veleminsky J. (1984): Inhibition of dimethylnitro-samine-induced mutagenesis in Arabidopsis thaliana by diethyl-dithiocarbamate and carbon monoxide, Mutation Res. 139, 29-33.

Gichner T., Pospisil F., Veleminsky J., Volkeova V. and Volke J. (1987): Two types of the antimutagenic effects of gallic and tannic acids towards N-nitroso compounds-induced mutagenicity in the Ames/Salmonella assay, Fol. Microbiol. 32, 55-62.

Gichner T. and Veleminsky J. (1988): Inhibitors of N-nitroso compounds-induced mutagenicity, Mutation Res. 195, 21-43.

Gichner T., Baburek I., Veleminsky J. and Kappas A. (1992): UV-irradiation potentiates the antimutagenicity of p-amino-benzoic and p-aminosalicylic acids in Salmonella typhimurium, Mutation Res. 249, 119-123.

Gichner T., Veleminsky J., Wagner E.D. and Plewa M.J. (1993): Inhibitory effects of acetaminophen, 7,8-benzoflavone and methimazole towards N-nitrosodimethylamine mutagenesis in Arabidopsis thaliana, Mutation Res. 300, 57-61.

Gichner T., Voutsinas G., Patrineli A., Kappas A. and Plewa M.J. (1994): Antimutagenicity of three isomers of aminobenzoic acid in Salmonella typhimurium, Mutation Res., in press.

Gold L.S., Sawyer C.B., Magaw R., Backman G.M., de Veciana M., Levinson R., Hooper N.K., Havender W.R., Bernstein L., Peto R., Pike M.C. and Ames B.N. (1984): A carcinogenic potency database of the standardized results of animal bioassays Environmental Health Perspectives, 58, 9-322.

Gold L.S., Slone T.H., Backman G.M., Magaw R., Lopipero P., Blumenthal M., and Ames B.N. (1987): Second chronological supplement to the Carcinogenic Potency Database: Standardized results of animal bioassays published through Decemember 1984 and by the National Toxicological Program through May, 1986 Environmental Health Perspectives, 74, 237-329.

Gold L.S., Slone T.H., and Bernstein L. (1989). Summary of carcinogenic potency and positivity for 492 rodent carcinogens in the carcinogenic potency database, Environmental Health Perspectives, 79, 259-272.

Goldin B. and Gorbach S.L. (1977): Alterations in fecal microflora enzymes related to diet, age, Lactobacillus supplements, and dimethylhydrazine, Cancer 40, 2421-2426.

Harris C.C. (1991): Chemical and physical carcinogenesis: advances and perspectives for the 1990s, Cancer Research, (Suppl.), 51, 5023s-5044s.

Harris P.J. and Ferguson L.R. (1993): Dietary fibre: its composition and the role in protection against colorectal cancer, Mutation Res. 290, 97-110.

Hartman P.E. and Shankel D.M. (1990): Antimutagens and anticarcinogens: a survey of putative interceptor molecules, Environ. Mol. Mutagen. 15, 145-182.

Hattis D. (1988): The use of biological markers in risk assessment, Statistical Science, 3(3), 358-366.

Hayatsu H., Arimoto S. and Negishi T. (1988): Dietary inhibitors of mutagenesis and carcinogenesis, Mutation Res. 202, 429-446.

Hayatsu H., Negishi T., Arimoto S. and Hayatsu T. (1993): Porphyrins as potential inhibitors against exposure to carcinogens and mutagens, Mutation Res. 290, 79-85.

Hemminki K. (1993): DNA adducts, mutations and cancer, Carcinogenesis 14, 2007-2012.

Henderson B.E., Ross R.K. and Pike M.C. (1991): Toward the primary prevention of cancer, Science 254, 1131-1138.

Hirose M., Yada H., Hakoi K., Takahashi S. and Ito N. (1993): Modification of carcinogenesis by α-tocopherol, t-butylhydroquinone, propyl gallate and butylated hydroxytoluene in a rat multi-organ carcinogenesis model, Carcinogenesis 14, 2359-2364.

Ho T.A., Coutts T.M., Rowland I.R. and Alldrick A.J. (1992): Inhibition of the metabolism of mutagens occurring in food by arachidonic acid, Mutation Res. 269, 279-284.

Hochstein P. and Atallah A.S. (1988): The nature of oxidants and antioxidant systems in the inhibition of mutation and cancer, Mutation Res. 202, 363-375.

Hollander P.M. and Ernster L. (1975): Studies on the reaction mechanism of DT Diaphorase action of dead-end inhibitors and effects of phospholipids, Arch. Biochem. Biophys. 169, 560-567.

Hong J.-Y., Smith T., Lee M.-J., Li W., Ma B.-L., Ning S.M., Brady J.F., Thomas P.E. and Yang C.S. (1991): Metabolism of carcinogenic nitrosamines by rat nasal mucosa and the effect of diallyl sulfide, Cancer Res. 51, 1509-1514.

Hozumi M., Ogawa M., Sugimura T., Takeuchi T. and Umezawa H. (1972): Inhibition of tumorigenesis in mouse skin by leupeptin a protease inhibitor from Actinomycetes, Cancer Res. 32, 1725-1728.

IARC (1986): The design and analysis of long-term animal experiments, Lyon.

IARC (1992): Mechanisms of carcinogenesis in risk identification. Vainio H., Magee P.N., McGregor D.B., McMichael A.J. (eds.). Lyon, publ. 116.

Idle J.R., Mahgoub A., Sloan T.P., Smith R.L., Mbanefo C.O. and Bababunmi E.A. (1981): Some observations on the oxidation phenotype satus of Nigerian patients presenting with cancer, Cancer Lett., 11, 331-338.

Inoue T., Morita K. and Kadar T. (1981): Purification and properties of a plant desmutagenic factor for the mutagenic principle of tryptophan pyrilysate, Agr. Biol. Chem. 45, 345-353.

Ip D. (1981): Factors influencing the anticarcinogenic efficacy of selenium in dimethylbenz(α)anthracene-induced mammary tumorigenesis in rats, Cancer Res. 41, 2683-2686.

Jain A.K., Shimoi K., Nakamura Y., Kada T., Hara Y. and Tomita I. (1989): Crude tea extracts decrease the mutagenic activity of N-methyl-N'-nitro-N-nitrosoguanidine in vitro and in intragastric tract of rats, Mutation Res. 210, 1-8.

Jones P.A. and Buckley J.D. (1990): The role of DNA methylation in cancer, Adv. Canc. Res. 54, 1-23.

Kaisary A., Smith P., Jaczq E., McAllister C.B., Wilkinson G.R., Ray W.A. and Branch R.A. (1987): Genetic predisposition to bladder cancer: ability to hydroxilate debrisoquine and mephenytoin as risk factors, Cancer Res., 47, 5488-5497.

Kako Y., Toyoda Y., Hatanaka Y., Suwa Y., Nukaya H. and Nagao M. (1992): Inhibition of mutagenesis by p-aminobenzoic acid as a nitrite scavenger, Mutation Res 282, 119-125.

Kappas A. and Patrineli A. (1992): Antimutagenicity of p-animobenzoic acid and ascorbic acid in MNNG-induced meth suppressors in Aspergillus (abstr.), Proc. 22nd Meeting EEMS, Berlin.

Kawahjiri K., Nakachi K., Imai K., Yoshii A., Shinoda N. and Watanabe J (1990): Identification of genetically hugh risk individuals to lung cancer by DNA polymorphism of the cytochrome P450IA1 gene, FEBS Lett., 263, 131-133.

Ketterer B. (1988): Protective role of glutathione and glutathione transferases in mutagenesis and carcinogenesis, Mutation Res. 202, 343-361.

Khan P.K. and Sinha S.P. (1993): Antimutagenic efficacy of higher doses of vitamin C, Mutation Res. 298, 157-161.

Knudson Jr. A.G. (1986): Genetics of human cancer, Ann. Rev. Genet. 20, 231-251.

Kojima H., Konishi H. and Kuroda Y. (1992): Effects of L-ascorbic acid on the mutagenicity of ethyl methanesulfonate in cultured mammalian cells, Mutation Res. 266, 85-91.

Krewski D., Sziskowicz M., and Rosenkranz H. (1990): Quantitative factors in chemical carcinogenesis: Variation in carcinogenic potency, Regulatory Toxicology and Pharmacology, 12, 13-29.

Kuenzig W., Chau J., Norkus E., Holowaschenko H., Newmark H., Mergens W. and Conney A.H. (1984): Caffeic and ferulic acids as blockers of nitrosamine formation, Carcinogenesis 5, 309-313.

Kuo M.-L., Lee K.-C. and Lin J.-K. (1992): Genotoxicities of nitropyrenes and their modulation by apigenin, tannic acid, ellagic acid and indole-3-carbinol in the Salmonella and CHO systems, Mutation Res. 270, 87-95.

Kuroda Y. and Inoue T. (1988): Antimutagenesis by factors affecting DNA repair in bacteria, Mutation Res. 202, 387-391.

Lawley P.D. (1989): Mutagens as carcinogens: development of current concepts, Mutation Res. 213, 3-25.

Lialiaris T., Mourelatos D. and Vassiliades J.D. (1987): Enhancement and attenuation of cytogenetic damage by vitamin C in cultured human lymphocytes exposed to thiotepa and L-ethionine, Cytogenet. Cell Genet. 44, 209-214.

Luebeck E.G., and Moolgavkar, S.H. (1991): Stocastic description of initiation and promotion in experimental carcinogenesis, in Galli G., Rossi L., Vineis P., and Zapponi G.A. (eds): Risk assessment of chemical carcinogens, Annali Istituto Superiore di Sanità, 27, 4, 575-580.

Lutz W. K.(1990). Dose-response relationships and low-dose extrapolation in chemical carcinogenesis, Carcinogenesis, 11, 8, 1243-1247.

Matsumura H., Watanabe K. and Ohta T. (1993): o-Vanillin enhances chromosome aberrations induced by alkylating agents in cultured Chinese hamster cells, Mutation Res. 298, 163-168.

Mawson M.I., Chao W.-R. and Helmes C.T. (1987): Inhibition by retinoids of anthralin-induced mouse epidermal ornithine decarboxylase activity and anthralin-promoted skin tumor formation, Cancer Res. 47, 6210-6215.

McGarrity T.J. and Peiffer L.P. (1993): Selenium and difluoromethylornithine additively inhibit DMH-induced distal colon tumor formation in rats fed a fiber-free diet, Carcinogenesis 14, 2335-2340.

Mehta P.P., Bertram J.S. and Lowenstein W.T. (1989): The actions of retinoids on cellular growth correlate with their actions on gap-junctional communication, J. Cell Biol. 108, 1053-1065.

Minnunni M., Wolleb U., Mueller O., Pfeifer A. and Aeschbacher H.U. (1992): Natural antioxidants as inhibitors of oxygen species induced mutagenicity, Mutation Res. 269, 193-200.

Mirvish S.S. (1981): Ascorbic acid inhibition of N-nitroso compound formation in chemical, food and biological systems, in: M.S. Zedeck and M. Lipkin (eds), Inhibition of Tumor Induction and Development, Plenum Press, New York, pp. 101-126.

Mitchel R.E.J. and McCann R. (1993): Vitamin E is a complete tumor promoter in mouse skin, Carcinogenesis 14, 659-662.

Monticello T.M., and Morgan K.T. (1993): Cell proliferation and formaldehyde-induced respiratory carcinogenesis, Risk Analysis, 14, 3, 313-319.

Moon R.C., McCormick D.L. and Mehta R.G. (1983): Inhibition of carcinogenesis by retinoids, Cancer Res. 43, 2469s-2475s.

Mori T., Takai Y., Minakuchi R., Yu B. and Nishizuka Y. (1980): Inhibitory action of chlorpromazine, dibucaine, and other phospholipid-interacting drugs on calcium-activated, phospholipid-dependent protein kinase, J. Biol. Chem 255, 8378-8380.

Morse M.A. and Stoner G.D. (1993): Cancer chemoprevention: principles and prospects, Carcinogenesis 14, 1737-1746.

Narisawa T., Sato M., Tani M., Kudo T., Takahishi T. and Goto A. (1981): Inhibition of development of methylnitrosourea-induced rat colon tumors by indomethacin, Cancer Res. 41, 1954-1957.

Nelson M.A., Futscher B.W., Kinsella T., Wymer J. and Bowden G.T. (1992): Detection of mutant Ha-ras genes in chemically initiated mouse skin epidermis before the development of benign tumors, Proc. Natl. Acad. Sci. USA 89, 6398-6402.

Nomura T., Hata S., Enomoto T., Tanaka H. and Shibata K. (1980): Inhibiting effects of antipain on urethane-induced lung neoplasia in mice, Br. J. Cancer 42, 624-626.

Oesch F. (1988): Antimutagenesis by shift in monooxygenase isoenzymes and induction of epoxide hydrolase, Mutation Res. 202, 335-342.

Ohta T., Watanabe K., Moriya M., Shirasu Y. and Kada T. (1983a): Antimutagenic effects of cinnamaldehyde on chemical mutagenesis in E. coli, Mutation Res. 107, 219-227.

Ohta T., Watanabe K., Moriya M., Shirasu Y. and Kada T. (1983b): Antimutagenic effects of coumarin and umbelliferone on mutagenesis induced by 4-nitroquinoline 1-oxide or UV-irradiation in E. coli, Mutation Res. 117, 135-138.

Ohta T., Watanabe M., Shirasu Y. and Inoue T. (1988): Post-replication repair and recombination in uvrA umuC strains in Escherichia coli are enhanced by vanillin and antimutagenic compounds, Mutation Res. 201, 107-112.

Okey A.B, Riddick D.S., and Harper P.A. (1994): The Ah receptor: Mediator of the toxicity of 2,3,7,8-tetrachlorodibenzo-p-dioxin (TCDD) and related compounds, Toxicology Letters, 70, 1-22.

Owens R.A. and Hartman P.E. (1986): Glutathione: A protective agent in Salmonella typhimurium and Escherichia coli as measured by mutagenicity and by growth delay assays, Environ. Mutagen. 8, 659-673.

Pegg A.E. (1988): Polyamine metabolism and its importance in neoplastic growth and as a target for chemotherapy, Cancer Res. 48, 759-774.

Perera F., Mayer J., Santella R.M., Brenner D., Tsay W.Y., Brandt-Rauf P. and Hemminki K. (1991). DNA adducts and other biological markers in risk assessment for environmental carcinogens, Ann. Ist. Super. Sanit, 27(4), 615-620.

Peryt B., Szymczyk T. and Lesca P. (1992): Mechanism of antimutagenicity of wheat sprout extracts, Mutation Res. 269, 201-215.

Pickett C.B. and Lu A.Y.H. (1989): Glutathione S-transferases: gene structure, regulation, and biological function, Annu. Rev. Biochem. 58, 743-764.

Pignatelli B., Bereziat J.-C., Descotes G. and Bartsch H. (1982): Catalysis of nitrosation in vitro and in vivo in rats by catechin and resorcinol and inhibition by chlorogenic acid, Carcinogenesis 3, 1045-1049.

Portier C.J., and Kopp-Schneider A. (1991): A multistage model of carcinogenesis incorporating DNA damage and repair, Risk Analysis, 11,3, 535-543.

Preston-Martin S., Pike M.C., Ross R.K., Jones P.A., and Henderson B.E. (1990): Increased cell division as a cause of human cancer, Cancer Research, 50, 7415-7421.

Ramel C. (1990): Mutation spectrum in carcinogenicity, in: A. Kappas (ed.) Mechanisms of Environmental Mutagenesis-Carcinogenesis, Plenum Press, New York, pp. 3-24.

Ramel C., Alekperov U.K., Ames B.N., Kada T. and Wattenberg L.W. (1986): Inhibitors of mutagenesis and their relevance to carcinogenesis, Mutation Res. 168, 47-65.

Reddy B.S. (1975): Role of bile metabolites in colon carcinogenesis, Cancer 36, 2401-2406.

Reddy B.S., Nayini J., Tokumo K., Rigotty J., Zang E. and Kelloff G. (1990): Chemoprevention of colon carcinogenesis by concurrent administration of piroxicam, a nonsteroidal antiinflammatory drug with D,L-α-difluoromethylornithine, an ornithine decarboxylase inhibitor, in diet, Cancer Res. 50, 2562-2568.

Reddy B.S. and Rivenson A. (1993): Inhibitory effect of Bifidobacterium longum on colon, mammary, and liver carcinogenesis induced by 2-amino-3-methylimidazo[4,5f]-quinoline, a food mutagen, Cancer Res. 53, 3914-3918.

Reddy B.S., Rao C.V., Rivenson A. and Kelloff G. (1993): Inhibitory effect of aspirin on azoxymethane-induced colon carcinogenesis in F344 rats, Carcinogenesis 14, 1493-1497.

Rogers A.E., Zeisel S.H. and Groopman J. (1993): Diet and carcinogenesis, Carcinogenesis 14, 2205-2217.

Rotstein J.B. and Slaga T.J. (1988): Anticarcinogenesis mechanisms, as evaluated in the multistage mouse skin model, Mutation Res. 202, 421-427.

Rowland I.R. and Grasso P. (1975): Degradation of N-nitrosamines by intestinal bacteria, App. Microbiol. 29, 7-12.

Sai K., Hayashi M., Takagi A., Hasegawa R., Sofuni T. and Kurokawa Y. (1992): Effects of antioxidants on induction of micronuclei in rat peripheral blood reticulocytes by potassium bromate, Mutation Res. 269, 113-118.

Sasaki Y.F., Yamada H., Shimoi K., Kator K. and Kinae N. (1993): The clastogen-suppressing effects of green tea, Po-lie tea and Rooibos tea in CHO cells and mice, Mutation Res. 286, 221-232.

Shibata M.-A., Hirose M., Kagawa M., Boonyaphiphat P. and Ito N. (1993): Enhancing effect of concomitant L-ascorbic acid administration on BHA-induced forestomach carcinogenesis in rats, Carcinogenesis 14, 275-280.

Shih C.-A. and Lin J.-K. (1993): Inhibition of 8-hydroxydeoxyguanosine formation by curcumin in mouse fibroblast cells, Carcinogenesis 14, 709-712.

Shimoi K., Nakamura Y., Tomita I. and Kada T. (1985): Bio-antimutagenic effects of tannic acid on UV and chemically induced mutagenesis in Escherichia coli B/r, Mutation Res. 149, 17-23.

Simic M.G. (1988): Mechanisms of inhibition of free-radical processes in mutagenesis and carcinogenesis, Mutation Res. 202, 377-386.

Slaga T.J., Solanki V. and Logani M. (1983): Studies on the mechanism of action of antitumor promoting agents: suggestive evidence for the involvment of free radicals in promotion, in: O.F. Nygaard and M.G. Simic (eds) Radioprotectors and Anticarcinogens, Academic Press, New York, pp. 471-485.

Sporn M.B. and Roberts A.B. (1983): The role of retinoids in differentiation and carcinogenesis, Cancer Res. 43, 3034-3040.

Stich H.F. (1991): The beneficial and hazardous effects of simple phenolic compounds, Mutation Res. 259, 307-324.

Stich H.F., Chan P.K.L. and Rosin M.P. (1982): Inhibitory effects of phenolics, teas and saliva on the formation of mutagenic nitrosation products of salted fish, Int. J. Cancer 30, 719-724.

Stocker R., Yamamoto Y., McDonagh A.F., Glazer A.N. and Ames B.N. (1987): Bilirubin is an antioxidant of possible physiological importance, Science 235, 1043-1046.

Strickland J.E., Dlugosz A.A., Hennings H. and Yuspa S.H. (1993): Inhibition of tumor formation from grafted murine papilloma cells by treatment of grafts with staurosporine, an inducer of squamous differentiation, Carcinogenesis 14, 205-209.

Sugimura T. (1988): Successful use of short-term tests for academic purposes: their use in identification of new environmental carcinogens with possible risk for humans, Mutation Res. 205, 33-39.

Tabor C.W. and Tabor H. (1984): Polyamines, Annu. Rev. Biochem. 53, 749-790.

Tanaka T., Kojima T., Kawamori T., Wang A., Suzui M., Okamoto K. and Mori K. (1993a): Inhibition of 4-nitroquinoline-1-oxide-induced rat tongue carcinogenesis by the naturally occurring plant phenolics caffeic, ellagic, chlorogenic and ferulic acids, Carcinogenesis 14, 1321-1325.

Tanaka T., Kojima T., Hara A., Sawada H. and Mori H. (1993b): Chemoprevention of oral carcinogenesis by DL-α-difluoromethylornithine, an ornithine decarboxylase inhibitor: dose-dependent reduction in 4-nitroquinoline 1-oxide-induced tongue neoplasms in rats, Cancer Res. 53, 772-776.

Thompson C. L., McCoy Z., Lambert J.M., Andries M.J. and Lucier G.W. (1988): Relationships among benzo(a)pyrene metabolism, Benzo(a)pyrene-diolepoxide: DNA adduct formation and sister chromatid exchanges in human lymphocytes from smokers and nonsmokers, Cancer Research, 49, 6503-6511.

Travis C.C., and Belefant H. (1992): Promotion as a factor in carcinogenesis, Toxicology Letters, 60, 1-9.

U.S. EPA Integrated Risk Information System (IRIS), EPA file online, (1995): U.S. EPA, Washington D.C.

Voutsinas G., Kappas A., Demopoulos N.A. and Catsoulacos P. (1993): Comparative study on the mutagenicity of three structurally related substituted aniline mustards in the Salmonella/microsome assay, Mutation Res. 298, 261-267.

Walker G.C. (1985): Inducible DNA repair systems, Ann. Rev. Biochem. 54, 425-457.

Wattenberg L.W. (1981): Inhibition of carcinogen-induced neoplasia by sodium cyanate, tert-butyl isocyanate and benzyl isothiocyanate administered subsequent to carcinogen exposure, Cancer Res. 41, 2992-2994.

Wattenberg L.W. (1985): Chemoprevention of cancer, Cancer Res. 45, 1-8.

Wattenberg L.W. and Lam L.K.T. (1983): Phenolic antioxidants as protective agents in chemical carcinogenesis, in: O.F. Nygaard and M.G. Simic (eds) Radioprotectors and Anticarcinogens, Academic Press, New York, pp. 461-469.

Weinberg R.A. (1991): Tumor suppressor genes, Science 254, 1138-1146.

Weinstein I.B. (1988): Strategies for inhibiting multistage carcinogenesis based on signal transduction pathways, Mutation Res. 202, 413-420.

Weinstein I. C. (1991): Mitogenesis is only one factor in carcinogenesis, Science, 251, 387-388.

Williams G.M., Iatropoulos M.J., Djordjevic M.V. and Kaltenberg O.P. (1993): The triphenylethylene drug tamoxifen is a strong liver carcinogen in the rat, Carcinogenesis 14, 315-317.

Wise J.P., Orenstein J.M. and Patierno S.R. (1993): Inhibition of lead chromate clastogenesis by ascorbate: relationship to particle dissolution and uptake, Carcinogenesis 14, 429-434.

Wood A.W., Huang M.-T., Chang R.L., Newmark H.L., Lehr R.E., Yagi H., Sayer J.M., Jerina D.M. and Conney A.H. (1982): Inhibition of the mutagenicity of bay-region diol-epoxides of polycyclic aromatic hydrocarbons by naturally occurring plant phenols: exceptional activity of ellagic acid, Proc. Natl. Acad. Sci. USA 79, 5513-5517.

Yavelow J., Finlay T.H., Kennedy A.R. and Troll W. (1983): Bowma-Birk soybean protease inhibitor as an anticarcinogen, Cancer Res. 43, 2454s-2459s.

Zhang Y., Talalay P., Cho C.-G and Posner G.H. (1992): A major inducer of anticarcinogenic protective enzymes from broccoli: isolation and elucidation of structure, Proc. Natl. Acad. Sci. USA 89, 23992-403.

Chapter 3

SOURCES OF DATA FOR CANCER RISK ASSESSMENT

A. Kappas[1], V.J. Cogliano[2], K. Watanabe[3], and G.A. Zapponi[4]

[1]National Centre for Scientific Research "Demokritus", Athens, Greece
[2]U.S. Environmental Protection Agency, Washington DC, USA
[3]Tulane University Medical Center, New Orleans, USA
[4]National Institute of Health, Rome, Italy

3.1. INTRODUCTION

Several sources of data for risk assessment exist and are important and very useful for the estimation of hazard caused by various chemical agents acting as either initiator or promoter carcinogens. Existed data are necessary to be reviewed and evaluated in order to identify whether an agent can and under what circumstances be carcinogenic.

For carcinogenicity, data refering to humans are sparse. In some cases epidemiological studies have shown the relation between exposures to certain agents and cancers, such as the vinyl chloride and angiosarcomas or asbestos and mesotheliomas but in most cases carcinogenicity testing have relied on the rodent carcinogenicity database although problems such as species specific responses exist in animal experiments.

In this chapter the different sources of data for risk assessment will be discussed.

3.2. *IN VITRO* AND SHORT TERM TESTING

The use of short term tests to identify the mutagenic properties of environmental chemicals is a promising approach for the control of human carcinogens. Since accumulated evidence supports the somatic mutation theory of carcinogenesis (Yunis, 1983; Bishop,

[2]The views expressed in this chapter are those of the authors and do not necessarily reflect the views or policies of the U.S. Environmental Protection Agency.

Perspectives on Biologically Based Cancer Risk Assessment, edited by Cogliano *et al.*
Kluwer Academic/Plenum Publishers, New York, 1999.

1991) information on the mutagenic potential of a chemical is necessary to provide the basis of data for risk assessment.

A very large number of mutagenicity assays have been developed for testing chemicals for their ability to induce gene mutation, chromosomal mutation and aneuploidy. Among them, *in vitro* testing systems have been widely used because of several advantages they offer (OECD, 1990).

First *in vitro* testing has the potential to be more rigorously standardized than *in vivo* testing, thus reliable, quality-controlled data can be generated. This is usually not possible in whole animal testing due to the prohibitive cost of including positive and negative controls. Secondly, *in vitro* systems are in general faster, easier and inexpensive, thus offering an economic advantage which is important because it will allow testing of a larger number of chemicals for the same cost. Another advantage is that the problem of species differences associated with extrapolation of *in vivo* animal data to man and other organisms can be eliminated by using cells from different species even humans in *in vitro* testing systems. Another important advantage of *in vitro* tests is that it is possible to exactly define the critical concentration of the genotoxic chemicals which is not easy in *in vivo* tests where toxicokinetic analyses are also required. Also important is that *in vitro* tests can utilize a large number of test organisms or cells per dose level and require smaller quantities of test chemicals, thus producing small quantities of toxic waste. And of course *in vitro* testing offers the advantage of reducing the use of live animals which is very important from the social point of view.

One of the problems of the *in vitro* test systems is that in order to simulate the complexity of the responses of the whole animal it is necessary to use a battery of *in vitro tests*. Since no single assay has proved capable of detecting mammalian mutagens and carcinogens with an acceptable level of precision and reproducibility, it is usual practice to apply the assays in batteries comprising from two to five tests. Such batteries contain tests on both prokaryotic and eukaryotic cells and cover the major genetic changes to be expected. Selection of the assays and the extent of testing may be influenced by the nature of the material, the extent of its eventual distribution and use, data from other toxicological tests and pharmacokinetic studies and, in some cases, the available technical expertise (OECD, 1987).

A number of *in vitro* and short term test systems have been developed in recent years and accepted by regulatory agencies.

These test systems are classified into three main categories according to the genetic end points they identify: Test systems for DNA damage , test systems for gene mutations and test systems for chromosomal aberrations (OECD, 1987).

1. Test systems for DNA effects

   One cellular response to chemically-induced genetic damage on DNA is the damage which involves degradation of the damaged part and subsequent synthesis of a new, relatively short, strand of DNA to replace the degraded region. Such repair could be identified in cultured mammalian cells by the "UDS" (Unscheduled DNA Synthesis) test system (Mitchell et al, 1983).

   Also mitotic crossing over and mitotic gene conversion are regarded as useful indicators of primary DNA damage and could be investigated in *Saccharomyces cerevisiae* (Zimmermann et al., 1984). The test system of Sister Chromatid Exchange (SCE) in cultured mammalian cells is also detecting chemicals that affect DNA (Perry et al., 1984).

2. Test systems for gene mutations

   The most widely used short term test system for detecting chemically-induced mutations is the Ames test based on the detection of histidine revertants in *Salmonella typhimurium* (Maron and Ames, 1983). The system is relatively simple to perform, reproducible and give reliable data on the ability of a chemical to interact with DNA and produce mutations.

   Other bacterial systems are also used for detecting gene mutations such as the *Escherichia coli.* In eukaryotic cells test systems are also available for gene mutations such as the system of the yeast and cultured mammalian cells.

3. Test systems for chromosomal aberrations

   Mammalian cell cultures are the most commonly used tests for investigating chromosomal aberrations (Adler, 1984). These tests identify chemicals that are capable of damaging mammalian chromosomes. Test systems are also available for detecting aneugenic chemicals which cause numerical chromosomal changes (Kafer and Kappas, 1990).

Table 3.1 shows a number of short term and *in vitro* test systems which are accepted and recommended for detecting mutagens - carcinogens (OECD, 1987).

The choice of appropriate short term test systems for screening chemical mutagens-carcinogens is made difficult because of the large number of system discussed in the literature. The tests shown in Table 1 are of the most commonly recommended not only by OECD but also by other Regulatory Agencies. A recommended scheme for proper mutagenicity testing includes 3 stages (Dept. of Health, UK, 1989):

- In the first stage two tests are required for initial screening. One bacterial assay for gene mutation and one test for clastogenicity in mammalian cells.

- In the second stage the compounds which have been found positive in at least one test of the first stage, are tested in an *in vivo* short term test namely the bone marrow assay for chromosome damage (metaphase analysis or micronucleus test).

- Finally in the third stage tests can be used to show either interaction with DNA and potential for inherited effects such as the dominant lethal assay or quantitative assessment of heritable effects such as the mouse specific locus test.

The Ad Hoc Group on Dangerous Chemicals-Carcinogens of the European Community has presented a number of summary reviews of the salient scientific evidence that underlies the assessment of a particular chemical in terms of carcinogenicity (Commission of the European Community, 1989, 1990, 1991, 1993). In all cases results on

For DNA effects
– *In vitro* Sister Chromatid exchange
– Unscheduled DNA Synthesis (UDS)
– Yeast mitotic recombination
– Gene conversion
For Gene Mutations
– Reverse mutation in *Salmonella typhimurium* (Ames test)
– Reverse mutation in *Escherichia coli*
– Gene mutation in cultured mammalian cells
– Gene mutation in *Saccharomyces cerevisiae*
– Mouse spot test
For Chromosomal Aberrations
– *In vitro* cytogenetics for chromosomal aberrations
– *In vivo* cytogenetics for chromosomal aberrations
– Micronucleus test
– Heritable translocation assay
– Dominant lethal assay
– Mammalian germ cell cytogenetics test

Table 3.1: *Short term testing systems for mutagen-carcinogen screening*

mutagenicity screening in short term and *in vitro* testing systems have been included and in most cases compounds which have been labeled as carcinogens were shown to be positive in at least one short term test system.

For example, Acrylonitrile an important monomer widely used in the plastic and rubber industry, was one of the 10 test chemicals in the International Programme on Chemical Safety's Collaborative study on *in vitro* assays (Ashby et al., 1985). In this study nearly 90 individual sets of data were provided for most of the test chemicals. Acrylonitrile displayed a broad spectrum of genotoxic activity in some *in vitro* assay systems ranging from gene mutations in bacteria to chromosomal aberrations and gene mutations in cultured mammalian cells.

Acrylonitrile is DNA damaging and mutagenic to bacteria and cultured mammalian cells. It is clastogenic and induces sister chromatid exchanges and cell transformations *in vitro* but not *in vivo*. A dominant lethal assay was also negative. Acrylonotrile is carcinogenic in rats after inhalation and ingestion exposures, producing an increased incidence of tumours of the central nervous system, Zymbal gland forestomach and mammary gland. The possibility that acrylonitrile could be a lung or prostatic carcinogen cannot be excluded (Commission of the European Communities, 1989, pp. 1-7).

Another example is the compound 4-amino biphenyl which has been evaluated as carcinogenic to humans (IARC, 1987). Because of the great interest in the carcinogenic aromatic amines there have been many studies in which 4-aminobiphenyl has been used as a model carcinogen in mutagenicity assay systems in the context of the study of metabolic aspects of carcinogencity. 4-Aminobiphenyl is mutagenic to *Salmonella typhimurium* after metabolic activation and in several eukaryotic cell lines *in vitro*. It induces unscheduled DNA synthesis in primary cultures of rat hepatocytes as does its N-hydroxy metabolite in cultures of human urothelial cells. In *in vivo* systems it reacts with DNA and induces sister chromatid exchanges and micronuclei (Commission of the European Communities, 1987, pp. 9-13).

Vinyl chloride which also has been evaluated as carcinogen to humans (IARC, 1987) has been examined in a large number of studies for genotoxicity. After metabolic activation, vinyl chloride was mutagenic to *Salmonella typhimurium* caused DNA damage in *Escherichia coli* and induced gene mutation and gene conversion in *Schizosaccharomyces pombe* and *Saccharomyces cerevisiae* (Commission of the European Communities, 1987, pp. 127-136).

3.3. TRENDS IN ANIMAL TOXICOLOGY TESTING

Currently, a standard test of carcinogenicity involves lifetime administration of high doses of the agent to laboratory animals. Such testing is based on two fundamental assumptions.

1. Results in experimental animals can be used to make inferences about results in humans.

2. Results at high doses can be extrapolated to lower doses.

The second assumption is an important one. The information value of the animals tested at the maximum tolerated dose alone may be rather low. There is the question of whether the predominant mechanism of carcinogenesis at the highest dose is also the predominant mechanism at lower doses; it is possible for a mechanism to be more or less important in different portions of the dose range.

Qualitatively, this can lead either to the inference of a low-dose risk where none exists, or to the inability to detect a low dose risk because a high-dose mechanism is predominant in the range of doses tested. Quantitatively, the magnitude of low-dose risk may, similarly, be either overestimated or underestimated.

High administered doses are used for several reasons. One objective of carcinogenicity testing is to serve as a screening tool to determine whether an agent has the capacity to induce cancer at some dose. High-dose testing provides a sensitive indicator to potential carcinogenic activity. If high doses are effective in inducing cancer, the dose-response relationship can be further investigated by subsequent testing at lower doses. Conversely, if the agent does not cause cancer at the maximum dose tolerated by the animals, then it would be unlikely to cause cancer at any dose level. In addition, high-dose testing is used to provide a balance between the level of sensitivity required of carcinogenicity experiments and the impracticality of using large numbers of animals. Regulatory agencies are interested in identifying exposures associated with an increased life time cancer risk of one in a thousand to one in a million. Thousands, or even millions, of animals would be required if the agent were administered at these exposure levels. To provide for a more practical sample size, higher exposure levels are administered to a smaller number of animals; thus, high dose is substituted for large numbers. Low-dose extrapolation models are then used to make inferences about the risks that could be expected at lower exposure levels.

The doses used in a carcinogenicity study are selected after a series of less-than-lifetime studies known as range-finding studies. For example, animals may be exposed to a wide range of high doses for, say, 14 days. The highest dose showing no overt toxicity becomes the highest of several doses tested for a longer term, say, 90 days. The highest dose showing no overt toxicity, called the maximum tolerated dose, becomes the highest dose tested in the chronic carcinogenicity study. One or two lower doses, for example one-half and one-quarter of the maximum tolerated dose, may also be tested in the chronic study.

Typically, four parallel experiments are conducted: in male rats, female rats, male mice, and female mice. In each experiment, animals are randomly assigned to groups exposed to different levels of the agent. Group sizes are typically about 50 animals of the same sex and species, although groups of 100 or more are occasionally used. One group typically is exposed to the maximum dose tolerated by the animal. Other groups receive doses that may be on the order of one-half, one-quarter, one-tenth, or one-hundredth of the maximum tolerated dose. A control group receives no exposure to the agent.

Exposure begins when the animals are nearly mature-typically at 2 or 3 months of age. Exposure continues at a constant level until the surviving animals are killed at the end of the experiment, typically at 24 months following the first exposure. This length of the experiment has been chosen to be a time after chemically induced tumors would be observable but before spontaneously arising tumors would be expected to appear in large numbers, optimizing the opportunity to observe effects. Microscope slides of the animals' organs are prepared and examined for tumors. Sometimes all major organs are examined, other times attention is restricted to one or more target organs. The incidence of cancer (number of tumors divided by number of animals examined) is reported for each group of animals. Because the occurrence of malignant tumors or related premalignant lesions may reflect the termination of an experiment before the end of the animals' natural lifespan, malignant and related premalignant lesions are often considered together.

In recent years, this basic experimental design has been extended to provide information on the time course of tumor development. Interim sacrifice studies add small auxiliary groups of animals that are scheduled to be killed before the end of the experiment (for example, at 12, 15, 18, or 21 months). These animals provide information on the time course of the development of cancer, including whether benign or other precursor lesions precede the development of malignant tumors and the duration of the latent period before the manifestation of cancer. Stop studies add parallel groups of animals for which exposure is stopped several months before the end of the experiment. These animals provide information on whether continued exposure plays a role in the progression of precursor lesions to malignant tumors. Intermittent exposure studies add groups of animals exposed to noncontinues dosing regiments to provide information on the relative effectiveness of long-term constant exposure as compared to short-term, more intense exposure. Early-life exposure studies add groups of animals exposed before the animals are mature. For example, Maltoni has studied the effects of vinyl chloride in animals exposed prenatally or in animals exposed for 5 weeks beginning at 1 day of age. Such studies provide information on whether early life may be a sensitive period leading to the subsequent development of cancer.

This basic experimental design and its extensions are not useful for obtaining the information necessary to specify a mechanism of carcinogenesis. More recently, as increased attention is being given to mechanisms of carcinogenic action, new bioassays are being designed to identify the role these mechanisms play in the induction of cancer by particular carcinogenic agents. These new bioassays will greatly increase the amount of information available on the carcinogenicity of an agent. These bioassays can provide both quantitative as well as qualitative descriptions of cellular and subcellular events leading to carcinogenesis.

For example, the National Toxicology Program of the United States develops and provides data used to estimate human health hazards of environmental exposures. Its carcinogenicity testing program currently uses the experimental design described above. These may be considerable redundancy in the current two-species, two-sex experimental design: Lai and Hughes (1992) found 75 percent concordance in cancer response when rats and mice were exposed by the same route. Expansion of the basic testing design is currently being considered, with the objectives of developing and validating alternative assays that may reduce the need for long-term testing in animals and to ensure that emphasis is placed on studies of the mechanisms of toxicity and carcinogenicity. Proposals include:

- Incorporating hypothesis-driven mechanistic research into the testing program. The research component would include pharmacokinetics/metabolism, genotoxic and nongenotoxic mechanisms, toxicity, cell proliferation, and unique susceptibility.

- Use of flexible protocols; for example, genotoxic and nongenotoxic agents may be evaluated using different tests.

- Continued use of standard, inbred rodent strains, which can provide a standard for comparison and allow reduction of the number of animals in future studies.

- Use of mechanistic studies and pharmacokinetics/metabolism studies before chronic studies are conducted, which may allow reduction of the number of chronic experiments from two species/two sexes to either two species/one sex each or one species/two sexes. If a positive bioassay is anticipated with confidence, it may even be possible to use only one species/one sex but test it over an extended range of doses.

- Exploration and validation of alternative systems, including nonmammalian species.

- Development of new sensitive test systems to reduce the number of animals needed and allow more agents to be tested. For example, transgenic animals containing mutated positive oncogenes or deleted tumor supressor genes.

Some of these proposals would require that existing methods be adapted. For example, cancer in transgenic animals may be modeled by multistage models with one fewer stage, reflecting the initiated state of transgenic animals. Other proposals would provide additional information that cannot be incorporated into currently used low-dose extrapolation models. In some cases, future protocols would not provide the information that is required by currently used models (that is, lifetime dose levels and tumor incidencies). Thus, low-dose extrapolation models will need to be developed to make use of experimental information likely to be developed in future years.

Other issues will arise when interpreting information from these expanded testing designs. For example, an apparently sublinear relationship between administered dose and tumor incidence may result from either pharmacokinetic or mechanistic considerations: it may reflect tumor promotion that is not very active at low doses; alternatively, it may reflect the linear tumor relationship of a mutagenic metabolite formed through a secondary metabolic pathway that becomes increasingly active at higher doses. The current standard test of carcinogenicity does not allow distinguishing the roles of pharmacokinetics and mechanisms. Expanded testing designs will provide information to permit testing of hypotheses about pharmacokinetics and mechanism.

3.4. CELL PROLIFERATION

There is a large body of epidemiologic evidence that implicates increased cell proliferation with higher cancer risk. For an overview of the role of cell division in the etiology of human cancers see Preston-Martin et al., 1991. Ample evidence exists also for the importance of cell proliferation in experimental carcinogenesis, as gathered from initiation-promotion (IP) experiments of papillomas in mouse skin and of enzyme altered foci (EAF) in the rat liver (see relevant articles in proceedings edited by Moolgavkar, 1990 and Butterworth et al., 1991).

To capture this body of evidence and to better understand the process of carcinogenesis, biologically motivated models are needed that incorporate the phenomenon of cell proliferation and its significance for determining cancer risk. One model that accounts explicitly for cellular kinetics of intermediate cells which have suffered at least one critical event on the pathway to cancer is the two-mutation clonal expansion model (Knudson, 1971; Moolgavkar, 1978, Moolgavkar and Knudson, 1981; Moolgavkar et al., 1988; Dewanji et al., 1989; Moolgavkar and Luebeck, 1990). This model is introduced in detail in chapter 6.

Before discussing the role of cell proliferation and its implication for cancer risk assessment we need to define what is meant by cell replication (division) and cell proliferation. Clear distinction between these two terms is, as we shall see later, important for our understanding of the mechanisms and the modes of action of non-genotoxic carcinogens.

Cell replication describes the process of cell division of a parental cell into two (not necessarily identical) daughter cells. However, if the population of cells of interest is homogeneous, then cell division can be said to occur with a certain rate, say α. In tissues that are under strong homeostatic control cell division needs to be balanced by cell death or differentiation. Assuming that the latter process proceeds with rate β, we expect $\alpha \cong \beta$ under normal conditions. Departures form equilibrium are best measured by the dimensionless ratio α/β.

Cell proliferation refers in general to the increase in number of a select population of cells, as observed in growing or regenerative tissues. Since either necrosis or programmed cell death (apoptosis) may also be present in a select cell population this term refers to the net cell proliferation and is measured by the difference $\alpha - \beta$. Net cell proliferation can be increased in different ways, namely by either increasing the cell division rate, by decreasing the cell death or differentiation rate or by both. However, if the increase is caused by an increase in cell division, and if this increase interferes with DNA repair processes, then fixation of accumulated genetic errors may occur, increasing the rate of irreversible (pre)malignant transformations. Thus, cell proliferation after cytotoxic insults is known to potentiate the initiation of normal cells (Columbano et al., 1981).

Different mechanisms have been identified by which genotoxic and non-genotoxic agents increase cell proliferation or cause weakening of homeostasis. For instance, 2,3,7,8- Tetrachlorodibenzo-p-dioxin (TCDD) is known to be a potent liver tumor promoter that appears to have no direct genotoxic effects. The action of TCDD, as well as HCDD (1,2,3,4,6,7,8-Heptachlorodibenzo-p-dioxin), is understood to be mediated through the aromatic hydrocarbon-responsive (Ah) receptor that appears to play a role in cell growth control and cell differentiation signal transduction pathways (Nebert et al., 1991). Still, it is not clear whether chronic dioxin exposure substantially increases the rate of cell division of hepatocytes (Buchmann et al., 1994). However, there is indication that such exposures rather disturb the delicate balance between cell division and cell death (Moolgavkar and Luebeck, 1995).

Human cancers in the breast, endometrium and ovary have also been strongly associated with hormonal factors, such as elevated steroid and polypeptide hormone levels that induce epithelial cell proliferation in these tissues (Preston-Martin et al., 1991). Breast cells, for instance, are known to respond positively to estrogen and progesterone increasing cell proliferation and cell differentiation (Key and Pike, 1988). Thus, early menarche and late menopause are considerable risk factors for breast cancer in women.

3.4.1. Quantitative Methods and Data Sources

Recognition of the importance of cell proliferation in multistage carcinogenesis has led to the adoption of models that incorporate explicitly cell kinetics of intermediate and malignant cell populations. Yet, unless data are obtained that provide information on such cellular processes as cell division and death, inferences from these models remain largely hypothetical and are hampered by the large number of unknown parameters in these models.

In order to quantitate the effects of a large body of putative non-genotoxic carcinogens, such as polychlorinated biphenyls (PCBs), dioxins and other P-450 inducers, a number of rat hepatocarcinogenesis experiments have been performed with the objective to assess the growth kinetics of enzyme altered foci and their relationship with primary subcellular effects (for instance Buchmann et al., 1987, 1991 and 1994).

Two types of measurements are often considered: The volume fraction, as estimated from the area fraction of the focal tissue seen on 2-dimensional histologic slides and the mean number of foci per unit volume estimated by use of the Fullman formula (Fullman, 1953). Measurement of the volume fraction of these lesions has been correlated with the amount of net cell proliferation of focal cells, although it is confounded with spontaneous or induced initiation of EAF under chronic exposures. Similarly, the mean number of foci observed is only indicative of the amount of initiation. It is confounded with cell death and clonal extinction. Thus, simultaneous measurements of cell division via autoradiographic or immunohistochemic labeling are of interest and should be obtained whenever possible (Goldsworthy et al., 1991). Alternatively, measurements of the number of EAF and their sizes on 2-dimensional microtome sections may, with suitable stereological assumptions, reveal much about cell proliferation, including cell division and death. The extraction of such information via explicit modeling of initiation and promotion of EAF is described in chapter 6. Examples are given in chapter 8.

To aid the statistical analysis and to allow for valid comparisons between treatment groups it is important that experimental protocols include all necessary control groups in the design. If a promoter is to be tested, that is not yet shown to be entirely non-genotoxic, then the design should include a regimen without acute initiation in order to control for the possibility of induced initiation.

3.4.1.1. Direct Measurements of Cell Division Pulse and continuous labeling methods: DNA synthesis can be measured directly through incorporation of DNA precursors such as ^{3}H-thymidine or its analogue bromeodeoxyuridine (BrdU) during S-phase of the cell cycle. In the case of pulse labeling, most often intraperitoneal injections are given repeatedly over a 24 hr period, or a shorter period that covers the diurnal peak of DNA synthesis in the tissue of question. If sufficient time is allowed for labeled cells to undergo mitosis then the cell division rate can be directly estimated from the labeling index (LI), i.e. the fraction of labeled cells in the target tissue. Some cells, however, may not divide but simply double their ploidy instead. Other disadvantages of the pulse method are described in the literature (see Goldsworthy et al., 1991).

Continuous labeling is administered through osmotic pumps that are implanted subcutaneously or intraperitoneally. Osmotic pumps can operate for up to several weeks. The obvious advantages of this method are that it is insensitive to diurnal variation of DNA synthesis and that essentially all cells that enter S-phase become labeled and accumulate in larger numbers. A simple method of analysis of labeling indices from continuous labeling experiments has been developed by Moolgavkar and Luebeck (1992). They showed that under the assumption of exponential growth the presence of cell death does not influence the estimation of cell division rates. Nuclear markers of cell proliferation: Using appropriate monoclonal antibodies, it is possible to detect different proliferation-associated nuclear antigens. These include the nuclear antigen identified by the Ki-67 MAb, the proliferating cell nuclear antigen (PCNA) identified by the PC10 MAb, several Cyclins, Topo isomerases; the TPA and TPS antigens have been proposed as serum biomarkers of cellular proliferation.

Ki-67 This antibody reacts with a nuclear antigen which is expressed only in proliferating cells which are in G1, S, G2 or M phase of the cell cycle; it is not expressed by resting cells in G0 (Gerdes et al, 1983). Ki-67 reactivity has been shown to correlate with other measures of cell proliferation (Isola et al, 1990). The related Ki-S1 marker has been shown to be closely linked to proliferation rates in cultured human breast carcinoma cells; Ki-S1 immunostaining also correlated well with the S-phase fraction determined from DNA profiles, in a series of breast carcinomas (Camplejohn et al, 1993).

PCNA Proliferating cell nuclear antigen functions as an auxiliary protein for DNA-polymerase-Ä and is an absolute requirement for semiconservative DNA synthesis (Bravo and Macdonald-Bravo, 1987; Bravo et al, 1987); it is expressed in all proliferating cells (Kamel et al, 1991). PCNA can be used as an S-phase marker (Landberg and Roos, 1991), but staining conditions are very stringent (Wilson et al, 1992). A complete correlation with Ki-67 has not been observed (Hall et al, 1994), due to the fact that PCNA is also involved in DNA nucleotide excision repair (Shivji et al, 1992) and has been shown to be up-regulated in non-cycling cells adjacent to pathological lesions (Harrison et al, 1993; Hall et al, 1994).

Cyclins Progression of cells through the cell cycle requires the interaction of a series of proteins, the cyclins, forming complexes with several enzymes, the cdK's (cyclin-dependent Kinases). Specific Cyclin/cdK complexes mediate the transition from G1 to S phase. The identification of different cyclins represents a novel tool for the evaluation of cell proliferation that might usefully complement the use of Ki-67 and PCNA markers (Paterlini et al., 1993).

3.4.1.2. Serum Biomarkers of Cellular Proliferation Tissue Polypeptide Antigen (TPA) and Tissue-Specific Polypeptide Antigen (TPS) have been reported to be serological indicators of tumor proliferation. The recent finding that cytosol levels of TPA and TPS are inversely correlated with the thymidine labeling index (Gion et al, 1994) leaves the exact significance of these markers open to discussion; this topic will be considered in another chapter of this book.

An increase in net cell proliferation can also come about by a decrease in apoptosis. Thus qualitative and quantitative measures of this process should also be considered. Morphologically, apoptosis proceeds in distinct phases. Early signs include separation of dying cells from neighboring cells, condensation of chromatin which is followed by fragmentation of the cell into apoptotic bodies. These bodies are then either digested by phagocytes or neighboring epithelial cells. Duration of apoptosis, as measured by the duration of removal of cell residues appears to be short, of the order of only a few hours (Bursch et al., 1990). Thus, in tissues that are turning over slowly, visible apoptosis is a rare event, and microscopic measurements of a significant number of events are laborious. For a thorough description of the effects and methods for the measurement of apoptosis see Bursch et al. (1984, 1985, 1990) and Schulte-Hermann et al. (1990).

Recently, a new method has been developed that detects DNA fragments *in situ* using terminal deoxyribonucleotidyl transferase (TDT)-mediated dUTP-digoxigenin nick end labeling (TUNEL). However, see the cautionary note by Grasl-Kraupp et al. (1995). For a simple and elegant morphological method using a transmitted light microscope on H&E-stained liver sections, see the work by Stinchcombe et al. (1995).

3.4.1.3. Cell kinetics of EAF Characteristic for hepatocarcinogenesis is the appearance of phenotypically altered lesions that correlate well with the incidence of neoplastic nodules and hepatocellular carcinomas (Friedrich-Freska et al., 1969; Scherer and Emmelot, 1976; Emmelot and Scherer, 1980, Goldfarb and Pugh, 1981; Kunz et al., 1983, 1985; Bannasch et al., 1986). The lesions can be identified by enzyme markers such as canalicular adenosine triphosphatase (ATPase), γ-glutamyl transpeptidase (GGT) or glucose-6-phosphatase (G6Pase).

The fact that these lesions are of monoclonal origin (Rabes et al., 1982; Williams et al., 1983) and that their geometric shape is approximately spherical, can be used to gain information about their growth kinetics. This effort, which will be described in more detail in chapter 6, is complicated by the stereological problem. Observations are obtained from 2-dimensional sections through the liver and are not from the 3-dimensional objects (the lesions) themselves However, given 2-dimensional observations that bear information on the number and size distribution of EAF during the course of time, inferences about initiation rates and cell kinetic parameters can be made. For a description of this method, see Moolgavkar et al. 1990. The method is based upon the premise that EAF expand clonally, according to a stochastic birth and death process with respective rates α and β (Kendall, 1960; Cox and Miller, 1972). Estimates of these parameters can be obtained through likelihood maximization as described in chapter 6.

Consistency and adequacy of the modeling effort of the growth of EAF must be checked against direct measurements of cell kinetic parameters. Models are only useful if they generate hypotheses that suggest new experiments to deepen our understanding of the biological processes involved. The interplay between quantitative modeling and experiments, in turn, drives on the scientific process necessary to better understand cancer and its risks.

3.5. SOURCES OF TOXICOKINETIC DATA

3.5.1. Introduction

Physiologically based toxicokinetic (PBTK) models compartmentalize the body into regions that have a notable effect on the disposition of a compound. Having some basis in biological reality, these models rely, as much as possible, on physiological and biochemical parameters independently measured in the population of interest.Traditional methods use population averaged model parameters and visual fitting of the toxicokinetic data by adjusting the parameters for which no independent measurements are available (Leung and Paustenbach, 1990; Paustenbach et al., 1988; Ramsey and Andersen, 1984; Reitz et al., 1990; Travis et al., 1990). An alternative is to allow for population variability in the model parameters using Monte Carlo simulations (Bois et al., 1991; Spear et al., 1991; Spear and Bois, 1992; Watanabe, 1993; Woodruff, 1991; Woodruff et al., 1992). In either approach, physiological and biochemical parameter data must be obtained in constructing the model. The first part of this section focuses on where these data can be found.

Estimation of model parameters and model validation requires toxicokinetic data. These data come from experiments where a drug or toxicant is administered and the concentration of the compound is measured over time in organ tissues, blood, expired air, and excreta. Animal studies can be comprehensive in the data collected. That is, concentrations can be measured in all of the biological media described above. In humans, a large number of the studies were intended for purposes other than physiologically based toxicokinetic modeling (e.g., investigating methods of biological monitoring, toxicity). As such, the reports often contain measurements made in blood, expired air and urine. The second part of this section focuses on toxicokinetic data with a list of references for carcinogenic compounds and the investigator(s) that used them for PBTK modeling.

3.5.2. Model Parameters

3.5.2.1. Physiologic Arms and Travis (1988) recommend reference values for risk assessment and document previously used parameter values as the basis for their reference values. Physiologic parameter values are reported for the vessel rich group, muscle and skin (muscle group), adipose tissue, and liver compartments with the caveat that compound specific PBTK models may have slightly different compartment definitions. The "physiologic" parameters of the vessel rich compartment are a weighted average of the organ and tissue values comprising the compartment.

The most recent compilation of physiologic toxicokinetic parameters is provided by Davies and Morris (1993). Tables of organ weights, volumes, blood flow rates, and other physiologic parameters are reported for six species (mouse, rat, rabbit, monkey, dog, and human). Only averages are listed in the tables, but references are given for the individual measurements used in calculating the average.

3.5.2.2. Biochemical Partition coefficients relate the equilibrium concentrations of a chemical in two media. For example, the blood to air (blood-gas) partition coefficient is the ratio of the equilibrium con centrations of the chemical in blood and air. Fiserova-Bergerova and Diaz (1986) measure human tissue-gas partition coefficients for hydrophilic chemicals. Measurement of tissue-gas partition coefficients for approximately 30 other compounds were made previously (Fiserova-Bergerova, 1983; Fiserova-Bergerova et al., 1984; Perbellini et al., 1985). In addition, Fiserova-Bergerova and Diaz cite the following studies reporting blood-gas partition coefficients of approximately 100 chemicals: Wagner et al. (1974), Dueck et al. (1978), Sato and Nakajima (1979a; 1979b), Fiserova-Bergerova (1983), Pezzagno et al. (1983), Fiserova-Bergerova et al. (1984), and Perbellini et al. (1985). In the absence of measured values, Kamlet et al. (1987) propose correlation equations to predict partition coefficients from solvatochromic parameters.

3.5.3. Toxicokinetic Data

Table 3.2 lists carcinogenic compounds for which animal PBTK models have been developed. The toxicokinetic data and the investigator(s) who used the data in a PBTK model are reported and separated according to the type of animal studied. In addition, the active agent and site of action for the compound are listed when the information could be found.

Human data can be found in both experimental and occupational studies. However, occupational studies generally do not contain the details of a worker's exposure, but rather a time weighted average of the exposure for a given work shift. If dose rate is important in the toxicokinetics, the use of occupational data becomes problematic. It is preferable to have controlled exposure conditions for modeling purposes since there are a number of approximations already used in the development of a PBTK model. However, some PBTK models have been validated with occupational data. Table 3.3 lists possible and known human carcinogens, toxicokinetic data and the investigator(s) that used the data to develop a PBTK model. In addition, the active agent and site of action in humans is reported if this information could be found.

3.6. INTER- AND INTRA-SPECIES VARIABILITY

3.6.1. Variability in Genetic Damage

In the estimation of the genetic hazards of environmental mutagens one of the main problems is the extrapolation from experimental data in animal species to humans.

Mutagens may cause genetic damage in any cell of the body. If the damage occurs in somatic cells it may lead to cancer or in the case of somatic cells of a foetus it may result in congenital abnormality. If the damage occurs in a germ cell, it may be transmitted to the following generations where it may cause hereditary disease.

Genes affect all aspects of the development of an individual and consequently genetic damage must be expected to affect all aspects of physical and mental qualities. Genetic differences among individuals may be responsible for differences in susceptibility to disease, including infective disease and cancer (ICPEMC, 1983).

In estimating the increase in mutation rate in man caused by chemicals, data are obtained from experiments in animals or other organisms. In some cases information may be available from somatic cells of exposed humans or cultured human cells. In any case the types of cells studied may not be those of greatest importance in relation to human hazards and the doses used experimentally may greatly differ from those man is

Parent Compound	Animal	Active Agent	Site of Action	Toxicokinetic Data	Model Development and Use
Benzene	mice and rats	muconaldehyde, benzoquinone	earduct, oral or nasal cavity, skin, squamous stomach, mammary gland, lung, angiosarcomas of the liver, lymphoreticular tumors (Goldstein, 1988; Maltoni and Selikoff, 1988; Mehlman, 1989)	Medinsky et al. (1989a), Sabourin et al. (1988; 1989; 1987)	Spear et al. (1991), Travis et al. (1990), Bois et al. (1991), Woodruff (1992), Cox and Ricci (1992), Medinsky et al. (1989a; 1989b; 1989c)
1,3-Butadiene	mice and rats		mice: heart, lung, stomach,liver mammary gland, ovary (IARC, 1986) rats: mammary gland thyroid, pancreas (Owen et al., 1987)	mice: Schmidt and Loeser (1985), Kreiling et al. (1986), Bond et al. (1986) rats: Bolt et al. (1984), Filser and Bolt (1984), Schmidt and Loeser (1985), Bond et al. (1986), Kreiling et al. (1986)	Hattis (1991), Johanson and Filser (1993)
Carbon Tetrachloride	mice and rats	trichloromethyl free radical (Amdur et al., 1991)	liver	mice: Bergman (1979) rats: Paul and Rubenstein (1963), Dambrauskas and Cornish (1970), Shimizu et al. (1973), Uemitsu (1986), Paustenbach et al. (1986a; 1986b), Veng-Pedersen et al. (1987)	mice: Paustenbach et al. (1988) rats: Veng-Pedersen (1984), Uemitsu (1986), Veng-Pedersen et al. (1987), Paustenbach et al. (1988)
Chloroform	mice and rats	probably phosgene (Pohl et al., 1977)	mice: liver rats: kidney (Amdur et al., 1991)	mice: Brown et al. (1974), Ilett et al. (1973) rats: Brown et al. (1974)	Corley et al. (1990)
1,2-dichloroethane or ethylene dichloride	mice and rats	2-(s-chloroethyl)-glutathione (D'Souza et al., 1988)	mice: liver, lung rats: angiosarcoma, adenocarcinoma	mice: D'Souza et al. (1988; 1987) rats: D'Souza et al. (1988; 1987)	D'Souza et al. (1988; 1987)

Table 3.2: *Animal toxicokinetic data by compound*

Parent Compound	Animal	Active Agent	Site of Action	Toxicokinetic Data	Model Development and Use
1,1-dichloroethylene or vinylidene chloride	rat	reactive metabolite	liver	McKenna et al. (1977; 1978a; 1978b), Jones and Hathaway, (1978), Reynolds et al. (1980), D'Souza (1984)	D'Souza and Andersen (1988)
Dieldrin	rats	liver (IARC, 1987)	Walker et al. (1969), Robinson and Roberts (1969)	Lindstrom et al. (1974)	
1,4-dioxane	mice and rats	p-dioxane-2-one (Woo et al., 1977)	mice: liver rats: liver, nasal turbinates	mice: none rats: Young et al. (1978)	mice: Reitz et al. (1990) rats: Leung and Paustenbach (1990), Reitz et al. (1990)
Ethyl Acrylate	rats		forestomach	Frederick et al. (1992)	Frederick et al. (1992)
Ethylene Oxide	mice and rats		mice: lung, Harderian gland, uterus, mammary rats: forestomach (IARC, 1987)	mice: Ehrenberg et al. (1974), Osterman-Golkar et al. (1976), Segerback (1983) rats: Tyler and McKelvey (1983)	Hattis (1991)
2,2',4,4',5,5'-hexabromobiphenyl	rats		liver (IARC, 1987)	Tuey and Matthews (1980a)	Tuey and Matthews (1980a)
Lead	rats	lead	kidney (Amdur et al., 1991)	Dalley et al. (1990)	Dalley et al. (1990)
Methylene Chloride or dichloromethane	mice and rats	phosgene (Amdur et al., 1991)	mice: lung, liver rats: mammary, ventral neck region, salivary gland	mice: Angelo et al. (1984) rats: Andersen et al. (1984), Angelo et al. (1984)	Andersen et al. (1987a)
Nickel	rats	nickel	tissue where deposited (IARC, 1987)	Menzel et al. (1988)	Menzel (1988)

Table 3.2: (cont.) *Animal toxicokinetic data by compound*

Parent Compound	Animal	Active Agent	Site of Action	Toxicokinetic Data	Model Development and Use
Polychlorinated Biphenyls	mice and rats		liver (IARC, 1987)	mice: Tuey and Matthews (1980b) rats: Matthews and Anderson (1975)	mice:Tuey and Matthews (1980b),Lutz et al. (1984) rats: Lutz et al.(1977;1984)
Styrene	rats	styrene oxide	lung, brain (IARC, 1987)	Young et al. (1979)	Ramsey and Andersen (1984)
2,3,7,8-tetrachlorodibenzo-p-dioxin	mice and rats		mice: liver, thyroid rats: liver, thyroid, lung, hard palate/nasal turbinates, tongue (IARC, 1987)	mice: Gasiewicz et al. (1983) rats: Kociba et al. (1976; 1978), Rose et al. (1976), McConnell et al. (1984), Leung et al. (1990b)	mice: Leung et al. (1988) rats: Leung et al. (1990a; 1990b)
Tetrachloroethylene or Perchloroethylene	mice and rats	epoxy intermediate	mice: liver rats: bone marrow	mice: Buben and O'Flaherty (1985), Schumann et al. (1980) rats: Pegg et al. (1979)	Ward et al. (1988), Travis et al. (1989), Hattis (1991)
1,1,1-trichloroethane	mice and rats		mice: liver rats: liver and kidney toxicity	mice: Schumann et al. (1982a; 1982b) rats: Schumann et al. (1982a; 1982b), Reitz et al. (1988), Dallas et al. (1989)	mice: Reitz et al. (1988) rats: Reitz et al. (1988), Dallas et al. (1989)
1,1,2-trichloroethylene	mice and rats	dichloroacetic acid, trichloroacetic acid	mice: liver rats: kidney	mice: Fisher et al. (1991) rats: Andersen et al. (1987b), Withey and Collins (1980), Koizumi (1989), Fisher et al. (1991)	mice: Fisher et al. (1991), Fisher and Allen (1993) rats: Andersen et al. (1987b), Fisher et al. (1989), Koizumi (1989)

Table 3.2: (cont.) *Animal toxicokinetic data by compound*

Parent Compound	Active Agent	Site of Action	Toxicokinetic Data	Model Development and Use
Benzene	muconaldehyde, benzoquinone	bone marrow (Amdur et al., 1991)	Srbova et al. (1950), Teisinger and Fiserova-Bergerova (1955), Berlin et al. (1980), Sato et al. (1974; 1975), Nomiyama and Nomiyama (1974a; 1974b), Sherwood (1972; 1988), Pekari et al. (1992)	Sato et al. (1974), Travis et al. (1990), Watanabe et al. (1994)
Carbon Tetrachloride	trichloromethyl free radical (Amdur et al., 1991)	inadequate evidence (IARC, 1987)	Stewart et al. (1961)	Paustenbach et al. (1988)
Chloroform	probably phosgene (Pohl et al., 1977)	inadequate evidence (IARC, 1987)	Fry et al. (1972)	Corley et al. (1990)
1,4-dioxane		inadequate evidence (IARC, 1987)	Young et al. (1976; 1977)	Leung and Paustenbach (1990), Reitz et al. (1990)
Ethylene Oxide		bone marrow	Calleman et al. (1978), Brugnone (1985)	Hattis (1991)
2,2',4,4',5,5'-hexa-bromobiphenyl		inadequate evidence (IARC, 1987)	Gladen and Rogan (1979), Wolff et al. (1979)	Tuey and Matthews (1980a)
Methylene Chloride or dichloromethane		inadequate evidence (IARC, 1987)	Dow Chemical Company study	Andersen et al. (1987a)
Styrene		inadequate evidence (IARC, 1987)	Ramsey et al. (1980), Stewart et al. (1968)	Ramsey and Andersen (1984)
Tetrachloroethylene	epoxy intermediate	inadequate evidence (IARC, 1987)	Fernandez (1976)	Travis et al. (1989), Hattis (1988), Koizumi (1989)
1,1,1-trichloroethane or methyl-chloroform		no adequate data (IARC, 1987)	Nolan et al. (1984)	Reitz et al. (1988)
1,1,2-trichloroethylene	trichloroacetic acid	inadequate evidence (IARC, 1987)	Stewart et al. (1970), Muller et al. (1974; 1975), Monster et al. (1976; 1979), Sato and Nakajima (1978)	Allen and Fisher (1993), Koizumi (1989)

Table 3.3: *Human toxicokinetic data by compound*

exposed to real environment. So it is necessary to extrapolate from experimental data to humans e.g. from one species to another.

A number of factors interfere in studies of a dose-response relationships in the chain of events from exposure or pharmacological dose to genetic end points (Ehrenberg et al. 1983). Such factors are the uptake, transport, metabolism and excretion of chemicals. The same factors also cause difficulties in extrapolating from one species to another.

In genetic toxicology experiments with whole mammals are both time and money consuming. On the other hand data from lower organisms (bacteria or insects) although valuable otherwise are of little value in attempts at quantitative risk estimation even when a hepatic microsomal preparation is incorporated to those organisms.

It has been claimed that Drosophila carries the same enzymes as mammals, thus extrapolation can be made form Drosophila germ cells to mammals. In practice however this is not true, since differences have been found in the genotoxic activity of certain chemicals in Drosophila and mammals. For example methylnitrosourea is effective in the fly but has little or no effect in the mouse (Ehling, 1982). This could be attributed to the fact that insect physiology is very different from that of the mammals.

Differences also exist among species of mammals in the metabolism and distribution in the body of some compounds. For example isoniazid in the mouse is hydrolyzed to the carcinogenic compound hydrazine whereas this is not the case in rats and Syrian hamsters (Jansen et al., 1980).

It is also possible in some cases that although the molecular dose at DNA is about similar in two different species the genotoxic damage may differ due to differences in the repair capacity of the two species or even other factors as it was the case with ionizing radiations (van Buul, 1980).

A dose of a chemical can be measured and expressed by different definitions such as exposure dose, pharmacological dose, tissue dose, target dose, molecular dose, genetically significant dose. The latter one is referred to the dose received by germ cells and risk estimates should be made on the basis of data obtained with mammalian germ cells only, because of the fact of the metabolic differences among species.

The problem of variability between species and the difficulty of extrapolation data from one species to another exists also within the same species where variability exists between the different types of cells and also between sexes.

Data on mutagenicity from somatic cells of various types are much easier to obtain than those from germ cells. However it is not possible to argue quantitatively from somatic to germ cells. In the case of cultured cells the normal metabolism of a chemical is bypassed and this may lead to a different result.

Regarding sexes, germ cells of males show varying sensitivities to chemicals according to their stage of spermatogenesis, while in females the relative sensitivities of various stages may differ among species (Caine and Lyon, 1979). In human lymphocytes it was found that higher Sister Chromatid Exchanges (SCE) were observed in females comparing to males (Lazutka et al. 1994). Also the micronucleus frequency in females was significantly higher than the micronucleus frequency in males in cultured peripheral blood lymphocytes (Fenech et al., 1994).

Physiological parameters such as nutrition, existence of certain hormones and diseases may influence the response of an organism to chemical exposure. Such influence could be either direct at the level of mechanism of response, or indirect through the kinetics of the chemical within the body. Since those parameters differ among species, also different responses are expected to the effects of genotoxic chemicals. Other factors such as sex, reproductive status, age and diet can also influence the response to chemical pollutants of many animal species (Stegeman et al., 1993).

3.6.2. The Parallelogram Model

In view of the difficulties in extrapolating from experimental data obtained in animals to effects on humans the "Parallelogram" method has been proposed (Sobels 1982, Anderson et al. 1994) where the idea is to find some suitable indicator of genetic damage in somatic cells which can be measured in both animals and man as is the DNA adducts. The principal in this method is to obtain information on genetic damage which is difficult to measure directly, for example mutation in germ cells, by comparison of endpoints that can be determined experimentally, e.g. alkylation per nucleotide in cultured mammalian cells (Sobels, 1982).

The basic assumption in the parallelogram method is that the ratio between somatic and germ cell mutation is the same in the experimental model and in man. But because of the existed variations in gene expression between tissues and species, there is no theoretical justification for this assumption (Wright, 1994).

In any case the extrapolation of data from experimental animals to humans remains a difficult approach even with the use of the parallelogram because of the exitting differences in exposure, toxicokinetics and genetic endpoints between animals and humans.

3.7. REFERENCES

Allen, B. C. and Fisher, J. W. (1993). Pharmacokinetic modeling of trichloroethylene and trichloroacetic acid in humans. Risk Anal. 13, 71-86.

Amdur, M. O., Doull, J. and Klaassen, C. D. (Eds.) (1991). Casarett and Doull's Toxicology (4th ed.). McGraw-Hill, Inc., New York.

Andersen, M. E., Archer, R. L., Clewell, H. J. and MacNaughton, M. G. (1984). A physiological model of the intravenous and inhalation pharmacokinetics of three dihalomethanes. Toxicologist 4, 443.

Andersen, M. E., Clewell III, H. J., Gargas, M. L., Smith, F. A. and Reitz, R. H. (1987a). Physiologically based pharmacokinetics and the risk assessment process for methylene chloride. Toxicol. Appl. Pharmacol. 87, 185-205.

Andersen, M. E., Gargas, M. L., Clewell, H. J., III and Severyn, K. M. (1987b). Quantitative evaluation of the metabolic interactions between trichloroethylene and 1,1-dichloroethylene in vivo using gas uptake methods. Toxicol. Appl. Pharmacol. 89, 149-157.

Anderson, D., Sorsa, M. and Waters M.D. (1994) The parallelogram aproach in studies of genotoxic effects, Mutation Res., 313, 101-115.

Angelo, M. F., Bischoff, K. B., Pritchard, A. B. and Presser, M. A. (1984). A physiological model for the pharmacokinetics of methylene chloride in B6C3F1 mice following i.v. administration. J. Pharmacol. Biopharmacol. 12, 413-436.

Arms, A. D. and Travis, C. C. (1988). Reference Physiological Parameters in Pharmacokinetic Modeling. (Report #EPA/600/6-88/004). United States Environmental Protection Agency.

Ashby, J., de Serres, F., Draper, J., Ishidate, M., Margolin, B.H., Matter, B.E. and Shelby,M.D. (1985) Evaluation of short-term tests for carcinogens. Report of the IPCS's collaborative study on in vitro assays. Prog. Mut. Res. 5, Elsevier Scientific, Amsterdam.

Bergman, K. (1979). Whole-body autoradiography and allied tracer techniques in distribution and elimination studies of some organic solvents (including carbon tetrachloride). Scand. J. Work Environ. Health 5, 1-163.

Berlin, M., Gage, J., Gullberg, B., Holm, S., Knutsson, P. and Tunek, A. (1980). Breath concentration as an index of the health risk from benzene. Scand. J. Work Environ. Health 6, 104-111.

Bishop, J.M. (1991) Molecular themes in oncogenesis, Cell 64, 235-248.

Bois, F. Y., Woodruff, T. J. and Spear, R. C. (1991). Comparison of three physiologically based pharmacokinetic models of benzene disposition. Toxicol. Appl. Pharmacol. 110, 79-88.

Bolt, H. M., Filser, J. G. and Störmer, F. (1984). Inhalation pharmacokinetics based on gas uptake studies. V. Comparative pharmacokinetics of ethylene and 1,3-butadiene in rats. Arch. Toxicol. 55, 213-218.

Bond, J. A., Dahl, A. R., Henderson, R. F., Dutcher, J. S., Mauderly, J. L. and Birnbaum, L. S. (1986). Species differences in the disposition of inhaled butadiene. Toxicol. Appl. Pharmacol. 84, 617-627.

Bravo, R. and Macdonald-Bravo, H. (1987): Existence of two populations of cyclin/proliferating cell nuclear antigen during the cell cycle: associated with DNA replication sites. J. Cell Biol., 105, 1549-1554.

Bravo, R., Frank, R., Blundell, P.A. and Macdonald-Bravo H.: Cyclin/PCNA is the auxiliary protein of DNA polymerase-α. Nature 326, 515-520, London.

Brown, B. R., Langley, P. F., Smith, D. and Taylor, D. C. (1974). Metabolism of chloroform. I. The metabolism of ^{14}C-chloroform by different species. Xenobiotica 4, 151-163.

Brugnone, F., Perbellini, L., Faccini, G. and Pasini, F. (1985). Concentration of ethylene oxide in the alveolar air of occupationally exposed workers. Am. J. Ind. Med. 8, 67-72.

Buben, J. A. and O'Flaherty, E. J. (1985). Delineation of the role of metabolism in the hepatotoxicity of trichloroethylene and perchloroethylene: A dose-effect study. Toxicol. Appl. Pharmacol. 78, 105-122.

Buchmann, A., Schwarz, M., Schmitt, R., Wolf, C.R., Oesch, F. and Kunz, W. (1987): Development of cytochrome P-450 altered preneoplastic and neoplastic lesions during nitrosoamine-induced hepatocarcinogenesis in the rat. Cancer Research, 47, 2911-2918.

Buchmann, A., Ziegler, S., Wolf, A., Robertson, L.W., Durham, S.K. and Schwarz, M. (1991): Effects of polychlorinated biphenyls in rat liver: Correlation between primary subcellular effects and promoting activity. Toxicol. Appl. Pharmacol. 111, 454-468.

Buchmann, A., Stinchcombe, S., Körner, W., Hagenmaier, H. and Bock, K.W. (1994). Effects of 2,3,7,8-tetrachloro- and 1,2,3,4,6,7,8-heptachlorodibenzo-p-dioxin on the proliferation of preneoplastic liver cells in the rat. Carcinogenesis 15, 1143-1150.

Bursch, W., Lauer, B., Timmermann-Trosiener, I., Barthel, G., Schuppler, J. and Schulte-Hermann, R. (1984): Controlled death (apoptosis) of normal and putative preneoplastic cells in rat liver following withdrawal of tumor promoters. Carcinogenesis, 5, 453-458.

Bursch, W., Taper, N.S., Lauer, B. and Schulte-Hermann, R. (1985): Quantitative histological and histochemical studies on the occurrence and stages of controlled cell death (apoptosis) during regression of rat liver hyperplasia. Virchows Archiv (Cell Pathol.), 50, 153-166.

Bursch, W., Putz, B., Barthel, G. and Schulte-Hermann, R. (1990): Determination of the length of the histological stages of apoptosis in normal liver and in altered hepatic foci of rats. Carcinogenesis, 11, 5, 847-853.

Butterworth, B.E., Slaga, T.J., Farland, W. and McClain, M. editors (1991): Chemically Induced Cell Proliferation - Implications for Risk Assessment, Progress in Clinical and Biological Research, 369, Wiley-Liss.

Van Buul, P.P.W. (1980) Dose-response relationship for X-ray-induced reciprocal translocation in stem cell spermatogonia of the Rhesus monkey (Macaca mulatta), Mutation Res., 73, 363-375.

Caine, A. and Lyon, M.F. (1979) Reproductive capacity and dominant lethal mutations in female guinea-pigs and Djungarian hamsters following X-rays or chemicals mutagens, Mutation Res., 59, 231-244.

Calabrese, E. J. (1988): Animal extrapolation and the challenge of human interindividual variation, in C.C. Travis (ed): Carcinogen risk assessment, Plenum Press, N.Y., pp. 115-122.

Calleman, C. J., Ehrenberg, L., Jansson, G., Osterman-Golkar, S., Segerback, D., Svensson, K. and Wachtmeister, C. A. (1978). Monitoring and risk assessment by means of alkylgroups in hemoglobin in persons occupationally exposed to ethylene oxide. J. Environ. Pathol. Toxicol. 2, 427-442.

Camplejohn, R.S., Brock, A., Barnes, D.M., Gillett, C., Raikun-Dalia, B., Kreipe, H. and Parwazeseh, M.R. (1993): Ki-S1 a novel proliferative marker: flow cytometric assessment of staining in human breast carcinoma cells. Brit J. Cancer 67, 657-662.

Caporaso, N., Hayes, R., Dosemini, M. et al. (1989): Lung cancer risk, occupational exposure and the debrisoquine metabolic phenotype, cancer res., 49, 3675-3679.

Caporaso, N., Tucker, M.A., Hoover, R.N., Hayes, R.B. et al. (1990): Lung cancer and debrisoquine metabolic phenotype, JNCI, 82, 1264-1272.

Caporaso, N. (1991): Study design and genetic susceptibility in the risk assessment of chemical carcinogens, Ann. Ist. Super. Sanita, 27(4), 621-630.

Carlson, G.P. (1987): Factors modifying toxicity, in R.G. Tardiff and G.V. Rodricks (eds): Toxic substances and human risk, Plenum Press, N.Y.

Columbano, A., Rajalakshmi, S., Sarma, D.S.R. (1981): Requirement of Cell Proliferation for the Initiation of Liver Carcinogenesis as Assayed by Three Different Procedures. Cancer Research, 41, 2079-2083.

Commission of the European Communities (1989, 1990, 1991, 1994), The Toxicology of Chemicals, Carcinogenicity Volumes 1-4.

Corley, R. A., Mendrala, A. M., Gargas, M. L., Andersen, M. E., Conolly, R. B., Staats, D. and Reitz, R. H. (1990). Development of a physiologically based pharmacokinetic based model for chloroform. Toxicol. Appl. Pharmacol. 103, 512-527.

Cox, D.R. and Miller, H.D. (1972): The theory of stochastic processes. Chapman and Hall Ltd..

Cox, L. A. and Ricci, P. F. (1992). Reassessing benzene cancer risks using internal doses. Risk Anal. 12, 401-410.

Dallas, C. E., Ramanathan, R., Muralidhara, S., Gallo, G. M. and Bruckner, J. V. (1989). The uptake and elimination of 1,1,1-trichloroethane during and following inhalation exposures in rats. Toxicol. Appl. Pharmacol. 98, 385-397.

Dalley, J. W., Gupta, P. K. and Hung, C. T. (1990). A physiological pharmacokinetic model describing the disposition of lead in the absence and presence of L-ascorbic acid in rats. Toxicol. Lett. 50, 337-348.

Dambrauskas, T. and Cornish, H. H. (1970). Effect of pretreatment of rats with carbon tetrachloride on tolerance development. Toxicol. Appl. Pharmacol. 17, 83-97.

Davies, B. D. and Morris, T. (1993). Physiological parameters in laboratory animals and humans.

Pharmaceut. Res. 10, 1093-1095.

Department of Health, UK (1989) Guidelines for the Testing of Chemicals for Mutagenicity, pp 1-99.

Dewanji, A., Venzon, D.J. and Moolgavkar, S.H. (1989): A stochastic two-stage model for cancer risk assessment. II. The number and size of premalignant clones. Risk Analysis 9, 179-187.

D'Souza, R. W. (1984). Pharmacokinetics of Halogenated Hydrocarbons in the Rat, Ph.D. dissertation, University of Houston.

D'Souza, R. W. and Andersen, M. E. (1988). Physiologically based pharmacokinetic model for vinylidene chloride. Toxicol. Appl. Pharmacol. 95, 230-240.

D'Souza, R. W., Francis, W. R. and Andersen, M. E. (1988). Physiological model for tissue glutathione depletion and increased resynthesis after ethylene dichloride exposure. J. Pharmacol. Exp. Ther. 245, 563-568.

D'Souza, R. W., Francis, W. R., Bruce, R. D. and Andersen, M. E. (1987). Physiologically-based pharmacokinetic model for ethylene dichloride and its application in risk assessment. In Pharmacokinetics in Risk Assessment, Drinking Water and Health, Vol. 8, pp. 286-301. National Academy Press, Washington, D.C.

Dueck, R., Rathbun, M. and Wagner, P. D. (1978). Chromatographic analysis of multiple tracer inert gases in the presence of anesthetic gases. Anesthesiology 49, 31-36.

Ehling, U.H (1982) Risk estimation based on germ cell mutations in mice, in: T. Sugimura, S. Kondo and H. Takebe (Eds.), Environmental Mutagens and Carcinogens (Proc. 3rd Intern. Conf. on Environmental Mutagens), University of Tokyo Press, Tokyo, and Alan R. Liss, New York, pp. 709-719.

Ehrenberg, L., Hiesche, K. D., Osterman-Golkar, S. and Wennberg, I. (1974). Evaluation of genetic risks of alkylating agents: tissue doses in the mouse from air contaminated with ethylene oxide. Mutat. Res. 24, 83-103.

Ehrenberg,L., Moustacchi,E. and Osterman-Golkar,S. (1983) Dosimetry of genotoxic agents and dose response relationships of their effects, ICPEMC Working Paper 4/4, Mutation Res. pp. 123, 121-182.

Emmelot, P. and Scherer, E. (1980): The first relevant cell stage in rat liver carcinogenesis: A quantitative approach. Biochemica et Biophysica Acta 605, 247-304.

Fenech, M., Neville,S. and Rinaldi, J. (1994) Sex is an important variable affecting spontaneous micronucleus frequency in cytokinesis-blocked lymphocytes, Mutation Res., 313, 203-207.

Fernandez, J., Guberan, E. and Caperos, J. (1976). Experimental human exposures to tetrachloroethylene vapor and elimination in breath after inhalation. Am. Ind. Hyg. Assoc. J. 37, 143-150.

Filser, J. G. and Bolt, H. M. (1984). Inhalation pharmacokinetics based on gas uptake studies. VI. Comparative evaluation of ethylene oxide and butadiene monoxide as exhaled reactive metabolites of ethylene and 1,3-butadiene in rats. Arch. Toxicol. 55, 219-223.

Finney, D.J. (1987): Statistical method in biological assay, Oxford University Press, Oxford.

Fiserova-Bergerova, V. (1983). Gases and their solubility: A review of fundamentals. In Modeling of Inhalation Exposure to Vapors: Uptake, Distribution, and Elimination, Vol. 1 (V. Fiserova-Bergerova, Ed.), pp. 3-28. CRC Press, Boca Raton.

Fiserova-Bergerova, V. and Diaz, M. L. (1986). Determination and prediction of tissue-gas partition coefficients. Int. Arch. Occup. Environ. Health 58, 75-87.

Fiserova-Bergerova, V., Tichy, M. and Di Carlo, F. J. (1984). Effects of biosolubility on pulmonary uptake and disposition of gases and vapors of lipophilic chemicals. Drug Metab. Rev. 15, 1033-1070.

Fisher, J. W. and Allen, B. C. (1993). Evaluating the risk of liver cancer in humans exposed to trichloroethylene using physiological models. Risk Anal. 13, 87-95.

Fisher, J. W., Gargas, M. L., Allen, B. C. and Andersen, M. E. (1991). Physiologically based pharmacokinetic modeling with trichloroethylene and its metabolite, trichloroacetic acid, in the rat and mouse. Toxicol. Appl. Pharmacol. 109, 183-195.

Fisher, J. W., Whittaker, T. A., Taylor, D. H., Chlewell, H. J., III and Andersen, M. E. (1989). Physiologically based pharmacokinetic modeling of the pregnant rat: A multiroute exposure model for trichloroethylene and its metabolite, trichloracetic acid. Toxicol. Appl. Pharmacol. 99, 395-414.

Frederick, C. B., Potter, D. W., Chang-Mateu, M. I. and Andersen, M. E. (1992). A physiologically based pharmacokinetic and pharmacodynamic model to describe the oral dosing of rats with ethyl acrylate and its implications for risk assessment. Toxicol. Appl. Pharmacol. 114, 246-260.

Friedrich-Freska, H., Gössner, W. and Börner, P. (1969): Histochemische Untersuchungen der Cancerogenese in der Rattenleber nach Dauergabe von Diäthylnitrosamin, Z. Krebsforsch., 72, 226-239.

Fry, B. J., Taylor, R. and Hathway, D. E. (1972). Pulmonary elimination of chloroform and its metabolite in man. Arch. Int. Pharmacodyn. 196, 98-111.

Fullman, R.L. (1953): Measurement of particle sizes in opaque bodies, Journal of Metals, 447-452.

Gasiewicz, T. A., Geiger, T. A., Rucci, G. and Neal, R. A. (1983). Distribution, excretion, and metabolism of 2,3,7,8-tetrachlorodibenzo-p-dioxin in C57BL/6J, DBA/2J and B6D2F1/J mice. Drug Metab. Dispos. 11, 397-403.

Gerdes, J., Schwab, U., Lemke, H. and Stein, H. (1983): Production of a mousemonoclonal antibody reactive with a human nuclear antigen associated with cell proliferation. Int. J. Cancer, 31: 13-20.

Gion, M., Mione, R., Becciolini, A., Balzi, M., Correale, M., Piffanelli, A.,Giovannini, G., Saccani-Jotti, G., Fontanesi, M. (1994): Relationship between cytosol TPS, TPA and cell proliferation. Int. J. Biol. Markers 9, 109-114.

Gladen, B. C. and Rogan, W. J. (1979). Misclassification and the design of environmental studies. American Journal of Epidemiology 109, 607-616.

Goldfarb, S. and Pugh, T.D. (1981): Enzyme histochemical phenotypes in primary hepatocellular carcinomas. Cancer Research 41, 2092-2095.

Goldstein, B. D. (Ed.) (1988). Benzene metabolism, toxicity and carcinogenesis. Environ. Health Perspect. 82, 3-307.

Goldsworthy, T.L., Morgan, K.T., Popp, J.A. and Butterworth, B.E. (1991): Guidelines for Measuring Chemically Induced Cell Proliferation in Specific Rodent Target Organs. In: Chemically Induced Cell Proliferation - Implications for Risk Assessment, edited by Butterworth, B.E., Slaga, T.J., Farland, W. and McClain, M., Progress in Clinical and Biological Research, 369, Wiley-Liss, 253-284.

Grasl-Kraupp, B., Ruttkay-Nedecky, B., Koudelka, H., Bukowska, K., Bursch, W. and Schulte-Hermann, R. (1995): *In situ* detection of fragmented DNA (TUNEL assay) fails to discriminate among apoptosis, necrosis, and autolytic cell death: A cautionary note. Hepatology 21, 1465-1468.

Hall, P.A., Coates, P.J., Goodlad, R.A., Hart, I.R. and Lane, D.P. (1994): Proliferating cell nuclear antigen expression in non-cycling cells may be induced by growth factors in vivo. Brit. J. Cancer 70, 244-247.

Harris,C.C. (1991): Chemical and physical carcinogenesis:advances and perspectives for the 1990s, Cancer Research, (Suppl.), 51, 5023s-5044s.

Harrison, R.F., Reynolds, G.M. and Rowlands, D.C. (1993): Immunohistochemical evidence for the expression of $PCNA$ by non-proliferating hepatocytes adjacent to metastatic tumours and inflammatory conditions. J. Pathol 171, 115-122.

Hattis, D.(1988): The use of biological markers in risk assessment, Statistical Science, 3, 358-366.

Hattis, D. (1991). Use of biological markers and pharmacokinetics in human health risk assessment. Environ. Health Perspect. 90, 229-238.

IARC (1986). Some chemicals used in plastics and elastomers. IARC Monographs on the Evaluation of the Carcinogenic Risk of Chemicals to Humans 39.

IARC (1986): The design and analysis of long-term animal experiments, IARC, Lyon.

IARC (1987). Overall evaluations of carcinogenicity: An updating of IARC Monographs volumes 1 to 42. IARC Monographs on the Evaluation of Carcinogenic Risks to Humans Supplement 7.

IARC (1987) IARC Monographs on the Evaluation of the Carcinogenic Risk to Humans. Suppl. 7, Lyon pp. 79-80.

ICPEMC (1983) Estimation of genetic risks and increased incidence of genetic disease due to environmental mutagens. Mutation Res., 115, 255-291.

Idle, J.R., Mahgoub, A., Sloan, T.P., Smith, R.L., Mbanefo, C.O. and Bababunmi, E.A. (1981): Some observations on the oxidation phenotype satus of Nigerian patients presenting with cancer, Cancer Lett., 11, 331-338.

Ilett, K. F., Reid, W. D., Sipes, I. G. and Krishna, G. (1973). Chloroform toxicity in mice: Correlation of renal and hepatic necrosis with covalent binding of metabolites to tissue macromolecules. Exp. Mol. Pathol. 19, 215-229.

Isola, J.J., Helin, H.J., Helle, M.J. and Kallioniemi, O.P. (1990): Evaluation of cell proliferation in breast carcinoma. Comparison of Ki-67 immunohistochemical study, DNA flow cytometric analysis and mitotic count. Cancer 65: 1180-1184.

J.D. Jansen, J. Clemmesen and K. Sundaram (1980) ICPEMC Publication No. 4, Isoniazid, an attempt at retrospective prediction, Mutation Res., 76, 85-112.

Johanson, G. and Filser, J. G. (1993). A physiologically based pharmacokinetic model for butadiene and its metabolite butadiene monoxide in rat and mouse and its significance for risk extrapolation. Arch. Toxicol. 67, 151-163.

Jones, B. K. and Hathway, D. E. (1978). The biological fate of vinylidene chloride in rats. Chem. Biol. Interact. 20, 27-41.

Kafer, E. and Kappas, A. (1990) Genetic analysis of genotoxic effects on chromosomes and cell division in lower eukaryotes. In: Kappas, A. (ed.) Mechanisms of Environmental Mutagenesis-Carcinogenesis. Plenum Press New York, pp. 49-68.

Kaisary, A., Smith, P., Jaczq, E., McAllister, C.B., Wilkinson, G.R., Ray, W.A. and Branch, R.A. (1987): Genetic predisposition to bladder cancer: ability to hydroxilate debrisoquine and mephenytoin as risk factors, Cancer Res., 47, 5488-5497.

Kamel, O.W., Lebrun, D.P., Davis, R.E., Berry, G.J. and Warnke, R.A. (1991): Growth fraction estimation of malignant lymphomas in formalin-fixed paraffin-embedded tissue using anti-PCNA/cyclin 1gA2. Amer. J. Pathol. 138, 1471-1477.

Kamlet, M. J., Doherty, R. M., Fiserova-Bergerova, V., Carr, P. W., Abraham, M. H. and Taft, R. W. (1987). Solubility properties in biological media: Prediction of solubility and partition of organic nonelectrolytes in blood and tissues from solvatochromic parameters. J. Pharm. Sci. 76, 14-17.

Kawahjiri, K., Nakachi, K., Imai, K., Yoshii, A., Shinoda, N. and Watanabe, J (1990): Identification of genetically hugh risk individuals to lung cancer by DNA polymorphism of the cytochrome P450IA1 gene, FEBS Lett., 263, 131-133.

Kendall, D.G. (1960): Birth-and-death processes, and the theory of carcinogenesis. Biometrika 47, 13-21.

Key, T.J.A. and Pike, M.C. (1988): The Role of Estrogens and Progestogens in the Epidemiology and Prevention of Breast Cancer, Europ. J. Cancer Clin. Oncol., 24, 29-43.

Knudson, A.G. (1971): Mutation and Cancer: Statistical study of retinoblastoma. Proc. Nat. Acad. Sci., USA, 68, 820-823.

Kociba, R. J., Keeler, P. A., Park, C. N. and Gehring, P. J. (1976). 2,3,7,8-tetrachlorodibenzo-p-dioxin (TCDD): Results of a 13-week oral toxicity study in rats. Toxicol. Appl. Pharmacol. 35, 553-574.

Kociba, R. J., Keys, D. G., Beyer, J. E., Carreon, R. M., Wade, C. E., Dittenber, D. A., Kalnins, R. P., Frauson, L. E., Park, C. N., Barnard, S. D., Hummel, R. A. and Humiston, C. G. (1978). Results of a two-year chronic toxicity an oncogenicity study of 2,3,7,8-tetrachlorodibenzo-p-dioxin in rats. Toxicol. Appl. Pharmacol. 46, 279-303.

Koizumi, A. (1989). Potential of physiologically based pharmacokinetics to amalgate kinetic data of trichloroethylene and tetrachloroethylene obtained in rats and man. Brit. J. Ind. Med. 46, 239-249.

Kopp-Schneider, A. and Portier, C.J. (1992): Birth and death/differentiation rates of papillomas in mouse skin. Carcinogenesis 13, 973-978.

Kreiling, R., Laib, R. J., Filser, J. G. and Bolt, H. M. (1986). Species differences in butadiene metabolism between mice and rats evaluated by inhalation pharmacokinetics. Arch. Toxicol. 58, 235-238.

Kunz, H.W., Tennekes, H.A., Port, R.E., Schwarz, M., Lorke, D. and Schaude, G. (1983): Quantitative Aspects of Chemical Carcinogenesis and Tumor Promotion in Liver. Environ. Health Perspect., 50, 113-122.

Kunz, H.W., Schwarz, M., Tennekes, H.A., Port, R.E. and Apple, K.E. (1985): Mechanism and Dose-time Characteristics of carcinogenic and tumor promoting xenobiotics in liver, in "Tumorpromotoren, Erkennung, Wirkungsmechanismen und Bedeutung", Appel, K.E. and Hildebrandt, A.G. (eds), MMV Medizin Verlag München, BGA-Schriften 6, 76-94.

Lai, D.Y. and Hughes, D. (1992). Feasibility of using less than two species, two sexes of rodents in carinogenicity testing of selected chemicals. Toxicologist 12(1):256.

Landberg, G. and Roos, G. (1991): Antibodies to proliferating cell nuclear antigen as S-phase probes in flow cytometric cell cycle analysis. Cancer Research 51, 4570-4574.

Lazutka, J.R., Dedonyte, V. and Krapavickaite, D. (1994) Sister-chromatid exchanges and their distribution in human lymphocytes in relation to age, sex and smoking, Mutation Res., 306, 173-180.

Leung, H. and Paustenbach, D. J. (1990). Cancer risk assessment for dioxane based upon a physiologically-based pharmacokinetic approach. Toxicol. Lett. 51, 147-162.

Leung, H. W., Ku, R. H., Paustenbach, D. J. and Andersen, M. E. (1988). A physiologically based pharmacokinetic model for 2,3,7,8-tetrachlorodibenzo-p-dioxin in C57BL/6J and DBA/2J mice. Toxicol. Lett. 42, 15-28.

Leung, H. W., Paustenbach, D. J., Murray, F. J. and Andersen, M. E. (1990a). A physiological pharmacokinetic description of the tissue distribution and enzyme inducing properties of 2,3,7,8-tetrachlorodibenzo-p-dioxin in the rat. Toxicol. Appl. Pharmacol. 103, 399-410.

Leung, H. W., Poland, A., Paustenbach, D. J., Murray, F. J. and Andersen, M. E. (1990b). Pharmacokinetics of [^{125}I]-2-iodo-3,7,8-trichlorodibenzo-p-dioxin in mice: Analysis with a physiological modeling approach. Toxicol. Appl. Pharmacol. 103, 411-419.

Lindstrom, F. T., Gillett, J. W. and Rodecap, S. E. (1974). Distribution of HEOD (dieldrin) in mammals: I. Preliminary model. Arch. Environ. Contam. Toxicol. 2, 9-42.

Lutz, R. J., Dedrick, R. L., Matthews, H. B., Eling, T. E. and Anderson, M. W. (1977). A preliminary pharmacokinetic model for several chlorinated biphenyls in the rat. Drug Metab. Dispos. 5, 386-396.

Lutz, R. J., Dedrick, R. L., Tuey, D., Sipes, I. G., Anderson, M. W. and Matthews, H. B. (1984). Comparison of the pharmacokinetics of several polychlorinated biphenyls in the mouse, rat, dog, and monkey by means of a physiological pharmacokinetic model. Drug Metab. Dispos. 12, 527-535.

Lutz, W. K. (1990). Dose-response relationships and low-dose extrapolation in chemical carcinogenesis, Carcinogenesis, 11, 8, 1243-1247.

Maltoni, C. and Selikoff, I. J. (Eds.) (1988). Living in a chemical world: Occupational and environmental significance of industrial carcinogens. Ann. NY Acad. Sci. 534, 1-1045.

Matthews, H. B. and Anderson, M. W. (1975). Drug Metab. Dispos. 3, 371.

McConnell, E. E., Lucier, G. W., Rumbaugh, R. C., Albro, P. W., Garvan, D. J., Hass, J. R. and Harris, M. W. (1984). Dioxin in soil: Bioavailability after ingestion by rats and guinea pigs. Science 223, 1077-1079.

McKenna, M. J., Watanabe, P. G. and Gehring, P. J. (1977). Pharmacokinetics of vinylidene chloride in the rat. Environ. Health Perspect. 21, 99-105.

McKenna, M. J., Zemple, J. A., Madrid, E. O., Brown, W. J. and Gehring, P. J. (1978a). Metabolism and pharmacokinetic profile of vinylidene chloride in rats following oral administration. Toxicol. Appl. Pharmacol. 45, 821-835.

McKenna, M. J., Zemple, J. A., Madrid, E. O. and Gehring, P. J. (1978b). The pharmacokinetics of [^{14}C]vinylidene chloride in rats following inhalation exposures. Toxicol. Appl. Pharmacol. 45, 599-610.

Medinsky, M. A., Sabourin, P. J., Henderson, R. F., Lucier, G. and Birnbaum, L. S. (1989a). Differences in the pathways for metabolism of benzene in rats and mice simulated by a physiological model. Environ. Health Perspect. 82, 43-49.

Medinsky, M. A., Sabourin, P. J., Lucier, G., Birnbaum, L. S. and Henderson, R. F. (1989b). A physiological model for simulation of benzene metabolism by rats and mice. Toxicol. Appl. Pharmacol. 99, 193-206.

Medinsky, M. A., Sabourin, P. J., Lucier, G., Birnbaum, L. S. and Henderson, R. F. (1989c). A toxicokinetic model for simulation of benzene metabolism. Exp. Pathol. 37, 150-154.

Mehlman, M. A. (Ed.) (1989). Benzene: Occupational and Environmental Hazards Scientific Update. Princeton Scientific Publishing Co., Princeton.

Menzel, D. B. (1988). Planning and using PB-PK models: an integrated inhalation and distribution model for nickel. Toxicol. Lett. 43, 67-83.

Menzel, D. B., Burke, A. M., Shoaf, C. R., Wolpert, R. L. and Boger, J. R. I. (1988). Integration of pharmacokinetic and genotoxicity damage to assessment of nickel exposure risks. Toxicologist 8, 193.

Mitchell, A.D., Cassiano, D.A., Meltz, A.L., Robinson, D.E., San, R.H.C. Williams, G.M., and Von Halle, E.S. (1983), Unscheduled DNA synthesis tests: A report of the US Environmental Protection Agency Gene-Tox Program, Mutation Res. 123, 363-410.

Monster, A., Boersma, G. and Duba, W. (1976). Pharmacokinetics of trichloroethylene in volunteers, influence of workload and exposure concentration. Int. Arch. Occup. Environ. Health 38, 87-102.

Monster, A. C., Boersma, G. and Steenweg, H. (1979). Kinetics of 1,1,1-trichloroethane in volunteers: Influence of exposure concentration and work load. Int. Arch. Occup. Environ. Health 42, 293-301.

Moolgavkar, S.H. (1978): The multistage theory of carcinogenesis and the age distribution of cancer in man. J. Natl. Cancer Inst., 61, 49-52.

Moolgavkar, S.H. and Knudson, A. (1981). Mutation and Cancer: A Model for Human Carcinogenesis. Journal of the National Cancer Institute 66, 1037-1052.

Moolgavkar, S.H., Dewanji, A., and Venzon, D.J. (1988): A stochastic two-stage model for cancer risk assessment. I. The hazard function and the probability of tumor. Risk Analysis 8, 383-392.

Moolgavkar, S.H. (editor) (1990): Scientific Issues in Quantitative Cancer Risk Assessment. Birkhauser, Boston.

Moolgavkar, S.H., Luebeck, E.G., De Gunst, M., Port, R.E. and Schwarz, M. (1990): Quantitative analysis of enzyme-altered foci in rat hepatocarcinogenesis experiments I: Single agent regimen. Carcinogenesis, 11, 8, 1271-1278.

Moolgavkar, S.H. and Luebeck, E.G. (1990): Two-event model for carcinogenesis: Biological, mathematical and statistical considerations. Risk Analysis 10, 323-341.

Moolgavkar, S.H. and Luebeck, E.G. (1992): Interpretation of labeling indices in the presence of cell death. Carcinogenesis, 13, 6, 1007-1010.

Moolgavkar, S.H., Luebeck, E.G., Buchmann, A., Bock, K.W. (1995): Quantitative analysis of enzyme-altered liver foci in rats initiated with diethylnitrosamine and promoted with 2,3,7,8-tetrachlorodibenzo-p-dioxin or 1,2,3,4,6,7,8-heptachlorodibenzo-p-dioxin. Toxicol. Appl. Pharmacol., in press.

Muller, G., Spassovski, M. and Henschler, D. (1974). Metabolism of trichloroethylene in man. II. Pharmacokinetics of metabolites. Arch. Toxicol. 32, 283.

Muller, G., Spassovski, M., and Henschler, D. (1975). Metabolism of trichloroethylene in man. III. Interaction of trichloroethylene and ethanol. Arch. Toxicol. 33, 173.

Nebert, D.W., Petersen, D.D. and Puga, A. (1991): Human AH locus polymorphism and cancer: inducibility of CYP1A1 and other genes by combustion products and dioxin. Pharmacogenetics, 1, 68-78.

Nolan, R. J., Freshour, N. L., Rick, D. L., McCarty, L. P. and Saunders, J. H. (1984). Kinetics and metabolism of inhaled methylchloroform (1,1,1-trichloromethane) in male volunteers. Fund. Appl. Toxicol. 4, 654-662.

Nomiyama, K. and Nomiyama, H. (1974a). Respiratory retention, uptake and excretion of organic solvents in man. Int. Arch. Arbeitsmed. 32, 75-83.

Nomiyama, K. and Nomiyama, H. (1974b). Respiratory elimination of organic solvents in man. Int. Arch. Arbeitsmed. 32, 85-91.

OECD (1987) Guidelines for Testing Chemicals 3rd Addendum 1-21.

OECD (1990) Scientific Criteria for validation of in vitro toxicity tests, Environment Monographs No 36 pp 1-61.

Osterman-Golkar, S., Ehrenberg, L., Segerback, D. and Hallstrom, I. (1976). Evaluation of genetic risks of alkylating agents. II. Haemoglobin as a dose monitor. Mutat. Res. 34, 1-10.

Owen, P. E., Glaister, J. R., Gaunt, I. F. and Pullinger, D. H. (1987). Inhalation toxicity studies with 1,3-butadiene. Am. Ind. Hyg. Assoc. J. 48, 407-413.

Paterlini, P., Suberville, A.M., Zindy, F., Melle, J., Sannier, M., Marie,J.P., Dzeyfus, F. and Brechot, C. (1993): Cyclin expression in human hematological malignancies: a new marker for cell proliferation. Cancer Research 53, 1-4.

Paul, B. B. and Rubenstein, D. (1963). Metabolism of carbon tetrachloride and chloroform by the rat. J. Pharmacol. Exp. Ther. 141, 141-148.

Paustenbach, D. J., Carlson, G. P., Christian, J. E. and Born, G. S. (1986a). A comparative study of the pharmacokinetics of carbon tetrachloride in the rat following repeated inhalation exposures of 8 and 11.5 hr/day. Fund. Appl. Toxicol. 6, 484-497.

Paustenbach, D. J., Christian, J. E., Carlson, G. P. and Born, G. S. (1986b). The effect of an 11.5 hr/day exposure schedule on the distribution and toxicity of inhaled carbon tetrachloride in the rat. Fund. Appl. Toxicol. 6, 472-483.

Paustenbach, D. J., Clewell III, H. J., Gargas, M. L. and Andersen, M. E. (1988). A physiologically based pharmacokinetic model for inhaled carbon tetrachloride. Toxicol. Appl. Pharmacol. 96, 191-211.

Pegg, D. G., Zempel, J. A., Braun, W. H. and Watanabe, P. G. (1979). Disposition of tetrachloro(^{14}C)ethylene following oral and inhalation exposure in rats. Toxicol. Appl. Pharmacol. 51, 465-474.

Pekari, K., Vainiotalo, S., Heikkilä, P., Palotie, A., Luotamo, M. and Riihimäki, V. (1992). Biological monitoring of occupational exposure to low levels of benzene. Scand. J. Work Environ. Health 18, 317-322.

Perbellini, L., Brugnone, F., Caretta, D. and Maranelli, G. (1985). Partition coefficients of some industrial aliphatic hydrocarbons (C5-C7) in blood and human tissues. Brit. J. Ind. Med. 42, 162-167.

Perera, F., Mayer, J., Santella, R.M., Brenner, D., Tsay, W.Y., Brandt-Rauf, P. and Hemminki K. (1991). DNA adducts and other biological markers in risk assessment for environmental carcinogens, Ann. Ist. Super. Sanita, 27(4), 615-620.

Perry, P.E. and Thomson,E.J. (1984), The Methodology of Sister Chromatid Exchange, in: Handbook of Mutagenicity Test Procedures, 2nd Edition, (edited by Kilbey, B.J., Legator, M., Nichols, W. and Ramel,C.), pp 495-530, Elsevier Scientific, Amsterdam .

Pezzagno, G., Ghittori, S., Imbriani, M. and Capodaglio, E. (1983). The measure of solubility coefficient of gases and vapours in blood. II. The largely used industrial solvents. G. Ital. Med. Lav. 5, 49-63.

Pohl, L. R., Bhooshan, B. and Whitaker, N. F. (1977). Phosgene: A metabolite of chloroform. Biochem. Biophys. Res. Comm. 79, 684-691.

Preston-Martin, S., Pike, M.C., Ross, R.K. and Henderson, B.E. (1991): Epidemiologic Evidence for the Increased Cell Proliferation Model of Carcinogenesis. In: Chemically Induced Cell Proliferation - Implications for Risk Assessment, edited by Butterworth, B.E., Slaga, T.J., Farland, W. and McClain, M., Progress in Clinical and Biological Research, 369, Wiley-Liss, 21-34.

Ramsey, J. C. and Andersen, M. (1984). A physiologically based description of the inhalation pharmacokinetics of styrene in rats and humans. Toxicol. Appl. Pharmacol. 73, 159-175.

Ramsey, J. C., Young, J. D., Karbowski, R., Chenoweth, M. B., McCarty, L. P. and Braun, W. H. (1980). Pharmacokinetics of inhaled styrene in human volunteers. Toxicol. Appl. Pharmacol. 53, 54-63.

Reitz, R. H., McCroskey, P. S., Park, C. N., Andersen, M. E., and Gargas, M. L. (1990). Development of a physiologically based pharmacokinetic model for risk assessment with 1,4-dioxane. Toxicol. Appl. Pharmacol. 105, 37-54.

Reitz, R. H., McDougal, J. N., Himmelstein, M. W., Nolan, R. J., and Schumann, A. M. (1988). Physiologically based pharmacokinetic modeling with methylchloroform: Implications for interspecies, high dose/low dose and dose route extrapolations. Toxicol. Appl. Pharmacol. 95, 185-199.

Reynolds, E. S., Moslen, M. T., Boor, P. J., and Jaeger, R. J. (1980). 1,1-dichloroethylene hepatotoxicity. Time course of GSH changes and biochemical aberrations. Amer. J. Pathol. 101, 331-343.

Robinson, J., and Roberts, M. (1969). Accumulation, distribution and elimination of organochlorine insecticides by vertebrates. Arch. Environ. Health 18, 106.

Rose, J. Q., Ramsey, J. C., Wentzler, T. H., Hummel, R. A., and Gehring, P. J. (1976). The fate of 2,3,7,8-tetrachlorodibenzo-p-dioxin following single and repeated oral doses to the rat. Toxicol. Appl. Pharmacol. 36, 209-226.

Sabourin, P. J., Bechtold, W. E., Birnbaum, L. S., Lucier, G., and Henderson, R. F. (1988). Differences in the metabolism and disposition of inhaled [^{3}H]benzene by F344/N rats and B6C3F1 mice. Toxicol. Appl. Pharmacol. 94, 128-140.

Sabourin, P. J., Bechtold, W. E., Griffith, W. C., Birnbaum, L. S., Lucier, G., and Henderson, R. F. (1989). Effect of exposure concentration, exposure rate, and route of administration on metabolism of benzene by F344 rats and B6C3F1 mice. Toxicol. Appl. Pharmacol. 99, 421-444.

Sabourin, P. J., Chen, B. T., Lucier, G., Birnbaum, L. S., Fisher, E., and Henderson, R. F. (1987). Effect of dose on the absorption and excretion of [^{14}C]benzene administered orally or by inhalation in rats and mice. Toxicol. Appl. Pharmacol. 87, 325-336.

Sato, A., and Nakajima, T. (1978). Differences following skin or inhalation exposure in the absorption and excretion kinetics of trichloroethylene and toluene. Brit. J. Ind. Med. 35, 43-49.

Sato, A., and Nakajima, T. (1979a). Partition coefficients of some aromatic hydrocarbons and ketones in water, blood and oil. Brit. J. Ind. Med. 36, 231-234.

Sato, A., and Nakajima, T. (1979b). A structure-activity relationship of some chlorinated hydrocarbons. Arch. Environ. Health 34, 69-75.

Sato, A., Nakajima, T., Fujiwara, Y., and Hirosawa, K. (1974). Pharmacokinetics of benzene and toluene. Int. Arch. Arbeitsmed. 33, 169-182.

Sato, A., Nakajima, T., Fujiwara, Y., and Murayama, N. (1975). Kinetic studies on sex difference in susceptibility to chronic benzene intoxication - with special reference to body fat content. Brit. J. Ind. Med. 32, 321-328.

Scherer, E. and Emmelot, P. (1976): Kinetics of Induction and Growth of Enzyme-deficient Islands Involved in Hepatocarcinogenesis. Cancer Research, 36, 2544-2554.

Schmidt, U., and Loeser, E. (1985). Species differences in the formation of butadiene monoxide from 1,3-butadiene and its reactive metabolites. Arch. Toxicol. 57, 222-225.

Schulte-Hermann, R., Timmermann-Trosiener, I., Barthel, G. and Bursch, W. (1990): DNA synthesis, apoptosis and phenotypic expression as determinants of growth of altered foci in rat liver during phenobarbital promotion. Cancer Research, 50, 5127-5135.

Schumann, A. M., Fox, T. R., and Watanabe, P. G. (1982a). [^{14}C]Methylchloroform (1,1,1-trichloroethane): Pharmacokinetics in rats and mice following inhalation exposure. Toxicol. Appl. Pharmacol. 62, 390-401.

Schumann, A. M., Fox, T. R., and Watanabe, P. G. (1982b). A comparison of the fate of inhaled methylchloroform (1,1,1-trichloroethane) following single or repeated exposure in rats and mice. Fund. Appl. Toxicol. 2, 27-32.

Schumann, A. M., Quast, J. F., and Watanabe, P. G. (1980). The pharmacokinetics and macromolecular interactions of perchloroethylene in mice and rats as related to oncogenicity. Toxicol. Appl. Pharmacol. 55, 207-219.

Segerback, D. (1983). Alkylation of DNA and hemoglobin in the mouse following exposure to ethene and ethene oxide. Chem. Biol. Interact. 45, 139-151.

Sherwood, R. J. (1972). Comparative methods of biologic monitoring of benzene exposures. The Annual Conference on Environmental Toxicology. Fairborn, Ohio.

Sherwood, R. J. (1988). Pharmacokinetics of benzene in a human after exposure at about the permissible limit. Ann. NY Acad. Sci. 534, 634-647.

Shimizu, Y., Nagase, C., and Kawai, K. (1973). Accumulation and toxicity of carbon tetrachloride after repeated inhalation in rats. Ind. Health 11, 48-54.

Shivji, M.K.K., Kenny, M.K. and Wood, R.D. (1992): Proliferating cell nuclear antigen (PCNA) is required for DNA excision repair. Cell 69, 657-676.

Sobels, F.H. (1982) The parallelogram; An indirect approach for the assessment of genetic risks from chemical mutagens, in: K.C. Bora, G.R. Douglas and E.R. Nestmann (Eds.), Progress in Mutation Research, Vol. 3, Elsevier Biomedical, Amsterdam, pp. 323-327.

Spear, R. C., Bois, F. Y., Woodruff, T., Auslander, D., Parker, J., and Selvin, S. (1991). Modeling benzene pharmacokinetics across three sets of animal data: parametric sensitivity and risk implications. Risk Anal. 11, 641-654.

Spear, R. D., and Bois, F. Y. (1992). Parameter variability and the interpretation of PBPK modeling results. Pharmacokinetics: Defining Dosimetry for Risk Assessment. Washington, D.C.

Srbova, J., Teisinger, J., and Skramovsky, S. (1950). Absorption and elimination of inhaled benzene in man. Arch. Ind. Hyg. Occup. Med. 2, 1-8.

Stegeman, J.J., Ballachey, B., Bickham, J., Hocker, B., Kennedy, S., Tompson, H. and Vethaak, A.D. (1993) Implementation of Biomarker-Based Studies. In: D.B. Peakall and L.R. Shugart (Eds.) NATO ASI Series, Vol. H 68 Biomarker, Springer-Verlag, Berlin pp. 31-48.

Stewart, R., Dodd, H., Gay, H., and al., ed. (1970). Experimental human exposure to trichloroethylene. Arch. Environ. Health 20, 64.

Stewart, R. D., Dodd, H. C., Baretta, E. D., and Schaffer, A. W. (1968). Human exposure to styrene vapors. Arch. Environ. Health 16, 656-662.

Stewart, R. D., Gay, H. H., Erley, D. S., Hake, C. L., and Peterson, J. E. (1961). Human exposure to carbon tetrachloride vapor - Relationship of expired air concentration to exposure and toxicity. J. Occup. Med. 3, 586-590.

Stinchcombe, S., Buchmann, A., Bock, K.W. and Schwarz, M. (1995): Inhibition of apoptosis during 2,3,7,8-tetrachlorodibenzo-p-dioxin-mediated tumor promotion in rat liver. Carcinogenesis 16, 6, 1271-1275.

Teisinger, J., and Fiserova-Bergerova, V. (1955). Valeur comparée de la détermination des sulfates et du phénol contenus dans l'urine pour l'évaluation de la concentration du benzène dans l'air. Arch. Mal. Prof. Med. Trav. 16, 221-232.

Thompson, C. L., McCoy, Z., Lambert, J.M., Andries, M.J. and Lucier, G.W. (1988): Relationships among benzo(a)pyrene metabolism, Benzo(a)pyrene-diolepoxide: DNA adduct formation and sister chromatid exchanges in human lypocytes from smokers and nonsmokers, Cancer Research, 49, 6503-6511.

Travis, C. C., Quillen, J. L., and Arms, A. (1990). Pharmacokinetics of benzene. Toxicol. Appl. Pharmacol. 102, 400-420.

Travis, C. C., White, R. K., and Arms, A. D. (1989). A physiologically based pharmacokinetic approach for assessing the cancer risk of tetrachloroethylene. In The Risk Assessment of Environmental and Human Health Hazards: A Textbook of Case Studies (D. J. Paustenbach, Ed.), pp. 769-796. John Wiley & Sons, New York.

Tuey, D. B., and Matthews, H. B. (1980a). Distribution and excretion of 2,2',4,4',5,5'-hexabromobiphenyl in rats and man: pharmacokinetic model predictions. Toxicol. Appl. Pharmacol. 53, 420-431.

Tuey, D. B., and Matthews, H. B. (1980b). Use of a physiological pharmacokinetic model for the rat to describe the pharmacokinetics of several chlorinated biphenyls in the mouse. Drug Metab. Dispos. 8, 397-403.

Tyler, T. R., and McKelvey, J. A. (1983). Dose Dependent Disposition of ^{14}C-labeled Ethylene Oxide in Rats. Bushy Run Research Center, Union Carbide, Export, PA.

Uemitsu, N. (1986). Inhalation pharmacokinetics of carbon tetrachloride in rats based on arterial blood: inhaled air concentration ratios. Toxicol. Appl. Pharmacol. 83, 20-29.

Veng-Pedersen, P. (1984). Pulmonary absorption and excretion of compounds in the gas phase. J. Pharm. Sci. 73, 1136-1141.

Veng-Pedersen, P., Paustenbach, D. J., Suarez, L., and Carlson, G. P. (1987). A linear systems approach to analyzing the pharmacokinetics in the rat following repeated exposures 8-11.5 hr/day. Arch. Toxicol. 60, 355-364.

Wagner, P. D., Naumann, P. F., and Laravuso, R. B. (1974). Simultaneous measurement of eight foreign gases in blood by gas chromatography. J. Appl. Physiol. 36, 600-605.

Walker, A. I. T., Stevenson, D. E., Robinson, J., Thorpe, E. and Roberts, M. (1969). The toxicology and pharmacodynamics of dieldrin (HEOD): Two-year oral exposures of rats and dogs. Toxicol. Appl. Pharmacol. 15, 345.

Ward, R. C., Travis, C. C., Hetrick, D. M., Andersen, M. E. and Gargas, M. L. (1988). Pharmacokinetics of tetrachloroethylene. Toxicol. Appl. Pharmacol. 93, 108-117.

Watanabe, K. H. (1993). Mathematical Modeling of Benzene Disposition: A Population Perspective, Ph.D. dissertation, University of California, Berkeley.

Watanabe, K. H., Bois, F. Y., Daisey, J. M., Auslander, D. M. and Spear, R. C. (1994). Benzene toxicokinetics in humans - bone marrow exposure to metabolites. Occupational and Environmental Medicine 51, 414-420.

Wilson, G.D., Camplejohn, R.S., Martindale, C.A., Brock, A., Lane, D.P. and Barnes, D.M. (1992): Flow cytometric characterization of proliferating cell nuclear antigen using the monoclonal antibody PC10. Eur. J. Cancer 28A, 2010-2017.

Withey, J. R. and Collins, B. T. (1980). Chlorinated aliphatic hydrocarbons used in the foods industry: the comparative pharmacokinetics of methylene chloride, 1,2-dichloroethane, chloroform and trichloroethylene after IV administration in the rat. J. Toxicol. Environ. Health 3, 313-332.

Wolff, M. S., Anderson, H. A., Rosenman, K. D. and Selikoff, I. J. (1979). Equilibrium of polybrominated biphenyl (PBB) residues in serum and fat of Michigan residents. Bull Environ. Contamin. Toxicol. 21, 775-781.

Woo, Y., Arcos, J. C., Argus, M. F., Griffin, G. W. and Nishiyama, K. (1977). Structural identification of p-dioxane-2-one as the major urinary metabolite of p-dioxane. Arch. Pharmacol. 299, 283-287.

Woodruff, T. J. (1991). Parameterization and Structure of Benzene Pharmacokinetic Models, Ph.D. dissertation, University of California at Berkeley.

Woodruff, T. J., Bois, F. Y., Auslander, D. and Spear, R. (1992). Structure and parametrization of pharmacokinetic models: Their impact on model predictions. Risk Anal. 12, 189-201.

Wright, A.S. (1994) Assessment of heritable mutations - the parallelogram approach. Proceedings of the EC/US workshop on risk assessment. Human genetic risks from exposure to chemicals focussing on the feasibility of a parallelogram approach October 11-14, 1993, Durham, NC, Health Effects Research Laboratory. Research Triangle Park, NC, EPA/600/R-94/042, EUR 15606 EN.

Young, J. D., Braun, W. H. and Gehring, P. J. (1978). The dose-dependent fate of 1,4-dioxane in rats. J. Toxicol. Environ. Health 4, 709-726.

Young, J. D., Braun, W. H., Gehring, P. J., Horvath, B. S. and Daniel, R. L. (1976). 1,4-Dioxane and α-hydroxyethoxyacetic acid excretion in urine of humans exposed to dioxane vapors. Toxicol. Appl. Pharmacol. 38, 643-646.

Young, J. D., Braun, W. H., Rampy, L. W., Chenoweth, M. B. and Blau, G. E. (1977). Pharmacokinetics of 1,4-dioxane in humans. J. Toxicol. Environ. Health 3, 507-520.

Young, J. D., Ramsey, J. C., Blau, G. E., Karbowski, R. J., Nitschke, K. D., Slauter, R. W. and Braun, W. H. (1979). Pharmacokinetics of inhaled or intraperitoneally administered styrene in rats. In Toxicology and Occupational Medicine. Proceedings of the Tenth Inter-America Conference on Toxicology and Occupational Medicine, pp. 297-310. Elsevier, New York.

Yunis,J.J. (1983) The chromosomal basis of human neoplasia, Science 221, 227-236.

Zimmermann, F.K., von Borstel, R.C., von Halle, E.S., Parry, J.M., Siebert, D., Zetterberg, G., Barale, R. and Loprieno, N. (1984), Testing of chemicals for genetic activity with Saccharomyces cerevisiae: report of the US Environmental Protection Agency Gene-Tox Program, Mutation Res. 133, 199-244.

Chapter 4

USE OF BIOCHEMICAL AND MOLECULAR BIOMARKERS FOR CANCER RISK ASSESSMENT IN HUMANS

J.J. Amaral-Mendes[1] and E. Pluygers[2]

[1]University of Evora, Evora, Portugal
[2]Oncology Department, Jolimont Hospital (honorary), La Louvière, Belgium

4.1. INTRODUCTION

Growing concern has arisen from the quasi-exponential increase in the numbers and quantities of man-made chemicals that presently are in current use, and their potential effects on human health, especially their delayed effects on degenerative diseases such as cancer. It is estimated that at least 50,000 chemicals have been introduced in the human environment since the end of the 40's and are presently in common use. However, only a few hundred have been submitted to thorough carcinogenicity studies in experimental animals, whereas relevant human data – mainly through epidemiological approaches – have been obtained for a few dozen compounds; on the other hand, several thousands of short-term assays have been performed in order to ascertain some of the more punctual effects of chemicals, such as genotoxicity.

For economical reasons, short-term bacterial mutagenicity or genotoxicity assays (not to say: nearly always) have often represented the first step in the evaluation of the suspected carcinogenicity of a given compound, based on the assumption that "carcinogens are mutagens" (Ames et al., 1973; Ames et al., 1975). The mutagenicity-genotoxicity concept of carcinogenesis has proven very successful indeed, correlations of 78-95% between mutagenicity in the Salmonella, or comparable, assays being currently reported (Mc Cann et al, 1975; Sugimura et al., 1976; Rinkus and Legator, 1979; Bartsch et al., 1980) and obviating – at least partially – the need for the massive recourse to the

Perspectives on Biologically Based Cancer Risk Assessment, edited by Cogliano *et al.*
Kluwer Academic/Plenum Publishers, New York, 1999.

considerably more expensive long-term animal experimentations. The huge amount of valuable information brought about by the short-term genotoxicity assays has for long, and still is, although to a lesser extent, dominating the field of cancer risk evaluation. It has somewhat obscured the flaws and shortcomings that, by the time, had become more and more obvious. As early as 1979, (Hollstein and Mc Cann) it has been observed that chlorinated as well as metal carcinogens were ineffectively reported by the Ames test. A clear trend of deteriorating performance with calendar year is reported by several authors (Zeiger, 1987; Tennant et al., 1987; Mendelsohn, 1988; Tennant, 1988; Ashby, 1988). Sensivity of the genotoxicity assays for carcinogens has dropped from 80-90 percent to about 60 or even 50 percent, and could have still been lower in selected classes of chemicals (Ashby 1988). In 1988, Trosko (1988) could entitle a paper "A failed paradigm: carcinogenesis is more than mutagenesis". During the 15 years between Ames' first report and Trosko's shaking statement, the complexity of carcinogenesis mechanisms had been better perceived and bacterial mutation assays clearly appeared as an oversimplification. As stated by Butterworth (1990), "simple plus/minus vs. carcinogen/ non-carcinogen comparisons used to validate the predictivity of bacterial and cell culture genotoxicity assays have revealed that a more comprehensive analysis will be required to account for the carcinogenicity of so many diverse chemical agents."

Indeed, progressive deciphering of the mechanisms of carcinogenesis revealed their extreme complexity, as well as the diversity of the pathways transforming an exposed (initiated) cell into a malignant cancer cell, after a long and complicated course, that could in no ways be reflected through the simplistic binary response of a bacterial assay. The major breakthrough in revealing the existence of a bulky group of carcinogenic agents that were not positive in the bacterial and cell culture genotoxicity assays came when the National Toxicity Program (NTP) of the US decided to evaluate the carcinogenicity of the chemicals of acute environmental relevance. It was also decided to base this evaluation on results of *in vivo* animal cancer bioassays rather than on those of short-term genotoxicity assessed in bacterial or related systems. In this way numerous animal carcinogens have been identified of which no more than 50 percent are genotoxic *in vitro*, thus emphasizing the importance of non-genotoxic (epigenetic) mechanisms in carcinogenesis, and contributing substantial additional information about the nonresponsiveness of genotoxicity assays.

Not only is genotoxicity related to the chemical class of the suspect carcinogen (e.g. higher with alkylating agents, low with chlorinated compounds), but it is also strongly dependent on the carcinogenic mechanisms involving sophisticated biological functions of a higher order than those in *in vitro* systems, as for instance immunological, neurological, endocrinological, physiological functions not found in organ tissue or cell culture systems (Trosko et al., 1983). It is therefore understandable that genotoxicity represents only one aspect of carcinogenesis, the other aspect being composed of the maze of facts and events known as tumour promotion in the multistage model of carcinogenesis.

As yet, the mechanisms of tumour promotion are far from being completely unraveled, although significant pieces of the puzzle are presentlly known and understood. They have but stressed the importance of the non-genotoxic mechanisms in carcinogenesis. The relative importance of both aspects is only a matter of speculation. Genotoxicity assays evaluate the exposure to potential carcinogens and its (very) early effects corresponding to the initiation phase of carcinogenesis. Numerous assays have been developed, also in humans, enabling the accurate evaluation of exposure. This is not true for the assessment of the events occurring during tumour promotion, and Butterworth pertinently writes that "meaningful new tests must be based on the actual mechanisms involved in the formation of tumours by these nongenotoxic carcinogens" (Butterworth, 1990); he adds that "much research remains to be done". This is also the opinion of C.C. Harris: "Methods to identify human tumour promoters and to predict responses to tumour promoters among different humans, need to be developed" (Harris, 1991; IB Weinstein, 1988; Travis and Belefant, 1992; F. Perera, 1987).

The present situation is one in which the very early events occurring after exposure to genotoxic carcinogens are known with reasonable accuracy. They may be adequately assessed by a series of methods and techniques based on that mechanistic knowledge. Thus exposure and initiation are fairly accurately circumvented nowadays, and a substantial amount of data is available to ascertain the value of the different approaches. As indicated by its very denomination, initiation is but the very first step of carcinogenesis; the fate of the initiated cell will then depend on the protracted and intermingling action of the numerous events composing promotion. Our knowledge of these events and their mechanisms is far from reaching the same level of certainty as exposure to genotoxicants and the ensuing initiation, notwithstanding the fact that considerable progress has been made in their understanding. So we have a rather accurate knowledge of the events that occur at the very initial stages of carcinogenesis and consequently are distant (in time) from the final outcome: the occurrence of a malignant cell. Hence it is foreseeable that these events will have nothing but a loose relation to this far-off outcome. Now paradoxically and to a large extent under the influence of occupational toxicologists and epidemiologists, these events and the very early changes induced by them, have been directly related to the occurrence of cancer, whereas the events occurring later in the process of carcinogenesis – hence probably more relevant to the final outcome, – are simply ignored. Conventional epidemiology with its simplistic exposure-outcome concept may therefore be considered as a kind of "black-box approach, that does not consider the intermediate mechanistic steps" (P.Vineis, 1992), as it only studies the relation between exposure and disease, the two extremes of the causal chain. This extremely important topic has recently received further emphasis from Sven Hernberg in his inaugural address at the twentieth International Symposium on Epidemiology in Occupational Health (S. Hernberg, 1994).

Nowadays, interest is shifting from initiating towards promoting agents in carcinogenesis, the importance of the latter being fully recognized. The extreme complexity of the mechanisms involved in promotion is also becoming more and more obvious. Whereas initiation, by initiating genotoxic carcinogens, is a rather simple phenomenon displaying a wide interspecies uniformity, including developmentally more primitive animals as well as higher eukaryotic plant (Sadowska et al., 1994), this is not any more true for non-genotoxic agents. Indeed, promotion proceeds through a wide array of different pathways, although resulting in the same outcome. It is a long-lasting process (decades in humans) and remains open to external influences acting both positively and negatively (the concept of "Invaders" and "Defenders", Sielken, 1987), many of them without any initiating potency and therefore unrecognizable by the methods that identify initiation. Moreover, the maze of pathways through which promotion proceeds may differ from one species to another and – in humans – not only depend on individual factors, but also on the type of the carcinogenic agent, the chemical structure, the target tissue, etc. This means that animal data will not be simply transposable to humans nor that any single marker will be able to identify all carcinogenic processes. Commenting on the use of markers of biological effect in cancer prevention studies, P. Greenwald pertinently states that "if there are different causal pathways leading to cancer, then a marker may be valid for an intervention working through one particular pathway but invalid for interventions affecting other pathways" (Greenwald et al., 1992). In practice, the diversity of pathways of promotion suggests that no single biomarker will be a common feature for all these pathways and that, instead, a panel of biomarkers, will be needed. The profile of the specific biomarkers composing a given panel as well as the sequence of their emergence are characteristic of a specific carcinogenesis pathway and may give a clue to the type of cancer that will finally develop, as shown by Pluygers et al. (1991-1992) in asbestos-exposed individuals.

These concepts are schematically represented in Figure 4.1.

Traditionally, carcinogenic chemicals are classified as initiators, promoters, complete carcinogens and progressing agents (Cohen and Ellwein, 1990). In the light of recent developments in the knowledge of the mechanisms underlying carcinogenesis, these distinctions are somewhat blurred out. It seems more useful to classify chemical carcinogens into those that directly interact with DNA (genotoxic), and those that act by other mechanisms (nongenotoxic, epigenetic).

Among the latter, are those which act mainly by increasing cell proliferation (Cohen and Ellwein, 1990; Preston-Martin et al., 1990; Travis and Belefant, 1992; Cohen and Ellwein, 1995), some do this specifically through interaction with a specific receptor, such as DES or TCDD and are not expected to demonstrate any threshold for activity whereas others induce proliferation non-specifically, mainly by three mechanisms:

1. Direct mitogenic stimulus

2. Toxicity and subsequent regeneration

3. Interruption of a physiological process.

These non-specific and non-genotoxic carcinogens are not expected to induce cell proliferation at non-toxic levels, thus demonstrating a definitive threshold, in contrast to the aforementioned non-cytotoxic promoters that do not appear to have a threshold level for effectiveness (Travis and Belefant, 1992; for details: Butterworth and Slaga, 1987). These concepts are summarized in Figure 4.2.

In our review of the results provided by biochemical and molecular biomarkers in cancer risk assessment in humans we have maintained the fundamental distinction between genotoxic and non-genotoxic effects, the latter corresponding to promotion.

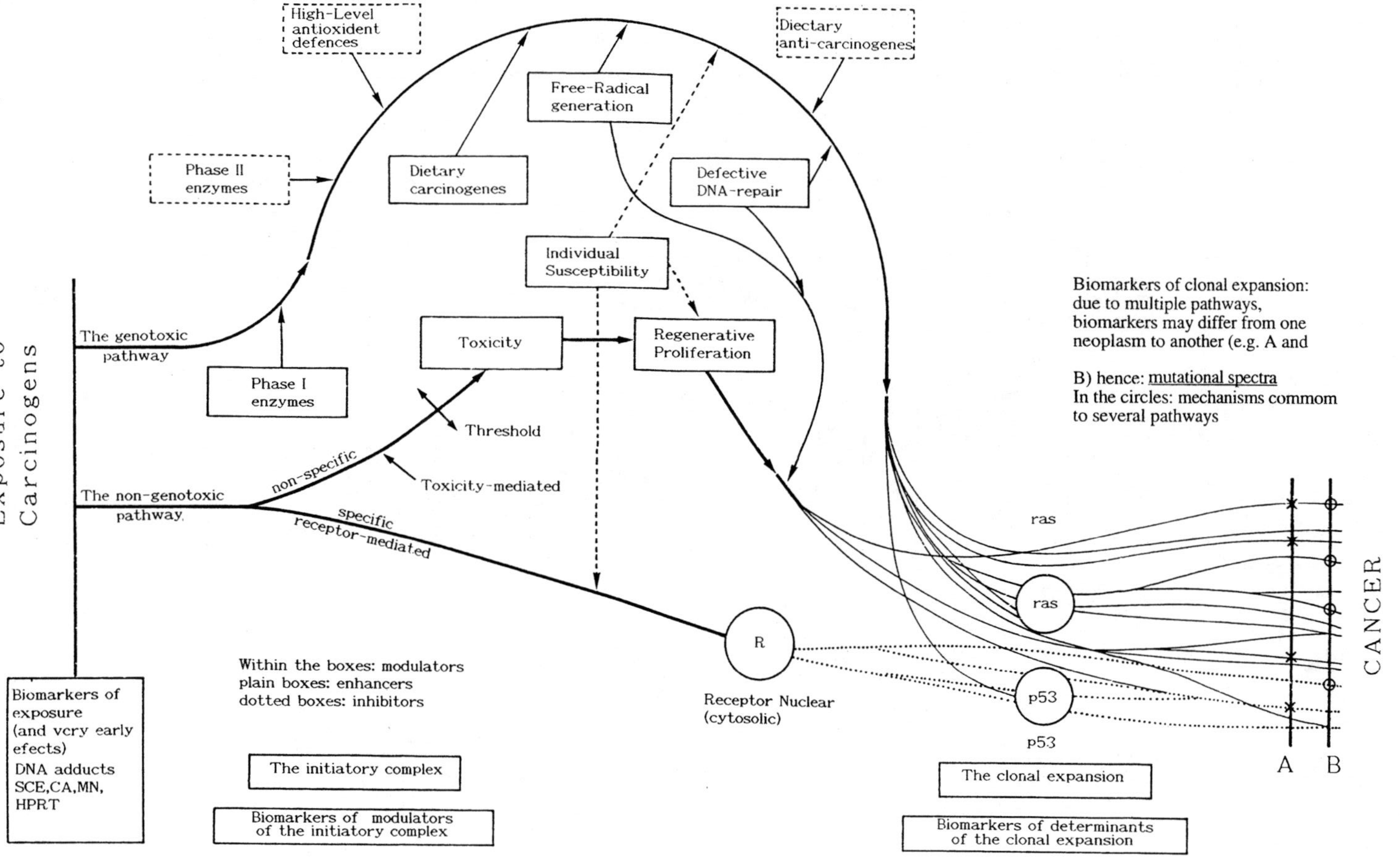

Figure 4.1: *Schematic representation of carcinogenesis*

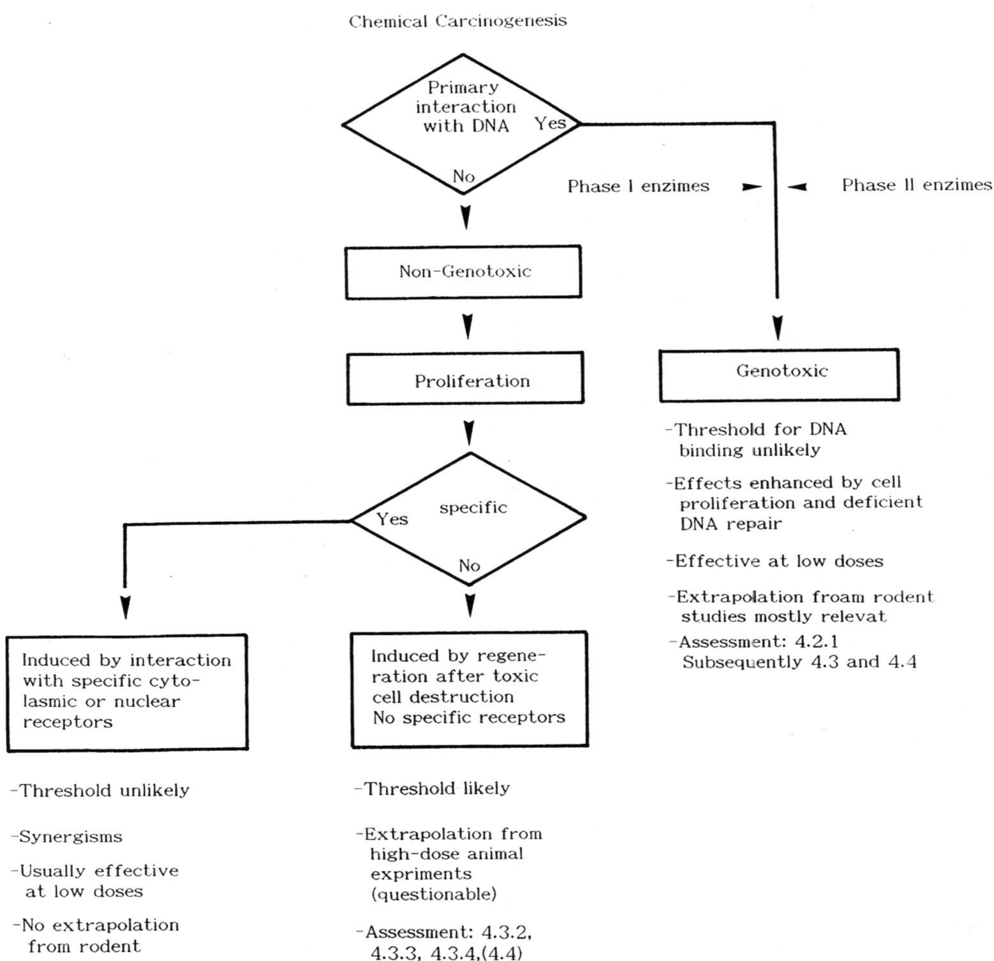

Figure 4.2: *Schematic mode of action of chemical carcinogens. (Modified from Cohen and Ellwein, 1990).*

In the Moolgavkar and Knudson (1981) model for characterization of the cancer dose-response relationship it is assumed that, after having been exposed to and "initiated" by a genotoxic carcinogen, the initiated cells, having acquired some selective growth advantage over the non-initiated cells, undergo the clonal expansion that will finally result in the formation of a malignant cell. The two major stages in this development are the initiation and the clonal expansion, with its proliferative advantage. Both of these stages may be assessed by a series of biomarkers, each of which will correspond to some peculiar step of the carcinogenic process.

Classically, biomarkers of cancer risk may be subdivided in three categories, according to the definitions given by the US National Academy of Sciences (NAS, 1989), identifying:

1. Biomarkers of exposure: such a marker is "an exogenous substance or its metabolite or the product of an interaction between a xenobiotic agent and some target molecule or cell that is measured in a compartment within an organism".

2. A biomarker of susceptibility is "an indicator of an inherent or acquired limitation of an organism's ability to respond to the challenge of exposure to a specific xenobiotic substance".

3. A biomarker of effect is "a measurable biochemical, physiological or other alteration within an organism that, depending on magnitude, can be recognized as an established or potential health impairment or disease".

Commenting on these definitions, we have added that "biomarkers of the promotional phase of carcinogenesis may be considered as markers of effect (in contrast to the markers of exposure), and represent an integrated expression of the effects induced not only by all the xenobiotics to which an organism is exposed, but also of their modulation (synergistic, or inhibitive) by endogenous or environmental factors" (Pluygers et al., 1993). We further noticed that such an integrated expression of effects, combined with the identification of the involved mechanisms, becomes especially decisive when an organism is exposed to complex mixtures of ill- or unidentified substances, a situation that usually prevails in the human environment. Moreover, considerable interindividual variations have been observed in humans with regard to the potency of e.g. enzymatic activation of pro-carcinogens to carcinogens or enzymatic detoxifying systems. Individual susceptibility therefore will be an important determinant of the ultimate cancer risk (NAS 1989; Schulte, 1990; Pluygers et al., 1992; Rhomberg, 1993). The capability of repairing damaged DNA also demonstrates considerable variability from one individual to another, a poor repair capacity being associated with higher cancer risk (Pero et al., 1990; Athas et al., 1991; Islas et al., 1991; Wei et al., 1994). Recently, the study of defective DNA repair has known spectacular developments with potentially far-reaching consequences (Heim et al., 1989; Digweed, 1993; Aaltonen et al., 1993; Thibodeau et al., 1993; Radman et al., 1994; Loeb, 1994). Further, exogenous nutritional factors may exert a considerable influence on the interaction between xenobiotics and important cellular macromolecules (Tell, 1986; Boothman et al., 1988; Wattenberg, 1985; Wattenberg, 1992).

On account of these considerations and although adhering to the general classification proposed by the NAS (1989), we have considered two distinct groups in this review of the biomarkers of cancer risk assessment. The first group forms what we have called "the initiatory complex", itself composed of markers of exposure-initiation, markers of individual susceptibility, markers of DNA repair capacity, and finally exogenous nutritional factors. The second group comprises the biomarkers characteristic of the mechanisms leading to the clonal expansion of the initiated cells, grouped together under the heading "the determinants of the clonal expansion".

Our aim is to critically consider in this review the relevance to cancer induction not only of the presently traditional biomarkers of exposure and early effect – mainly related to genotoxic carcinogens, but also the available evidence suggestive of later events in carcinogenesis, mainly – but not solely – induced by non-genotoxic agents; in the long run, the latter might prove more relevant to the ultimate cancer risk.

4.2. THE INITIATORY COMPLEX AND ITS MODULATORS

4.2.1. Biomarkers of Exposure

4.2.1.1. The External Dose This corresponds to the concentration of potential carcinogens in the surrounding environment (most often: atmosphere, but water and soil as well). This phase involves the identification of potential carcinogens as well as their concentration in the environment, and represents a major step in toxicology studies. Unfortunately, these assessments remain practically unrelated to the final cancer risk. Moreover, in the case of an exposure to complex mixtures – the most commonly occurring situation – generally only a few of the components are identified, and not necessarily the most relevant for carcinogenesis.

Nevertheless, the accurate identification of a potential carcinogen is important because this knowledge may give a clue to the particular cascade of events that will occur during carcinogenesis, and enable to select the appropriate panel of biomarkers. This is illustrated for instance, by the occurrence of chemical class-specific mutations in oncogenes (Jones, P.A. et al., 1991; Essigmann and Wood, 1993). The mechanisms of carcinogenesis are extremely complex and do depend on the involved carcinogens: hence it is important to identify them.

4.2.1.2. The Internal Dose This represents the concentration of a given substance in body fluids, such as blood or urine, or in tissues such as adipose tissue. Contrarily to a widespread believe, this is not a biologically effective dose, as it does not involve any interaction between the suspected carcinogen and relevant cellular macromolecules. Consequently, and at least for all those that are concerned with genotoxic carcinogens, their internal concentration in blood, urine or tissues may well bear no relation at all with future cancer incidence. To quote C. Garner, "molecular epidemiology should not be confused with the measurement of internal dose (the dose of a pollutant, that an individual absorbs, for example). Here the measurement made may have absolutely nothing to do with the eventual biological outcome – cancer". (Garner C., 1992). Many misleading conclusions have unfortunately been drawn for ignorance of this evidence and much confusion has arisen from the use of equivocal terminology. The target exposure (or target dose), should be defined as the biological effective dose of the chemical i.e. the concentration of the chemical, in the surroundings of the target tissue. It is related to the proportion of the internal dose which evades detoxification and penetrates to the critical target in the form of the ultimate toxic agent.

We have somewhat expanded on this topic because we do not believe that, in the field of genotoxic initiation of carcinogenesis, the mere concentration of a carcinogen, e.g. in blood, represents a biological effective dose. Biological effectiveness requires interaction with relevant cellular targets, as will be considered in the next section of this chapter, and even the effects of such interaction should be very critically considered. Be that as it may, to relate the concentration of a xenobiotic to its potential carcinogenic effect as an inducer of carcinogenesis initiation may well be an oversimplification.

However, in the case of exposure to non-genotoxic carcinogens without threshold, it might be considered that their cancer-promoting potency is directly related to their concentration in body fluids, or subsequently in tissues, although implying that in many cases it will still be receptor-dependent (with the ensuing interindividual variability). For instance, the concentration of some organochlorines, such as TCDD, in adipose tissue, is directly related to its concentration in the blood, or to the duration of exposure (Dewailly et al., 1994; Flesch-Janys et al., 1993), and to the subsequent incidence of some forms of cancer: breast and, possibly, pancreas, after exposure to DDT (Garabrant et al., 1992).

4.2.1.3. The Biologically Effective Dose Biological effectiveness may be inferred from observable interaction of the suspected carcinogen with relevant cellular macromolecules of which the most conspicuous is DNA, but also proteins such as hemoglobin and albumin. The excretion of altered nucleotides and their assessment in urine is still another means of evaluating the exposure to genotoxic carcinogens. The biologically effective dose may also be assessed through the evaluation of a series of early cytogenetic events, resulting themselves from an impairment of DNA function. We shall then consider DNA-adducts (and their surrogate protein and albumin adducts), and the urinary excretion of modified nucleotides as biomarkers of carcinogen exposure. We shall also consider a series of cytogenetic changes, including Sister Chromatid Exchanges (SCEs), Single Strand Breaks (SSBs) and other Chromosome Aberrations (CAs), Micronuclei (MN), as well as some specific mutations such as the Hypoxanthine Phosphoribosyl Transferase (HPRT) gene in lymphocytes and the mutant glycophorin in erythrocytes. Mutations of other genes (among them oncogenes, tumour suppressor genes, DNA-repair genes) may be evidenced at this stage of very early effects, but will be considered in the section on the determinants of the clonal expansion.

The events featured in the present section are related to carcinogen exposure; they bear little relation to the final outcome – cancer, as will be critically discussed.

4.2.1.4. Interaction with Relevant Macromolecules

DNA-adducts DNA-adducts result from the covalent binding to DNA of reactive electrophilic intermediates, most often produced by the enzymatic activation of (inactive) pro-carcinogens. As DNA is the presumed target molecule after exposure to genotoxic carcinogens, the rationale for this approach seems well established; indeed a quantitative relationship between dose, DNA-adduct level and animal carcinogenicity has been established in a number of tests (Autrup, 1991). Autrup mentions that the estimation of carcinogen DNA-adducts in target cell DNA "is considered the most biologically relevant measure of exposure" (Autrup, 1991). The assessment techniques have been developed over the past decade and are extremely sensitive; they include immunological, biochemical and physical methods; for instance the 32 P-postlabeling assay developed by Randerath et al. (1985) is able to detect one adduct per 10^9 normal nucleotides, representing about 3 adducts per genome (Kadlubar, 1992). The findings in experimental animals have been confirmed in humans and numerous studies have been published in validation of the method for exposure assessment (for reviews, see Wogan, 1989; Autrup, 1991; Santella, 1991; Perera, 1993).

The DNA damage resulting from the carcinogen binding may be repaired or may lead to programmed cell death; these processes will be later considered. DNA adducts do not, of course, participate in cell reproduction, but they can result in mutations in genes involved in cell proliferation and trigger carcinogenesis. Several classes of initiating carcinogens that bind to DNA, produce identifiable adducts and are evaluated in humans, in specific occupational or environmental settings, or in particular life-style conditions such as smoking or consumption of aflatoxin B1 contaminated food. Polycyclic Aromatic Hydrocarbons PAH have ranked among the first studied compounds (Perera et al., 1982; Shamsuddin et al., 1985; Vähäkangas et al, 1985; Harris et al., 1985, and many others). Others include aromatic and heterocyclic amines, nitrosamines (Hecht et al., 1994) chemotherapeutic anticancer drugs (Reed et al., 1987; Reed et al., 1988; Terheggen et al., 1988) and aflatoxin B1 (Groopman et al., 1984). An interesting investigation has been carried out in the population of a highly industrialized region in Poland, in order to identify and quantify the exposure to environmental carcinogens (Perera et al., 1992); global DNA adducts and PAH-DNA adducts have been determined in the peripheral blood of exposed inhabitants, together with a series of other biomarkers; this paper will be discussed.

With very few exceptions, such as their search in bronchial biopsies (Dunn et al., 1991), the assessment of the DNA-adducts is carried out in peripheral white blood cells (Harris et al., 1985; Shamsuddin et al., 1985; Reed et al., 1987; Perera et al., 1992; Schoket et al., 1991, and many others); these blood cells are not the usual target cells on which the carcinogen exerts its effects and this creates a serious problem in interpreting the results and correlating them to the target tissue in which eventually cancer will develop. Even in smokers, there is no correlation between adduct levels in the lung and in the bladder, two unquestionable target tissues (Routledge et al., 1992). There is no unequivocal correlation between adduct levels in the lung and in white blood cells of the same individual smoker (Van Schooten et al., 1992). It was observed, in tissue samples obtained at autopsy, that there was no strong correlation between an individual's adduct levels in different organs (Cuzick et al., 1990). These authors state further that "there are large variations in adduct levels in different organs and in different individuals". This represents a serious limitation to the usefulness of DNA levels in evaluating final cancer risk.

It is by far not the only reservation that can be made. Many factors are apt to influence the final significance of DNA adducts. For instance, adducts are randomly distributed over the genomic DNA, but only those occurring at genomic hotspots will induce mutations that will influence cell proliferation; these assays do not differentiate among these.

Several important factors do markedely influence the adduct levels: interindividual variation in carcinogen metabolism, more particularly the activation of procarcinogens to active metabolites induced by members of the cytochrome P450 family; interindividual variations in the DNA-repair capacity; modifications of carcinogen metabolism under the influence of dietary and environmental factors (Wogan, 1989; Autrup, 1991). For all these reasons, the assessment of carcinogen DNA adducts is a good qualitative measure of exposure, a rather inaccurate quantitative measure of exposure and an irrelevant predictor of cancer risk. Moreover, adduct determinations are technically rather difficult (for discussion, see Marzin, 1989; Autrup, 1991) and give information only about recent exposures; DNA sequences coding for important cellular functions are repaired within hours, and easily escape identification.

Urinary DNA adducts and DNA repair products To obviate some of the disadvantages of using carcinogen DNA adducts as exposure markers alternative methods have been developed, assessing the urinary excretion of altered nucleic acids. The method has been applied to the identification of aflatoxin B1 adducts in the urine of exposed populations in Guangxi Province of China (Groopman et al., 1985) and Kenya (Autrup et al., 1987). Whereas the levels of total immunoreactive aflatoxin equivalents appeared not to be related to intake levels (making this assay inappropriate for exposure assessment), AFB-N7-Gua and the aflatoxin M1 metabolite showed a dose-dependent relationship between intake and urinary levels, making this a good exposure meter (Groopman et al., 1994). Unfortunately, the analytical methods need sophisticated instrumentation (Wogan, 1989) and only reflect the exposure within the last 24 hrs. (Autrup, 1991). The influence of the urinary excretion of aflatoxin metabolites (in combination with hepatitis B virus surface antigen) on the subsequent risk of developing liver cancer has been evaluated and a high increase in relative risk has been observed when urinary aflatoxins were present (Ross at al, 1992) or in individuals testing positive for HBV surface antigen, with clearly multiplicative effects when both biomarkers were positive. The results by Groopman et al. (1994), "show for the first time a relationship between the presence of carcinogen-specific biomarkers and cancer risk". Indeed, the presence of AFB-N7-Gua in urine always resulted in a 2-3-fold elevation in risk of developing liver cancer (Groopman et al., 1994).

Other potential applications of the measure of altered bases in urine are: the assessment of 3-methyladenine, proposed as a marker of DNA methylation *in vivo* (Shuker et al., 1987); the determination of free thymidine glycol, proposed as a non-invasive assay for oxidative DNA damage (Cathcart et al., 1984); the assessment of

8-hydroxydeoxyguanosine (8OHdG) as a marker of oxidative DNA damage. This DNA repair product has interesting characteristics as it is excreted without being further metabolized (Fraga et al., 1990) and without being influenced by exogenous (dietary) DNA (Shigenaga et al., 1989); its level will therefore reflect the current oxidative DNA damage and repair (Loft et al., 1992). The assessment of 8OHdG is carried out using HPLC technology; this topic will be considered in more details in the section on oxidative damage.

Protein Adducts Several classes of carcinogens react with protein amino-acids such as valine, histidine, cysteine and lysine and high sensivity techniques are available to assess carcinogen-protein adducts. An advantage of protein adducts proceeds from the long half-lives of the involved serum protein molecules: 120 days for haemoglobin adducts in erythrocytes, 3 weeks for albumin adducts. As a result, an acute exposure to a genotoxic carcinogen can be detected many weeks after the exposure, and in the case of chronic exposures, haemoglobin adducts will give an integrated measure of multiple exposures occurring over a prolonged time period (Wogan, 1989, Autrup, 1991). Protein adducts are markers of exposure, but not of carcinogenic effects, as "erythrocytes are not a target cell for the carcinogenic effect and albumin is not a target molecule" (Autrup, 1991). There is no unequivocal relation between the levels of DNA-adducts and of haemoglobin adducts, both varying independently for compounds belonging to different chemical classes.

As no "repair" occurs in protein adducts, this factor will not influence haemoglobin (and to some extent serum albumin) adduct levels, making them more useful biomarkers than leucocyte DNA adducts for *in vivo* dose monitoring (Ehrenberg, 1993); adequate and sensitive methods for the measurement of Hb-adducts have been developed (Törnqvist et al., 1986). The measured levels of Hb-adducts (exposure assessment) have been related to the final risk of developing cancer, using a reference standard with well-known cancer risk per unit of *in vivo* dose.

The application of haemoglobin adducts to exposure assessments (and later to risk evaluations) has been initiated as early as 1978 by Ehrenberg and his team in workers exposed to ethylene oxide (EtO) (Calleman et al., 1978); the average tissue dose, evaluated through the measure of EtO-histidine adducts, was then converted to radiation risk equivalents and an excess cancer risk (for leukaemia) predicted; this proved to be similar to the excess risk in the follow-up epidemiological studies of the same cohort (Hogstedt, 1986; also reported in Perera, 1987). This methodology has been applied to a series of compounds including alkylating agents, aldehydes, aromatic amines, nitrosamines, polycyclic compounds (for complete list and references see Törnqvist, 1993). Attempts to correlate Hb-EtO levels with cytogenetic alterations have been recently published (Mayer et al., 1991; Schulte et al., 1992, Perera, 1993); EtO workplace exposure has been found to be significantly associated with EtO-Hb adducts and two measures of SCEs (Sister Chromatid Exchanges), "providing evidence of a direct link between a marker of biologically effective dose and markers of genotoxic effect" (Perera, 1993); no correlation was observed with micronuclei, CAs and SSBs. In the next section, we shall consider the significance of these cytogenetic alterations. Furthermore, EtO exposure was correlated with reduced DNA repair capacity (Mayer et al., 1993; Pero et al., 1989). This study has emphasized the importance of combining multiple complementary biomarkers in the exposure assessment to low doses of environmental or occupational carcinogens; we shall further stress this point when discussing the assessment of the multiple mechanisms intervening during the clonal expansion phase.

The methodology of serum-albumin adduct detection has been developed and used in an endeavour to correlate the adduct levels with dietary aflatoxin intake (Wild et al., 1980).

4.2.1.5. Cytogenetic Biomarkers of Early Effects Among the earliest effects of exposure to genotoxicants, structural changes in chromosomes have long been identified, initially after exposure to ionizing radiation. A linear relation has been observed between radiation dose and frequency of chromosome aberrations in circulating lymphocytes of exposed individuals, making this technique applicable to biological monitoring and dosimetry (Evans et al., 1979). The identification of chromosome damage in somatic cells has found wide application in the monitoring of exposure, especially in occupational settings, since the study by Vainio et al. (1983). The methodology has also been applied to the environmental monitoring of potentially exposed populations (see for instance: Perera et al., 1992); also Vleminckx et al., 1994). According to Wogan and Tannenbaum (1987), cytogenetic biomarkers may be subdivided into several classes: Sister Chromatid Exchanges (SCEs), structural aberrations and numerical alterations leading to aneuploidy; not all of these alterations carry the same significance, as will be considered later.

Sister Chromatid Exchanges (SCEs) This chromosome damage is characterized by the intrachromosomal exchange of sister chromatids; this process represents the breakage and rejoining of four DNA strands without any observable distortion of chromosome structure and without any mutational component. This peculiarity should be borne in mind, when evaluating the delayed effects of this kind of damage, and its eventual relation to the development of cancer.

A significant rise in the relative numbers of SCEs has been observed in the peripheral blood lymphocytes of several potentially exposed population groups, mainly in occupational settings. As early as 1979, Garry et al. (1979) reported an increased SCE frequency in workers exposed to Ethylene Oxide (EtO). The SCE assay has been adequately standardized (Perry and Wolff, 1974, Carrano and Moore, 1982) and has been further upgraded by the development of the High Frequency Cell (HFC) technique, identifying the most sensitive lymphocytes (Moore and Carrano, 1984). Garry's initial observations in EtO-exposed populations have been confirmed by many studies (for a review, see Mayer et al., 1991). The findings of the latter study (Mayer et al., 1991) demonstrated the high sensitivity of SCE's (higher than that of CAs) at exposure levels near or below 1 ppm, as well as a highly significant correlation between SCE-HFC and EtO-Hb adduct levels, thus showing a direct link between a marker of genotoxic response and a marker of biologically effective dose. Furthermore in this study there was no significant relation between exposure levels and frequency of CAs, SSBs and

MN. The long persistence – as long as two years – of elevated SCE levels after exposure to EtO, when compared to controls, has been mentioned in several studies (Stolley et al., 1984; Galloway et al., 1986); this was especially true for SCE-HFCs in primates exposed to EtO, in which the HFCs persisted for up to six years (Kelsey et al., 1988).

The assessment of SCEs has found further applications in individuals exposed to Styrene (Yager et al., 1989; Sorsa et al., 1991), PAH (Hemmink, 1992), welding fumes (Knudsen et al., 1992), diverse pesticides (Rupa et al., 1989; De Ferrari et al, 1991; Schulte et al., 1992), cytostatic drugs (Sorsa et al., 1988; Thiringer et al, 1991) and other occupational exposures. In all these situations, elevated frequencies of SCEs or SCE-HFCs have been observed; however the levels of exposure eliciting a respose may differ considerably from one compound (or group of compounds) to another; for instance much higher concentrations of styrene are needed than of EtO (Brenner et al., 1991). The situation is further complicated by the fact that SCE values are significantly influenced by factors such as season of blood sampling (higher values in Spring than Autumn), age, smoking status (Sinha et al., 1986) and possibly others. Several studies have brought evidence that the SCE and SCE-HFC frequency is significantly increased in active smokers (Husgafvel-Pursiainen, 1987; Husgafvel-Pursiainen et al., 1987) and is related to the pack-years of smoking (Kao-Shan et al., 1987; Perera et al., 1989). On the other hand it is not increased in passive smokers nor in non-smokers (Husgafvel-Pursiainen et al., 1987), whereas significant levels of PAH-DNA adducts are detected in non-smokers. As a result SCE frequency and DNA-adduct levels are not significantly correlated (Perera et al., 1989). These data have to be borne in mind when interpreting and comparing results, as the composition of side-stream smoke is very different from main-stream smoke; it might indicate that not all environmental genotoxic pollutants are effective in eliciting SCE responses.

This may in turn influence the interpretation of the results of environmental monitoring, as in the aforementioned studies (Perera et al., 1992; Vleminck et al., 1994) in which, for instance, an interpretation bias may be introduced as the result of sample collections in different seasons. Nevertheless, SCE and SCE-HFC indices in peripheral blood lymphocytes may be considered as adequate indicators of exposure to some genotoxicants; their relevance to ultimate cancer risk will be considered later, together with genetic markers.

Chromosome Aberrations (CAs) and Single Strand Breaks (SSBs) Contrarily to SCEs, chromosomal aberrations constitute a true damage to the genetic material and represent mutations, of which the final impact on health may be presumed to be more important. CAs are frequent in human tumours and tend to become more extensive with progression of the disease (Knudson, 1985; Heim et al., 1989; Weinberg 1987; Mitelman, 1988). A cascade of mutational events has presently been characterized in a number of human tumours, and available techniques allow for the accurate identification of these mutations and the mapping of "mutational spectra". This approach has been initiated by Vogelstein et al. (1988) in the study of colorectal tumour development and is now widely applied. These techniques and their results will be considered in the second part of this study (determinants of the clonal expansion).

The chromosome aberrations referred to in this section are observable with "simple" microscopic techniques and complementary techniques such as singe-cell microgel electrophoresis (Singh et al., 1988); they allow the identification of a wide array of chromosomal aberrations, extending from Single Strands Breaks (SSBs) to large deletions, translocations, chromosome rearrangements and amplifications. Mostly, these studies have been combined with SCEs and Micronuclei (MN) assays; exposure to genotoxic carcinogens results in increased rates of CAs. The overall sensivity of this evaluation seems to be somewhat less than that of the SCE index. However, the relevance of CAs in peripheral blood lymphocytes to the subsequent probability of the onset of cancer may be greater; indeed S. Bonassi (1994) reviewed a large cohort of 1455 subjects screened for CAs and followed for prolonged periods; according to CA levels, the cohort was split in three groups of low, medium and high structural CA levels using the 33rd and 66th percentiles as threshold values. A significantly increased Standardized Mortality Ratio (SMR) was found for all subjects with medium (SMR: 178.5) or high (SMR: 182) CA levels. In subjects with the highest levels of CAs, an excess mortality was observed for respiratory tract cancers (SMR: 250.8) and haematopoietic tissue cancers (SMR: 548.8). When comparing high and medium levels of CAs with the lowest level, a doubling of mortality for all cancers was observed; for respiratory tract cancers the RR was 4.36 (95%CI = 0.50 - 38.3) for medium and 7.96 (95% CI 1.04 - 61.8) for high CA levels. These results will be further considered below.

Micronuclei (MN) Micronuclei may arise either from acentric chromosome fragments or from entire whole chromosomes; they reflect not only the action of chromosome-damaging chemicals (Clastogens), but also of spindle poisons resulting in aneuploidy; the area covered by a micronucleus might give a point as to its origin: clastogenic or oncogenic (Vanparys et al., 1990)

The micronucleus test (MNT) was first developed in bone marrow erythrocytes in mammals (Matter and Schmid, 1971), a technique that could not be used for human monitoring because of sampling difficulties. The MNT was later proposed in cultured human lymphocytes (Countryman and Heddle, 1976) and the technique improved to yield lymphocytes with intact cytoplasm; this improved technique was then applied to the assessment of MN in styrene-exposed workers (Hogstedt, 1984; Maki-Paakkanen, 1987). Comparative studies in workers exposed to low concentrations of styrene have shown MN to be significantly elevated in the exposed group, whereas no effect was observed on SCEs (Brenner et al., 1991). For MN, a dose-response relationship was observed in the high exposure category; gender, education and smoking did not influence results. Several studies have confirmed these results.

A drawback common to all the reviewed cytogenetic techniques is the necessity to score large numbers of cells in order to detect low-dose effects; moreover culture conditions are stringent, and the techniques are laborious and expensive, hence unsuitable for the monitoring of large populations. An *in vivo* test in lymphocytes from human capillary blood has been developed and can be used for large-scale investigations (Xue et al., 1988); 2000 lymphocytes per person have to be scored and the observed MN frequencies are in the 0.010 - 0.030% range in healthy subjects, the higher frequencies being found in older subjects (Xue et al., 1992a). The results may also be expressed as the Micronucleus Positive Rate (MNPR) representing the rate of persons with MN in their lymphocytes; here the range in healthy persons is around 35% (Xue et al., 1992), with higher rates in elderly persons, but with no influence of gender. Smoking and a variety of occupational exposures bring on significantly elevated frequencies of MN; the presence of a higher MN frequency in some smokers might be indicative of increased susceptibility (Xue et al., 1992 b). A positive correlation has been found between MN frequency and Chromosome Aberrations.

The formation of micronuclei in several target tissues has been used as a biological marker of the early mutational events in carcinogenesis. For instance, in the buccal cavity higher MN counts are observed in premalignant lesions and in the normal appearing tissue adjacent to the lesions (Stich et al., 1982); Stich and Rosin, 1984, and other subsequent publications of the same team); similar observations pertain to gastrointestinal lesions (Lipkin, 1988), to bronchial carcinogenesis (Lippman et al., 1990a) and to several tissues in smokers, with or without premalignant lesions: sputum (Fontham et al., 1986), urine (Reali et al., 1987), buccal smears (Stich et al., 1992) and cervical smears.

Many of the aforementioned studies on MN frequency in selected target tissues have demonstrated a significant correlation with the subsequent risk of developing cancer in these tissues; hence the MN test is readily being used to assess the efficacy of chemoprevention trials (Rosin et al., 1987; Lippman et al., 1990b; Benner et al. , 1994). Chemopreventive agents that have reversed premalignancy have resulted in significant reductions in MN frequency. One advantage of the MN test is its non-invasiveness, making repeated measurements possible; on the other hand, among the drawbacks, the low frequency of the MN and the ensuing statistical problems as well as the labour intensive technique, should be mentioned (Benner et al., 1994). MN reflect only recent DNA damage.

In opposition to observations in target tissues, the predictive value of MN frequency in circulating blood lymphocytes on cancer risk has not been established. This point will be discussed later.

HPRT mutations in lymphocytes The study of somatic mutations in humans is important in order to evaluate mutation frequencies in relation with exposure to known or suspected mutagens, to monitor the effects of primary prevention, and eventually to identify individuals at risk, for instance due to genetic causes (Tates et al., 1989). Two assays have been developed, involving peripheral blood lymphocytes. The first, the *hprt* mutation assay, detects and quantifies mutants in lymphocytes deficient in the enzyme Hypoxanthine-Phospho-Ribosyl-Transferase (HPRT); the second detects mutations at the autosomal locus for human leukocyte antigen-A (HLA-A).

Technical difficulties in the HPRT assay have been largely overcome (Albertini et al., 1985); marked interindividual variations in mutation frequency have been observed, possibly in relation with individual DNA repair capacities, as very high mutation frequencies come along with DNA repair diseases such as xeroderma pigmentosa and ataxiatelangiectasia (Cole et al., 1988). A marked elevation in mutant T-cells has been reported after radiochemotherapy, as well as in subjects exposed to indoor radon (Bridges et al., 1991).

Comparable observations are available for mutations at the HLA-A locus and both procedures have recently been critically reviewed (Lambert, 1992; Autrup, 1991). In contrast to DNA-adducts, and to a lesser extent to SCE's, which give evidence of recent exposures to carcinogens, HPRT mutations are long-lasting, even a lifetime.

Indeed, increased HPRT mutation rates are still observed in survivors of the Hiroshima and Nagasaki atomic blasts, more than 40 years after the radiation exposures (Hakoda et al., 1988).

Hemoglobin mutations in erythrocytes The cell surface glycoprotein Glycophorin A is expressed as two allelic forms M and N that can be identified by highly specific monoclonal antibodies in circulating erythrocytes. By linking the specific MoAbs to fluorescent dyes, mutant erythrocytes, characterized by the loss of one of the alleles, can be identified and quantitated (Langlois et al., 1986).

Again, significant increases in mutation rates have been observed in atomic bomb survivors (Langlois et al., 1987).

In another approach, the single aminoacid change characteristic of sickle cell hemoglobin (HbS), induced by a transversion mutation GAG to GTG in the globin gene, is identified using fluorescent MoAbs (Stamatoyannopoulos et al., 1984; Tates et al., 1989).

4.2.1.6. Discussion about the Biomarkers of Exposure It is essential to bear in mind that the biomarkers that have been hitherto considered are biomarkers of exposure, simply providing evidence that an organism has been exposed to a (geno)toxic agent, but providing no evidence that this expression of an exposure is unquestionably correlated with later cancer occurrence. Lack of appreciation, of this fact has led to many improper conclusions; as judiciously stressed by Vineis (1992), conventional epidemiology has long acted as a "black-box" discipline, considering only exposure and the so much delayed outcome: cancer and ignoring, the intermediate mechanistic steps which in fact represent the clue of the ongoing process. Therefore we feel it advisable to summarize the potentialities of each of the sofar mentioned biomarkers, in order to better define their scope.

The *external dose*, consisting in the concentration of potential carcinogens in the ambient environment, bears no direct relation with the final cancer incidence in the exposed populations (Autrup, 1991; Garner, 1992); moreover, the effects are unpredictable after exposure to complex mixtures. One of the major contributions of these assessments, in addition to classical toxicity evaluations, is their capacity to provide hints about the involved agent-specific carcinogenesis mechanisms. Similar considerations apply to what is called the *internal dose* and has been discussed in the text.

The *biologically effective dose* implies that an interaction between the potential carcinogenic agent and relevant cellular targets has indeed taken place, making these biomarkers theoretically better suited to reveal the onset of the carcinogenic process. DNA-adducts represent excellent exposure markers, but their relation to final cancer incidence is less straightforward, because of several shortcomings. To recall a few of them: the random distribution of the adducts over the genome, leaving many adducts "silent" when occurring in non-coding DNA; the fast repair of adducts occurring at genomic hot-spots, before the cell divides and fixes the damage; the fact that adducts are assessed in peripheral blood white cells, very different of the usual target cells of the carcinogen, etc. DNA-adducts also reflect only recent exposures. These insufficiencies can be partly alleviated by the determination of DNA-adducts (and other DNA repair products) in the urine, or of protein adducts, mainly in the form of haemoglobin adducts. However, the relation of the latter to the final cancer risk is difficult to evaluate.

A series of cytogenetic effects have been identified after exposure to carcinogens and extensively studied as to their predictive value on cancer incidence. Although chromosome alterations truly represent early effects of the interaction between carcinogens and the genomic material, these biomarkers rather have proved to be valuable exposure markers, whereas their predictive value for cancer incidence has long remained questionable. Presently, however, the follow-up of a large cohort (3182 subjects) followed by the Nordic Study Group have reached the conclusion that Chromosome Aberrations (breakage) represent a relevant biomarker for future cancer risk (Reuterwall and the Nordic Study Group, 1994; Bonassi, 1994), while no relation is found for SCEs; the data are too limited to evaluate the relevance of MNs (Knudsen, Sorsa and the Nordic Study Group, 1994; Sorsa et al., 1992). These important findings should be borne in mind when assessing cancer risk: CAs have a predictive value, whereas SCEs are no more than sensitive exposure markers; many erroneous conclusions have sprung up for ignorance of this evidence.

4.2.2. Biomarkers of Individual Susceptibility

In human populations, large interindividual differences in cancer susceptibility are observed, due to genetic, host and environmental factors mediating the expression of enzymes that metabolize xenobiotics, among them carcinogens or procarcinogens. Marked polymorphisms in these metabolizing enzymes have been ascertained in relation with allelic differences in specific gene loci, resulting in quite common 30- or even 100-fold variations in activity (Vähäkangas and Peltonen, 1990). Many chemical carcinogens require metabolic activation to electrophilic intermediates capable of reacting with DNA; this is carried out by several members of the cytochrome P-450 family, including CYP1A1, CYP1A2, CYP2A6, CYP2D6, CYP2E1 and CYP3A4, called Phase I enzymes. Phase II enzymes ensure detoxification by conjugation with endogenous ligands such as glucuronic acid and comprise e.g. glutathione transferases, epoxide hydrolases, NAD(P)H: quinone reductase; N-acetyl-transferases, glucuronyl transferases. For several of these enzymes, genetic polymorphisms have been demonstrated and inducers identified; moreover individual human CYPs activate selected procarcinogens (for a review, see Pelkonen and Raunio, 1995) in such a way that the particular enzyme(s) to be assessed is carcinogen-specific.

4.2.2.1. Phase I Enzymes and Related Markers

Cytochrome P450 1A1 CYP1A1 is responsible for the metabolic activation of polyaromatic hydrocarbons, e.g. benzo(a)pyrene to the active carcinogen benzo(a) pyrene-diol-epoxide; due to the presence of PAHs in tobacco smoke CYP1A1 activity has been related to the incidence of lung cancer. Indeed, Aryl Hydrocarbon Hydroxylase (AHH) – an inducible phenotype of CYP1A1 – activity has been correlated with the risk of developing smoking-related bronchogenic carcinoma (Kellermann et al., 1973; Kouri et al., 1982).

Restriction Fragment Length Polymorphisms (RFLPs) of the human CYP1A1 gene have been identified; using the restriction enzyme MspI, (Kawajiri et al., 1990) 49% predominant homozygotes, 40% heterozygotes and 11% carriers of the homozygous rare (Val/Val) allele in a healthy Japanese population; the frequency of the latter was about 3-fold higher among lung cancer patients. It was then investigated whether MspI polymorphism is genetically associated with differences in structure of the encoded protein, and a novel point mutation from adenine to guanine was detected in exon 7 of the CYP1A1 gene, resulting in an isoleucine to valine substitution at the aminoacid level (Hayashi et al., 1991); both loci are very closely linked and the respective frequencies of the combined genotypes have been determined. The rare Val/Val homozygote is 2.6-fold more frequent in lung cancer patients than in healthy controls, and this polymorphism is particularly conspicuous in carriers of Kreyberg I type carcinomas (squamous cell carcinoma, undifferentiated cell carcinomas) – known to be strongly associated with tobacco consumption – while carriers of Kreyberg II type carcinomas (adenocarcinomas) did not show any significant difference (Hayashi et al., 1992); this polymorphism has been further linked to glutathione transferase genotypes; this will be later considered. The Japanese findings have not been substantiated in Norwegians, in Finnish subjects nor American Caucasians or Blacks, in whom homozygosity for the susceptible genotype is about ten times less frequent (Cosma et al., 1993); however a specific African-American CYP1A1 polymorphism has been found to be associated with adenocarcinoma of the lung (Taioli et al., 1995). On the other hand the consistency of the findings of increased cancer risk in subjects of Japanese ancestry has been further confirmed in Hawaii, where individuals homozygous for the Msp II mutant genotype had an odds ratio of 7.9 for the development of *in situ* colorectal cancer, compared to heterozygous and wild-type genotypes (Sivaraman et al., 1994). This study also opens interesting avenues with regard to etiologic agents in colorectal cancer, as the differences in odds ratios associated with Msp1 polymorphism of the CYP1A1 gene might point at a role for PAHs.

Ah receptor gene and Arnt gene polymorphism The individual susceptibility to chemical carcinogenesis, as described above, depends on the transcriptional regulation of the CYP1A1 gene, which has two kinds of CIS-acting regulatory elements: the xenobiotic responsive element (XRE) and the basal transcription element (BTE) (Kubota et al., 1991). The binding of xenobiotics (PAHs, Dioxins) to the XRE is mediated by a cytosolic arylhydrocarbon receptor Ahr, present in an inactive form and bound to a 90 Kda Heatshock protein (Hsp) (Landers and Bunce, 1991). After binding of the ligand, the Hsp is released and a heterodimer is formed with the aryl hydrocarbon receptor nuclear translator (Arnt) protein; this complex is translocated into the nucleus, binds to the target genes and activates transcription.

Polymorphisms in the human Ah receptor have been suggested and believed to be potentially very important in determining individual susceptibility to environmental toxicants and carcinogens. (Nebert et al., 1991). Confirmation of this hypothesis was obtained after the development of a quantitative RT-PCR analysis for Ahr and Arnt mRNAs, that demonstrated a close association between mRNA levels of Ahr and Arnt, and CYP1A1 expression levels; these correlated with cigarette consumption. In subjects with high mRNA levels, heavy cigarette consumption was burdened with a 30-fold odds ratio (Hayashi et al., 1994).

Apart from enhancing the transcription of the CYP1A1 (and also CYP1A2-activating heterocyclic amines) gene, the Ahr also mediates the expression of several other genes, among which genes regulating cell growth such as epidermal growth factor receptor, plasminogen activator inhibitor-2, interleukin 1ß, c-*fos* and c-*jun* (reported in Okey et al., 1994).

Cytochrome P450 2D6 First to be identified is the genetic polymorphism of the debrisoquine/sparteine oxidation mediated by CYP2D6, resulting in the identification of about 7% poor metabolizers (PM) in Caucasians, because of defective CYP2D6 alleles, opposed to extensive metabolizers (EM). PMs have the recessive homozygous (dd) genotype.

The metabolic rate is assessed after administration of the tester drug (debrisoquine, sparteine, a few others) and determination of the ratio between mother compound and metabolite in urine. Genotyping by means of PCR and RFLP of leucocyte DNA is also available. After having detected a polymorphism for the 4-oxidation of the anti-hypertensive drug debrisoquine in white British subjects, Idle et al. (1981) observed a "disproportionately large number" of EMs in a group of Nigerian patients presenting with carcinoma of the liver and gastro-intestinal tract. The results of this study prompted the initiation of a larger study in Britsh lung cancer patients (n = 245; controls n = 234).

In the lung cancer group, 78.8% were (probable) homozygous EMS, versus 27.8% in the control group (Ayesh et al., 1984). These results have been confirmed in a rigorously planned and controlled "biochemical epidemiology" study, in which EMs were found to be at a 6-fold increase of lung cancer compared to poor and intermediate metabolizers (odds ration 4.5 for Blacks; 10.2 for Whites) (Caporaso et al., 1990). In a study involving asbestos-exposed subjects, about a 10-fold increased risk for lung cancer has been found for EMs at each asbestos exposure level (Caporaso et al., 1988; Idle, 1989; Caporaso, 1991).

In other malignancies, evidence for a straightforward relation between CYP2D6 polymorphisms and cancer incidence has not been established. Even in lung cancer, a few puzzling questions remain unanswered. For instance, no potential carcinogen is activated by CYP2D6 *in vitro*; also the enzyme is mainly expressed in the liver, and its role in pulmonary carcinogenesis by inhaled substances is conceptually uneasy. It has been suggested that CYP2D6 polymorphism is linked to another determinant of carcinogenesis as will be considered later in this review (Poulsen et al., 1993).

Other phase I Cytochromes A restriction fragment lenght polymorphism of the human P450 2E1 gene has been detected (Uematsu et al., 1991); the enzyme is involved in the metabolic activation of the nitrosamines, aniline and benzene; significant differences from normal controls are found in lung cancer patients, thus confirming experimental data related to liver cancer (Aitio et al., 1991).

Complex interactions, may occur between several activating and detoxifying enzymes to finally determine individual susceptibility, as illustrated by the bioactivation of Aflatoxin B1, a major dietary carcinogen (Gallagher et al., 1994) and, possibly, of dietary heterocyclic amines (Boobis et al., 1994).

4.2.2.2. Phase II Enzymes

N-Acetylation polymorphism The N-acetylation of amines is one of their major detoxification pathways, catalyzed by the non-inducible enzyme N-acetyltransferase, present in the liver and probably in the bladder mucosa, that is under autosomal recessive genetic control, in such a way that the population can be segregated into 2 subgroups of "slow" and "rapid" acetylators, according to their efficiency in N-acetylation. The acetylator phenotype may be evaluated by administering an amine drug (e.g. dapsone or sulfadimidine) and measuring the recovery ratios in plasma or urine. Recently, the acetylation of a dietary caffeine metabolite has proven as accurate as the sulfadimidine assay (Grant et al., 1984), and the genetic alterations have been described, making PCR and RFLP assays available (Blum et al., 1991).

Arylamines (such as benzidine, 2-naphtylamine and 4-aminobiphenyl) are recognized bladder carcinogens, and slow acetylators are at increased risk. Reviewing a large number of studies, Hein (1988) found an odds ratio of 1.5 for slow acetylators among a total of 981 cancer cases and 1244 controls. In smokers, 4-aminobiphenyl-hemoglobin adducts have been shown to be significantly more frequent in slow acetylators (Vineis et al., 1990), and in textile industry workers exposed to arylamines, urinary mutagenicity also correlates with the slow acetylator phenotype (Sinnes et al., 1992).

Conversely, it has been proposed by several studies that fast acetylators were at higher risk of developing colon carcinoma; these findings have not been confirmed by more recent studies (Ladero et al., 1991; Rodriguez et al., 1993). No correlation seems to exist between acetylator phenotype and breast or lung cancer.

Glutathione transferases One of the major cellular detoxification systems involves the conjugation of (carcinogenic) electrophilic intermediates with the tripeptide glutathione, and the excretion of the resulting hydrophilic compound into urine; this reaction is catalysed by Glutathione-S Transferases (GSTs). Human GSTs can be classified into several distinct classes based on their isoelectric point: the basic GST *alpha*, the near neutral GST *mu* and the acidic GST *pi* (Mannervik et al., 1985); recently a fourth isoform – GST *theta* – has also been identified; all these classes are genetically distinct. The *mu* class enzymes – GST *mu* s – detoxify PAH-diol-epoxides as well as offering protection against reactive oxygen species and products of free radical-initiated lipid peroxidation (Berhane et al., 1994). Due to a genetic polymorphism occurring at the GSTM1 locus, where about 50% of Caucasians have a homozygous null allele, resulting in the null phenotype, considerable interindividual variations in sensivity is observed (Seidegård et al., 1988). Indeed, the null phenotype is more frequent in lung cancer patients (Seidegård et al., 1990; Nazar-Stewart et al., 1993) and seems to be specially associated with the squamous cell carcinomas of smokers (Hirvonen et al., 1993). The relative risk of the GST M-null genotype (compared with GSTM+ genotypes) has been estimated to be 1.44 for lung cancer, and 1.87 for Kreyberg I types (Hayashi et al., 1992). Remarkably high odds ratios of respectively 16.00 and 41.00 have been observed in individuals simultaneously carrying the GSTM-null genotype and the susceptible MspI or Val/Val genotyopes of CYP1A1, (Nakachi et al., 1993) (see page 99); this susceptibility is conspicuous at low cigarette consumption.

The GSTM-null genotype also conferred a 70% increased risk of bladder cancer (OR 1.7; 95% confidence interval 1.2 - 2.5), specially in persons exposed to tobacco smoke (OR 1.8) (Bell et al., 1993). In heavy smokers, e.g. exposure of more than 50 pack-years, GSTM-null carriers had a sixfold greater risk relative to the lowest risk group, i.e. non smokers with GSTM+/+ or +/0 genotype. Altogether, Bell's group (1993) considers 25% of all bladder cancers to be attributable to the high risk GSTM-null (0/0) genotype, a figure in accordance with the 17% proposed by Brockmöller et al. (1994). It has been suggested that the GSTM-null genotype might favour the development of gastro-intestinal adenocarcinomas. On the other hand, no correlation could be demonstrated between the GSTM1-null genotype and the susceptibility to squamous cell carcinoma of the cervix (Warwick et al., 1994) nor to breast cancer in Caucasian women (Ambrosone et al., 1995). However in the former of the studies, women who were smokers as well, CYP2D6 extensive metabolizers had an increased susceptibility to high-grade cervical intraepithelial neoplasia but were less likely to progress to squamous cell carcinoma; in the latter study, concomitant CYP1A1 polymorphism carried an OR of 1.53 for the heterozygous Ile/Val subjects and of 2.85 for the homozygous Val/Val; the GSTM1-null genotype used to be more frequent among the younger post-menopausal women (Ambrosone et al., 1995).

4.2.3. DNA Repair and its Variability

The importance of DNA repair in the development of cancer is clearly demonstrated by the observation that diseases characterized by DNA repair deficiencies often carry much higher cancer burdens, the example of which is Xeroderma Pigmentosum (XP) and its 1000- to 4000-fold increase in skin cancer incidence in UV exposed integuments. First identified in 1968 (Cleaver, 1968), the DNA repair defect in XP patients has become the prototypic example of the involvement of DNA repair efficiency in carcinogenesis, the importance of which has been extended well beyond the relatively rare cases of primary repair-deficiency diseases such as XP, Cockayne Syndrome (CS), Trichothiodystrophy (TTD), and others. Since the first identification of these disorders, the extreme complexity of DNA repair mechanisms has been largely deciphered and has opened, lately, unexpected and spectacular novel avenues in the conceptual knowledge and understanding of carcinogenesis. This has mainly sprouted from the very recent elucidation of the mechanisms of DNA excision repair and DNA mismatch repair – two major processes that will presently be considered, after recalling some of the alternative techniques that have been used. This analysis is relevant to carcinogenesis, as considerable interindividual differences in DNA repair capacity have been observed and may contribute to wide variations in the genetic susceptibility to cancer.

4.2.3.1. Assessment of DNA Repair

Unscheduled DNA synthesis (USD) Removal of the damaged DNA sequences leads to reparative DNA synthesis, of which the rate is indicative of the intensity of DNA repair (Trosko and Yager, 1974); this "unscheduled DNA synthesis" in target tissues, of cultured human cells and of human peripheral blood mononuclear leukocytes has been widely used to identify genotoxic carcinogens (e.g. Lake et al., 1980; Ide et al., 1982). Sophisticated methods allow for the differentiation of several different types of DNA damage and their repair (for a review see Smith et al., 1981; Hanawalt and Sarasin, 1986), and Hanawalt's team has demonstrated the preferential repair of psoralen-adducts in an actively expressed gene rather than in a transcriptionally inactive one (Islas et al., 1991). Pero et al. have attempted to evaluate DNA repair deficiencies associated with the most common dominantly inherited cancers, (i.e. breast, colon and lung) by assessing UDS in peripheral blood mononuclear leukocytes after exposure to pro-oxidant generating system (Pero et al., 1990). Odds ratios ranging from 6.2 to 11.7, relative to controls, are reported for cancer cases or high risk groups; a family history of cancer still bears a 2.9 ratio, as evaluated from UDS in blood mononuclear leukocytes (Pero et al., 1990). Enhanced repair, e.g. of photoproducts in melanoma cells has been reported and considered to be responsible for the resistance of these cell types both to radiotherapy and chemotherapy (Hatton et al., 1995). One shortcoming of UDS is that it allows the determination of the rate, but not of the fidelity of DNA repair.

DNA repair-mediating enzymes ADPRT (adenosine diphosphate ribosyl transferase) is a DNA repair enzyme, of which the ribosylation regulates the ligation steps completing the process of base excision repair (for description of the mechanism, see Satoh and Lindahl, 1994); its overexpression parallels DNA repair activity. As for UDS, repair deficiencies assessed by ADPRT levels have been observed in cancer patients (breast and lung) or in individuals predisposed for colon cancer, with odds ratios ranging from 3.7 to 13.8 (Pero et al., 1990). The interindividual variation in DNA repair, estimated as the ADPRT activity induced by pro-oxidant radical generating systems, reaches about one order of magnitude and indicates that this variation is common throughout the population, and might be involved in the risk for most of the major cancers (Pero et al., 1990). An interindividual variation of about 40-fold has been noted in the activity of O^6-alkyldeoxyguanine-DNA alkyltransferase (AT), an enzyme repairing alkylation damage to O^6-deoxyguanine (Grafstrom et al, 1984), and furthermore wide variations in this DNA repair activity have been noted in different types of tissues

(Myrnes et al., 1983; Krokan, 1994). Similar observations relate to the repair enzyme Uracil-DNA glycosylase (UDG) (Krokan, 1994). A decrease in AT repair activity in fibroblasts of lung cancer patients has been reported (Rudiger et al., 1989) and AT deficiency might be a risk factor for lung cancer. A high level of AT expression in cancer cells confers resistance to alkylating drugs, that may be alleviated by the administration of the AT antagonist O6-benzylguanine (Thomale et al., 1994).

While no differences in blood leukocyte levels of AT have been observed between smokers and non-smokers, in contrast the mean activities of both methylpurine (MeP)-DNA glycosylase and 2-6-diamino-4-hydroxy-5N formamido-pyrimidine (FaPy)-DNA glycosylase have been found to be elevated in smokers (Hall et al., 1993); the former of these enzymes repairs 3-methyladenine, 7-methylguanine and 3-methylguanine, and the latter, imidazole-ring-opened guanine, adenine, 7-methylguanine and 8-hydroxyguanine; both enzymes are the first to be involved in the multi-step repair cascade. It is concluded from these observations that the constitutive levels of AT present in the leukocytes of smokers are sufficient to cope with the smoke-induced DNA damage; however other exposures may reduce the AT levels (Oesch and Klein, 1992). On the other hand, MeP and Fapy-DNA glycosylases being first line enzymes in the repair process are not necessarily its rate-limiting step and will not give a measure of the overall efficiency of the repair process (Hall et al., 1993). Negative slopes for all 3 enzymes have been observed in relation with age, and Wei et al. (1993) have reported a steady decrease in the repair capacity of lymphocytes to UV-induced DNA damage of approximately 0.63% per year from 20 to 60 years of age.

Excision Repair (ER) The excision of damaged nucleotides followed by repair synthesis represents the most common and also the most effective repair system to eliminate a majority of DNA lesions. As mentioned above, failures in this repair system lead to the development of "diseases of DNA repair deficiency" characterized, among others, by a high incidence of (often specific) cancers. XP is – by far – the most studied of these diseases and several complete descriptions of its features are available; the disease is characterized by an extreme sensivity to ultra-violet (U-V) rays, the mechanism of which has enabled the isolation of the first human genes of DNA repair (Sarasin, 1994a). Interestingly, the mechanism of action of these genes is closely related to the repair mechanisms in *Escherichia coli*, and repair genes and protein functions are highly conserved between humans and *E. coli*; human genes have been found able to complement mutant yeast genes (Sarasin, 1994b). By fusing somatic cells of two XP patients, it is possible to constitute hybrids capable of repairing UV-induced DNA damage and to identify a series of complementation groups; so far, classical XP mutants fall into eight or nine complementation groups, of which six correpond to complementation groups identified in UV-sensitive rodent mutants (Thompson, 1989). This suggested that at least eight or nine genes are involved in the recognition, excision and repair of DNA damage in the human syndrome (Poulsen et al., 1993); this is not a surprise, considering the extreme complexity of the excision repair process, requiring the participation of diverse actors and actions such as identification of damage, helicases, glycosylase(s) (incision of the base-sugar bond), endonuclease (excision of the damaged DNA and flanking nucleotides), elimination of the damaged chunk, DNA polymerase for repairative synthesis, and ligase for the ligation of the neo-synthesized DNA. Six ERCC1-ERCC6 (excision repair cross-complementing) genes, as well as the XPAC gene (for XP type A correcting factor) and the XPCC gene (for XP type C complementing), as well as a few others, have been cloned and the function(s) of the encoded proteins determined, thus enabling the understanding of the mechanisms underlying the defective DNA repair diseases. The majority of these genes shared a considerable homology with DNA repair genes in yeast, in *E. coli* and in *Drosophila*, and it is the understanding of their precise functions in yeast (or bacteria or drosophila) that has brought clues to their roles in humans.

The characterization of the different steps involved in excision repair has made possible to allocate specific roles to the different gene products of the cloned genes, and to identify the deficiencies responsible for the emergence of certain pathological conditions. Therefore we shall successively consider the repair mechanisms, the genes and their products, and the diseases resulting from impairments.

Repair mechanisms The major steps of the repair process have already been mentioned above; two different paths are taken depending on the location of the DNA damage: in "silent" inactive-genes, or in those that are actively replicating. In the former, overall genomic repair implies the following steps: In *overall genomic repair*

1. Identification of the DNA distortion, as the result of a non-coding lesion, by a composite enzymatic complex encompassing the products of the XPAC, XPCC and XPEC genes.

2. This is followed by the separation of the two strands of the damaged DNA, by two DNA helicases, products of the ERCC2 and ERCC3 genes.

3. The products of the ERCC1, ERCC4 and ERCC5 genes, together with other proteins, cooperate in forming a large sized complex with endonuclease activity; this complex cuts a chunk out of the damaged strand, 22 - 24 nucleotides in 5' from the lesion and 4 - 6 nucleotides in 3'.

4. As a result, the remaining strand lies bare and is immediately covered by HSSB, human single strand binding protein, a protecting protein.

5. The breach is filled by a newly synthesized DNA, a process governed by DNA polymerase δ or ϵ, in the presence of specific proteins: PCNA, Proliferating Cell Nuclear Antigen (see further, subsection 4.3.5) and RF-C, replication Factor-C.

6. The newly synthesized strand is ligated to intact DNA by a ligase. This overall genomic repair, occurring in "silent" DNA, is a slow process that might seem of accessory importance as its failure will not result in immediate visible effects; however deficiencies in this slow repair imply that unrepaired damage may be fixed after DNA replication and trigger the presence of increasing numbers of permanent mutations, one of the features of the mutator phenotype in cancer, that will be taken up again in the subsection on mismatch repair.

The *active gene repair* proceeds somewhat differently:

1. DNA transcription is governed by RNA polymerase II, in the presence of the minimal basic transcription complex TFIIH of which the ERCC3 product is a component. This 3'-5' helicase separates the DNA strands in order to initiate transcription (Schaeffer et al., 1993).

2. RNA polymerase proceeds by sliding along DNA and gets blocked when encountering a DNA lesion, and is then identified by a complex formed by the products of ERCC6 and ERCC3, and possibly ERCC2.

3. The RNA helicase activity of these three enzymes displaces RNA polymerase from its substrates, as well as the mRNA being synthesized.

4. The endonuclease complex described under 3 in the overall genomic repair can then undertake the excision as described before.

One extremely important finding proceeding from the decipherment of these repair mechanisms is the implication of the ERCC3 gene product, a helicase, both in repair and transcription (through the TFIIH complex) and possibly in replication. This allows us to imagine that the other repair helicases, the products of the ERCC2 and ERCC6 genes, might also be implicated in transcription (Sarasin 1994a); in this respect these mechanisms might bear far reaching consequences in carcinogenesis. Mutations of the repair genes of XP patients have been correlated *in vivo* with the frequency of *ras* mutations in XP tumours (Daya-Grosjean et al., 1993) and the typical UV-induced mutational spectrum is found in the ras oncogene and the p53 tumour suppressor of XP tumours (Dumaz et al., 1993).

Genes and gene products Among the gene products of which the function has been elucidated, three are helicases:

1. The ERCC2 Product is a DNA/RNA helicase with 5'-3' polarity, recognizing modified DNA structure; its integrity is vital to yeast; its inactivation is lethal. It complements the cells of XP group D patients.

2. The ERCC3 product also is a DNA/RNA helicase with 3'-5' polarity. It is vital to yeast and might be vital in humans, explaining the small numbers of XP group B subjects whose cells it complements. It is also mutated in Cockayne Syndrome (group C) and is a component of the basic transcription factor TFIIH.

3. The ERCC6 product is involved solely in the repair of the actively transcribed DNA; hence its mutation is the major defect in cells of patients with CS group B.

Others of these gene products have endonuclease activity and participate in the mentioned ERCC1-ERCC4-(ERCC5) complex common to both repair pathways. The XPAC gene product is a DNA binding protein with very strong affinity for UV irradiated DNA; mutations in its yeast homologue completly prevent incision of the damaged

DNA strand.XP group A patients present with severe symptons including neurological deficiencies. This group is very common in Japan, with a majority of the patients carrying the same single point mutation (Satokata et al., 1990) deriving from a common ancestor. The XPCC gene codes for a DNA-binding protein involved in the repair of inactive DNA, that complements the cells in XP group C patients.

Diseases resulting from impairment in excision repair genes Among the commonest forms of XP, XP complementation group A patients, deficient in the XPAC product, are totally unable to repair any UV-induced DNA damage, both in resting and actively transcribed DNA; neurologic symptons are frequent, and so are skin cancers.

In XP-C, the XPCC gene is mutated; actively transcribed genes are integrally repaired, but repair of genomic DNA is pratically nonexistent; no neurologic symptoms; frequent skin cancers.

In XP-D, ERCC2 is deficient; both transcribed genes and genomic DNA are partially repaired; skin cancers are frequent, neurologic symptoms rare. In Cockayne Syndrome group B (CS-B), ERCC6 is deficient; the repair of genomic DNA is complete, but no repair of activately transcribed gene is observed, making this syndrome the reverse of XP-C. No skin cancers are noted, but neurologic involvement is frequent.

The other XP and CS complementation groups are but rarely observed and will not be considered; for details, see Sarasin (1994a).

Schematic summary of the excision repair mechanisms and related diseases These complex mechanisms are summarized in Figure 4.3; the diseases resulting from deficiencies are mentioned within the boxes; the figures within the circles refer to the different repair steps as described in the text.

4.2.3.2. Mismatch Repair, Microsatellite Instability and Mutator Phenotype

Microsatellites are short repetitive nucleotide sequences composed of two, three or four nucleotides, most often located between genes in non-coding ("junk") DNA; they are dispersed throughout the genome and are very numerous; for instance there are about 100.000 CA/GT repeats, each with a chain length greater than 24 (Weber and May, 1989). During DNA replication, DNA polymerases can increase the length of oligonucleotides consisting of repeats by slippage of one strand over the other; this results in a mismatch of opposing bases, creating regions of non-complementarity. These errors are normally detected and corrected by the Mismatch Repair System (MRS). Failures in the MRS, due to mutations in the system's genes, will result in defective proteins incapable of correcting the errors; as a result, base pairs may be substituted, but also dinucleotides may be inverted or deleted, leading to microsatellite instability, i.e. variations in the number of repeats (and consequently variations in lenght) of this microsatellite (Loeb, 1994). As a result, changes occur in the fingerprint pattern of DNA cancers (Matsumura and Tarin, 1992). Mutations are frequently observed in microsatellite repeats, making them sensitive indicators for genetic instability in tumours (Loeb, 1994).

While mismatch repair was arousing scientific rather than practical interest due

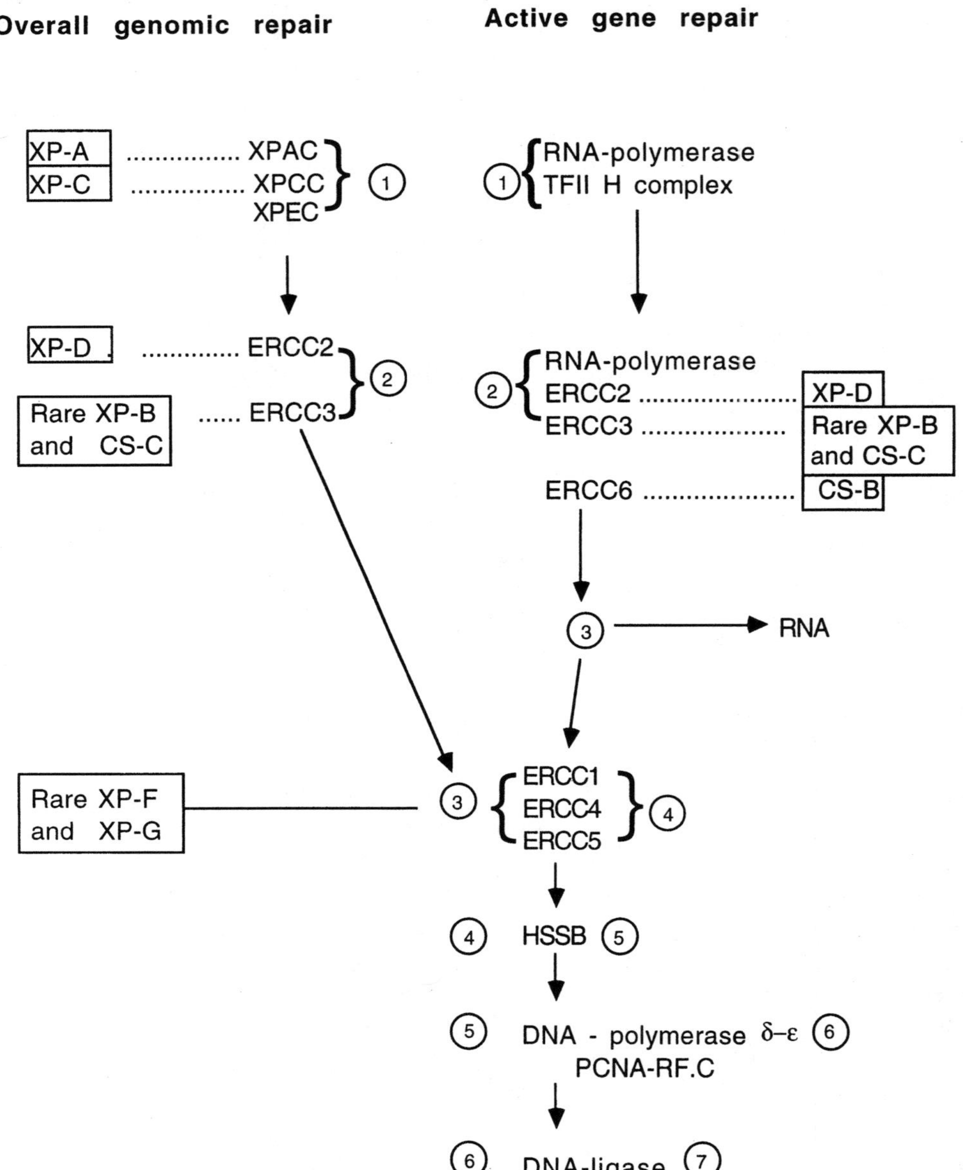

Figure 4.3: *DNA excision repair mechanisms*

to the relative rarity of the induced pathology, recent discoveries have completely overthrown this concept and tend to confer a central role to the MRS in carcinogenesis. The story started with the finding that bacteria deficient in the MRS, called *mut bacteria*, carry a 100-to 1000-fold excess mutation rate relative to corresponding wild-type bacteria and present with a *mutator phenotype* (Radman and Wagner, 1986; Modrich, 1991). The proteins involved in this bacterial repair system are termed *Mut*S, *Mut*L, *Mut*U and *Mut*H and equivalents have been found in yeast, e.g. the MSH2 gene (mutS homologue). The surprise came, unexpectedly, when it was detected that the human homologous genes hMLH1 (human mutant L homologue) and hMSH2 were implicated in the hereditary predisposition to colon cancer (and other cancers as well) in the Lynch II syndrome, also called HNPCC (Hereditary Non Polyposis Colorectal Cancer) (Lynch et al., 1993), a syndrome characterized by the early onset – before age 50 – of cancers of the proximal colon, unrelated to pre-existing polyposis and to alterations in the tumour suppressor genes FAP and DCC, known to be involved in polyposis-related familial colon cancer. By genetic linkage studies in HNPCC families, the teams of de la Chapelle at Helsinki University, Finland and of Volgelstein, Johns Hopkins University School of Medicine, spotted the new gene to chromosome 2 (Peltomaki et al., 1993; Aaltonen et al, 1993). The search for a deletion (common in tumour suppressor genes) at the suspected locus remained vain, but instead the analysis of the tumour DNA revealed - after painstaking efforts - variations in the length of a microsatellite, characteristic of instability. Simultaneously, two other teams (Thibodeau et al., 1993; Ionov et al., 1993) reported the discovery of microsatellite instability not only on chromosome 2, but also on other chromosomes in 12 to 28% of the familial and sporadic colon tumours that they had analyzed. At the time, the responsible gene was not characterized, but it was suggested that its mutation would entail genetic alterations disseminated throughout the genome and confer the *mutator phenotype*. This hypothesis was confirmed when it was demonstrated that the gene on chromosome 2 was hMSH2, the human homologue of the bacterial mutS, one of the mismatch repair genes (Fishel et al., 1993; Leach et al., 1993). This proved to be one of the most dramatic findings in recent genetic research, as mutations in the hMSH2 gene are considered to be responsible for 60% of the hereditary colon cancer cases. Another 30% were found to be related to mutations in the hMLH1 gene, another homolog of a bacterial mismatch repair gene, located on chromosome 3 (Bronner et al., 1994; Papadopoulos et al., 1994). It is anticipated that the remaining 10% might be related to mutations in other mismatch repair genes.

In HNPCC families, an elevated incidence of other cancers is also observed, including cancers of the endometrium, urinary tract, stomach, gallbladder and pancreas, and these tumours also display microsatellite instability, which seems to be prevalent in many familial cancers (Loeb, 1994). Microsatellite instability is also reported in sporadic tumours such as colon, endometrium, pancreas, lung, as well as in a series of neurodegenerative diseases, including the fragile X syndrome (from 20 to 200 CGG repeats, Ya et al., 1991), Huntington's disease and others.

The importance of these observations proceeds from the relative frequences of mutations in the HNPCC genes, estimated to be related to one in 200 people in Caucasians, and to about 10% of all colon cancers, a very frequent malignancy. The functions of the different components of the Mismatch Repair System have been elucidated (Radman et al., 1994), an *in vitro* repair system constructed (Lahue et al., 1989) and practical assessment methods developed.

4.2.3.3. Other Genetic Instability Syndromes Several other genetic instability syndromes have been identified from a clinical point of view; the underlying genetic alterations begin to be deciphered. These conditions will simply be mentioned; for a more completed description, see Digweed (1993) and references therein.

Fanconi's Anaemia is characterized by bone marrow deficiency and skeletal anomalies; the frequency of heterozygotes is reported to be about 1 in 300, of homozygotes about a 1000fold less. The basic defect seems to be an incapacity in FA cells to repair DNA interstrand crosslinks; the condition predisposes to leukemia.

Bloom syndrome is a rare condition characterized by photosensivity and growth retardation, and an extremely high frequency of SCEs; the condition predisposes to the development of various malignancies. While being very rare in the general population, the heterozygote frequency is an estimated 1 in 120 Ashkenazy Jews. The basic defect is a reduced DNA ligase I activity (see preceding schema) (Mezzina et al., 1989).

Ataxia Telangiectasia (AT) is a severe and rather frequent (heterozygote frequency 1:70 to 1:150, Digweed, 1993) condition, characterized by a considerably increased sensitivity to X-Ray exposure (and exposure to radiomimetic agents). Clinically the disease is characterized by brain degeneration starting with the *cerebellum* and causing *ataxia*, development of *telangiectasia* in the eyes and general immunodeficiency causing an acute predisposition to lymphoproliferative malignancies, of which the frequency is 500- to 1000-fold higher than in the general population. Repair of double-strand breaks is error-prone in AT cells; deletions around the break point are frequent (Cox et al., 1986). The high frequency of AT heterozygotes in the general population could have far reaching consequences, for instance with regard to breast cancer risk after very low dose X-Ray exposure. It has been calculated that A-T heterozygotes could account for 9 to 18% of all cases in the US (Swift et al., 1987); similar estimations carried out more recently in Britain impute about 4% of breast cancer cases to the A-T gene and have been confirmed in Norway and Italy (Gatti and McConville, 1994). A significant breakthrough has been recently achieved by finding that the mutated AT (ATM) gene product shares considerable homology with phosphatidylinosilol 3-kinases (PI 3Ks) (Savitsky et al., 1995). PI 3Ks are involved in the generation of early signals in the signal transduction pathway, as well as in the regulation of the actin cytoskeleton (Fry, 1994). This raises interesting insights about the function of the ATM protein, that might not only induce deficiencies in cell cycle control, and DNA repair, but also intervene in signal transduction (Kastan et al., 1992; Zakian, 1995).

4.2.3.4. Restatement of the DNA Repair Problem Although sometimes being associated with a high susceptibility to cancer (XP, FA, BS, AT), as mentioned above, DNA repair deficiencies have mostly been considered unimportant in carcinogenesis, due to the rarity of the homozygotes in the general population.

It seems that the frequency of the heterozygotes, carrying one modified allele in one of the numerous involved genes, has been understimated. It is presently admitted that deficiencies in the DNA repair processes represent a fairly common mechanism in carcinogenesis, since it has been demonstrated that a mutation in a repair gene – possibly also involved in replication and transduction – might lead to widespread mutations dispersed all over the genome, the mutator phenotype so frequently observed in cancer patients. Since the startling discoveries in HNPCC, it has become obvious that mutations in DNA repair genes represent a major mechanism of carcinogenesis, in addition to the "classical" mechanism of oncogene activation and tumour suppressor gene inactivation or deletion. Further developments may be anticipated in the near future.

4.2.4. Exogenous Nutritional Factors

Only nutritional factors contributing to the "initiatory complex" will be considered presently and briefly. Nutritional factors involved in "promotion" will be mentioned in section 4.4.5, and comprise both, macro and micronutrients. Several micronutrients exert a direct influence on the initiation phase of carcinogenesis; they have been repeatedly reviewed by Wattenberg (1992).

Several minor dietary constituents have long been shown to inhibit carcinogenesis; Wattenberg has classed them in blocking agents and suppressing agents. The former inhibit carcinogenesis by preventing the metabolic activation of inactive precursors to the final carcinogen, or by preventing the carcinogens to react with critical target macromolecules. Suppressing agents intervene at later stages when the carcinogenic process has already been triggered.

Metabolic activation of procarcinogens is prevented, e.g. by benzyl isothiocyanate found in cruciferous vegetables, by diallyl disulfide and other organosulfur compounds from *Allium* species (Wargowich et al., 1988), by monoterpenes found in citrus fruit oils (Wattenberg et al., 1989), by glucosinolates from cruciferous vegetables.

Carcinogen detoxification can also be enhanced by dietary components, after increasing the activity of phase 2 enzymes. Several organosulfur compounds from Allium species exert this activity (Sparnins et al., 1988), as well as flavonoids (Siess et al., 1992) and reducing agents.

Many effects of dietary components have presently been identified; as an example indole derivatives from cruciferous vegetables stimulate the 2-hydroxylation of oestrogens, leading to the formation of the biologically inactive 2-hydro-oestrone, whereas the normal pathway involves 16-α-hydroxylation, with the formation of 16-α-hydroxyoestrone which is both an initiator and promoter (Michnovicz and Bradlow, 1990). Such effects might have the potential to modulate mammary carcinogenesis.

It is anticipated that better knowledge of the multifaceted influences of dietary components on carcinogenesis will result in actions to reduce the risk of cancer (Thorling, 1993).

4.3. THE DETERMINANTS OF THE CLONAL EXPANSION OF THE INITIATED CELLS

4.3.1. Basic Mechanisms

Uncontrolled cellular proliferation – potentially leading to transformation – proceeds from the disruption of the regulatory cascades governing the normal progression through the cell cycle, characterized by the sequence of states G1 (Gap 1), S phase (DNA synthesis), G2 (Gap 2) and finaly M phase (mitosis), and formation of two daughter cells. The most critical checkpoint for the cell is the one governing the G1 to S transition, as overriding it corresponds to the irrevocable decision of growth, as opposed to non-growth (Pardee, 1989). Consequently, several control mechanisms bolt this checkpoint (called R for restriction) very tightly; however, any failure in the involved mechanisms may lead to uncontrolled growth and transformation.

The initial regulators of proliferation are extracellular stimuli, mainly protein and steroid growth factors that typically bind (at least the protein GFs) to specific trans-membrane receptors, thus activating their intracellular domain that usually has Protein Tyrosine Kinase activity (PTK) and acts as a first component of a signal transduction pathway, further relaying on a series of second messengers to convey the signal to the nucleus. Targets for these signals are the "immediate early" proto-oncogens c-*fos* and c-*jun* of which the protein products form an hetero-dimer binding specific DNA sequences (the AP-1, Activating Protein 1 - complex) (Curran and Franz, 1988) and activating transcription. The exposure to carcinogens has been shown to induce c-*jun* (Heintz et al., 1993) and it has also been observed that the DNA-binding activity of *fos* and *jun* is exquisitely sensitive to reduction-oxidation (redox) (Abate et al., 1990).

These events occur within 10 minutes after the application of the external stimuli and are followed, about 1 hour later, by the synthesis of the transcription factor c-*myc*; this triggers the transcriptional machinery in other genes of which the products are required for escape from quiescence (G0 state) and later for passing the G1-S checkpoint.

The effects of the transcription of the c-*fos*, c-*jun* and c-*myc* proto-oncogenes on the cell cycle are mediated by a series of cyclin-cdk (cyclin dependent kinases) complexes. Their oscillations throughout the cell-cycle are rate-limiting for progression through the key checkpoint(s), including G1-S transition at R (Hunter and Pines, 1991; Motokura and Arnold, 1993; Bartkova et al., 1994). Of particular importance is the Cyclin D1-cdk 4 complex, and probably to a lesser extent the Cyclin E-cdk 2 complex, both governing the G1-S transition and passage through the restriction point.

Cyclin D1 deregulation occurs in numerous malignancies through translocation or amplification of the chromosome band 11 q 13 to which the Cyclin D1 gene has been assigned (Lammie and Peters, 1991; Motokura et al., 1991). Amplification of this gene occurs in a series of common cancers such as breast, urinary bladder, oesophagus, and also lung (Berenson et al., 1990) and may be detected by immunohistochemical staining (Gillett et al., 1994; Lukas et al., 1994). The Cyclin E-cdk2 complex appears early in G1, reaches maximal levels near G1/S border and then disappears; it controls the expression of the Rb protein, inactivating it by phosphorylation.

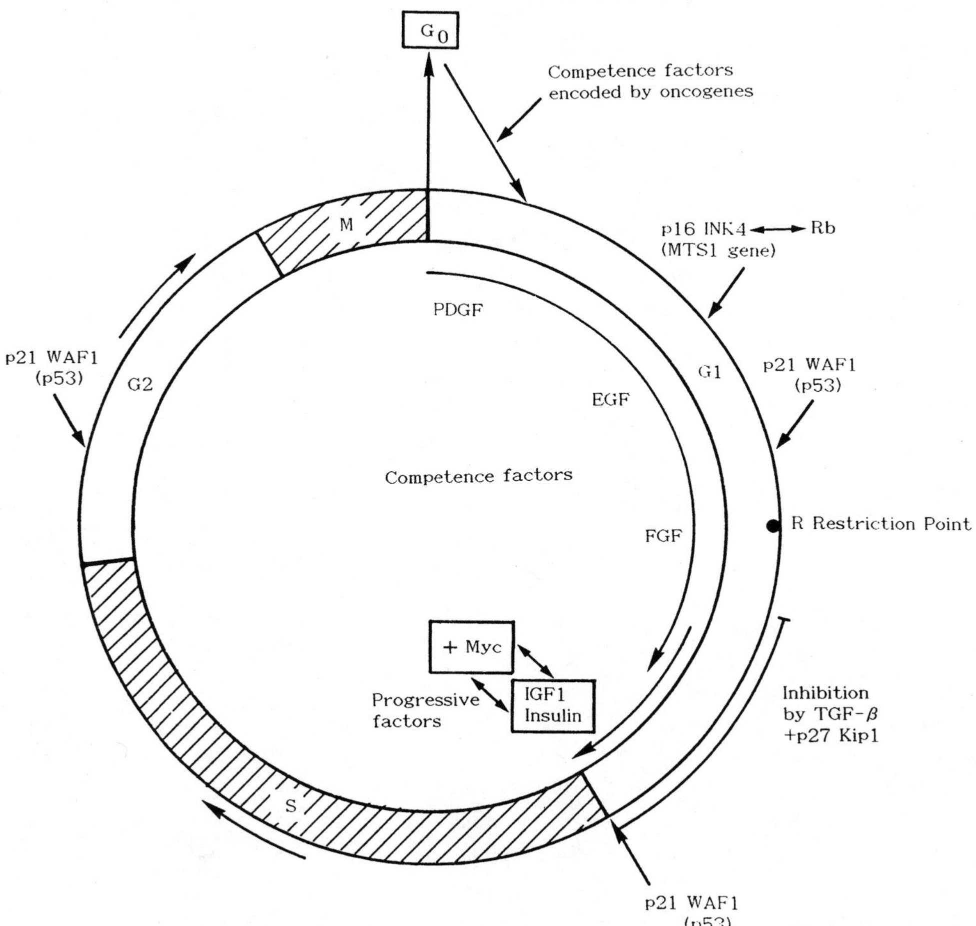

Figure 4.4: *The cell cycle and some of its control mechanisms. (Modified from Aaronson, 1990, for details see text)*

4.3.2. Cell Cycle Control Mechanisms

The cell has recourse to a battery of control mechanisms to prevent the inadvertent passage of checkpoint R in the late G1 phase, including the p53 protein, the Rb protein, the *myc* protein and *bcl*-2, as well as a series of low molecular weight inhibitory proteins. The review of the abundant literature covering this topic would go far beyond the scope of this introduction to the use of biomarkers in cancer risk assessment. Major data – believed to be relevant to the biomarker approach – will be presented and summarized in Figure 4.5.

4.3.2.1. p53 p53 is considered as "the guardian of the genome" (Lane, 1992); this tumour suppressor gene acts by blocking progression through checkpoint R in cells that have sustained DNA damage, until the damage is repaired. If no timely DNA repair takes place, p53 will trigger cell death by apoptosis (Lane, 1993). Wild-type (normal) p53 stimulates the transcription of the WAF1/CIP1 gene (El-Deiry et al., 1993; Harper et al., 1993) of which the p21 protein product inhibits the G1/S transition after fixation on the Cyclin D1/cdk 4 and Cyclin E-cdk 2 complexes. Simultaneously, the p21 WAF1/Cyclin D/cdk4 complex prevents the inactivation (by cdk4) of the Rb tumour suppressor gene product $p105^{Rb}$ (Kato et al., 1993). When p53 is mutated, it loses its capability of activating WAF1/CIP1 and in the absence of p21 WAF, no arrest occurs at checkpoint R, carrying the risk of DNA replication before damage is repaired and of definitive fixation of the damage (mutation). Mutated p53 is observed in a majority of human cancers; considering only the 10 most frequent cancers worldwide, p53 gene alterations are present in 40 - 45% of all cases, making this the most frequent alteration (Soussi et al., 1994); by comparison, ras mutations occur in 10 - 15% of all cancers. In lung carcinomas, p53 abnormalities have been found in 66% of cases, with a slight predominance in NSCLC (Gazzeri et al, 1994); alterations have also been observed in preneoplastic lesions such as bronchial metaplasia and dysplasia, suggesting that p53 mutations might be early events in lung carcinogenesis (Sundaresan et al., 1992; Klein et al., 1993). Many studies – too numerous to be individually cited – support the evidence for p53 alterations in lung carcinomas. Wild-type p53 protein is very short-lived (half-life less than 10 minutes), making it undetectable in the cell nucleus. By contrast the altered protein resulting from p53 mutation has a half-life of over half an hour and accumulates in the nucleus where it may be detected. The assessment of p53 alterations proceeds by three main approaches:

1. *The molecular analysis of the p53 gene*, after PCR amplification and DNA sequencing, leading to the identification of specific mutations. More than 2500 different mutations, spreading all over four of the five highly conserved exons of the gene, have been described (Hollstein et al., 1991; Greenblatt et al., 1994; Soussi et al., 1990). While opening fascinating avenues on cancer etiology and pathogenesis, this approach could not yet be considered affordable in routine risk assessment.

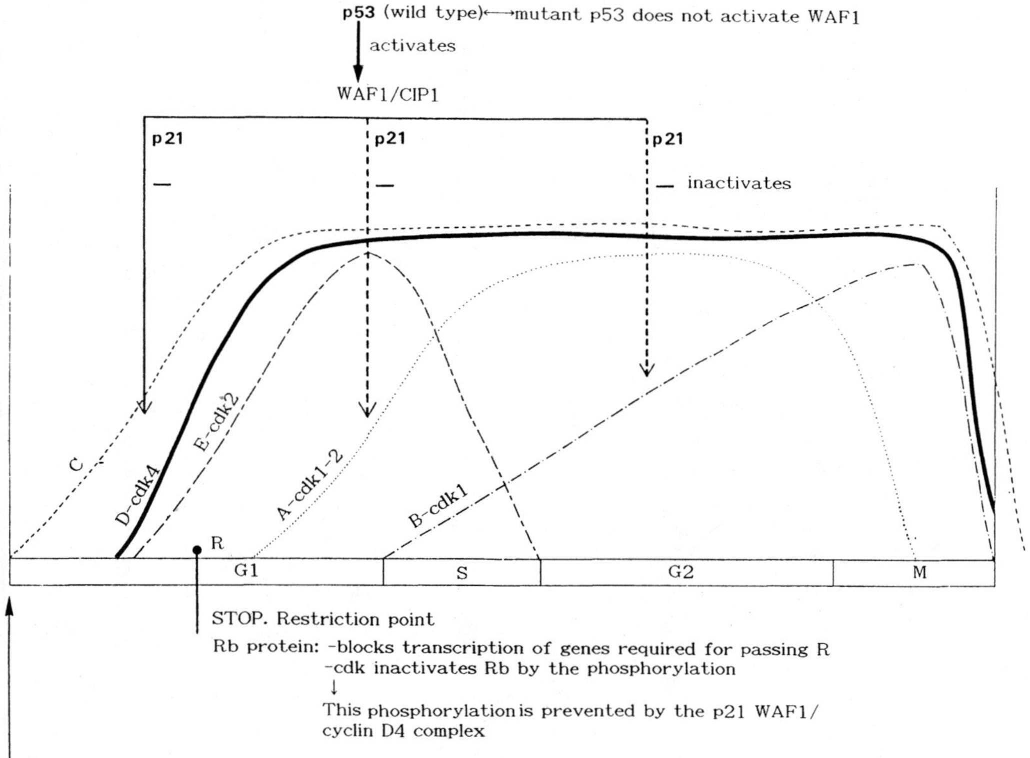

Growth factors

1) Normal c-myc ⊕ GFs (serum IGF1) = switched on → proliferation
⊖ Mitogenic stimulus = switched off → apoptosis
↑
blocked by bcl2

2) Mutated c-myc: cannot be switched off → proliferation

Figure 4.5: *The cell cycle and its major control mechanisms.*

2. *The immunohistochemical analysis*, based on the nuclear accumulation of the modified protein (see above) (Gannon et al., 1990); extensive studies demonstrate the good agreement between immunohistochemical posivity and mutations detected by DNA sequencing (Bartek et al., 1990; Hall et al., 1991; and many others). Positive staining has been observed in premalignant lesions of the bronchial epithelium (Vähäkangas et al., 1992) and has been considered to be an early event in lung tumourigenesis (Sozzi et al., 1991; Sozzi et al., 1992); increased p53 expression has been shown to correlate with the severity of dysplasia and to parallel PCNA expression (see below) (Walker et al., 1994). Finally, there is evidence that individuals homozygous for the GSTm null allele, a marker of susceptibility, also are at a higher risk of p53 mutations caused by exposure to PAHs, at least when highly exposed (Ryberg et al., 1994).

3. *Serological analysis.* The detection of the wild-type or mutant p53 proteins would represent an easy approach for its evaluation. However, the p53 protein, mutated or not, is a nuclear protein that is not normally released into the circulation, except for very minute quantities or after cell death, the situation being further complicated by its short half-life. Moreover, when there is release, this seems to be discontinuous and irregular, precluding its use in the assessment of the carcinogenic process. Recently, however, p53 has been detected in the fresh serum of NSCLC patients (Fontanini et al, 1994), but the significance of this finding needs further confirmation.

These difficulties have been – at least partly – circumvented by the finding of circulating p53 antibodies in the sera of patients with various cancer types (Crawford et al., 1982; Caron de Fromentel et al., 1987). The development of antibodies against p53 appears to be dependent on the type of p53 mutation (Winter et al., 1992), implying that it will not parallel the overall mutation rate; indeed in lung cancer the prevalence of circulating antibodies is reported to be from 8% (Angelopoulou et al., 1994) to 24% (Schlichtholz et al., 1994). This humoral response has been proposed to be the result of a self-immunization process which is the consequence of p53 protein accumulation in tumour cells (Lubin et al., 1993); the antigenic response seems to be conditioned by the formation of a p53-70 KDa Heatshock Protein Complex (Davidoff et al., 1992).

The interest of the assessment of p53 antibodies is further emphasized by their detection in the serum of subjects without any history of cancer, who later developed overt cancer (Schlichtholz et al., 1994). According to these authors, the presence of these antibodies may be related to the presence of occult cancers, that remain undetected by traditional diagnostic procedures; they suggest that the presence of p53 antibodies may constitute an earlier marker of lung tumours. They propose that "both immunohistochemical and serological analyses be simultaneously and routinely performed to diagnose p53 alterations" (Soussi et al., 1994). Ishioka et al. (1993) have described a functional assay for p53 mutations, by assaying the transactivational activity of p53 protein in yeast (reported by Soussi et al., 1994).

4.3.2.2. The Rb tumour suppressor gene The retinoblastoma gene located on chromosome band 13q14 and its protein product pRb105 are implicated in the tumourigenesis of retinoblastoma in such a way that simultaneous deletion or inactivation of the gene on both alleles leads to homozygosity, consequent loss of function and tumour development (Knudson, 1985). Originally believed to be restricted to retinoblastoma, chromosome band 13q14 alterations have been detected in a series of different cancers, including osteosarcoma and lung cancer (Yokota et al., 1987; Harbour et al., 1988). Rb inactivation is common in SCLC (Yokota et al.), with reported frequencies in excess of 90% (Kaye et al., 1990). In relatives of retinoblastoma cases, known to carry the retinoblastoma susceptibility, a 15-fold excess incidence of lung tumours has also been reported (Sanders et al., 1989).

pRb105 blocks the transcription of genes required for passing the G1 checkpoint R; the protein is inactivated by phosphorylation by cdk4 in response to overexpression of Cyclin D1; in turn this mechanism is inhibited by the p21WAF/Cyclin D1/cdk 4 complex. Progression of cells through the cell-cycle requires continuous phosphorylation of pRb by several Cdks (Sherr, 1994); moreover a reciprocal inactivation of Rb and p16INK4 (see later) expression is observed in lung cancer (Shapiro et al., 1995).

Alterations of the Rb gene can be detected by molecular analysis; no routine applications have been developed so far.

4.3.2.3. The *myc* Oncogene The *myc* family consists of at least six functional members, among which is c-*myc*, mapped to the long arm of chromosome 8 at 8q24; L-*myc* located at 1p32 and N-*myc* located at 2p23-24 (reported in Bergh, 1990); interesting to mention, c-*jun* has been mapped to the same chromosomal band as L-*myc* (Birrer and Minna, 1989).

Among many cancers, C-*myc* is frequently overexpressed (with or without amplification) in lung cancer, more commonly in NSCLC (48%) than in SCLC (24%) (Gazzeri et al., 1994). On the other hand, L-*myc* and N-*myc* amplification and overexpression are restricted to SCLC (Gazzeri et al., 1991) and were observed in 26% of cases (Gazzeri et al., 1994). According to these studies, *myc* deregulation is an occurrence independent of p53 mutation, both genes playing a major role in tumour formation; indeed only 25% of all lung cancers displayed no alteration of p53 nor *myc*. The best candidates for genetic cooperation with p53 and *myc* in NSCLC seem to be the *ras* gene family, c-*erb*B-1, c-*erb*B-2 and *fos* genes (Volm et al., 1992, 1993), as well as mutations in the Rb tumour suppressor gene and the putative anti-oncogenes located on chromosome 3. The specific time of occurrence of p53 and *myc* alterations in the carcinogenesis of lung tumours is not cleary established (Iggo, 1990).

The mechanism of action of *myc* appears to be extremely complex and it is clear that deregulation of c-*myc* expression plays a pivotal role in oncogenesis (Kato and Dang, 1992). The activation of transcription by *myc* occurs after heterodimerization with the *max* protein, the latter enabling DNA binding, and is further regulated by Mad protein (Ayer et al., 1993) (for a review, see Västrik et al., 1994). It has been established that in the presence of mitogenic stimuli, e.g. growth factors, deregulation or overexpression of c-*myc* induces oncogene activation and cellular proliferation; when the latter is blocked – e.g. by growth factor or metabolite depletion, or by the action of a drug or chalone – *myc* deregulation induces programmed cell death (apoptosis) (Evan et al., 1992); this can be blocked by the activated *bcl*-2 proto-oncogene (Hockenbery et al., 1990). Definite targets for the *myc* protein have not been identified so far, but Ornithine-Decarboxylase (ODC) gene is a good candidate (Bello-Fernandez et al., 1993) and so is p53 (Reisman et al., 1993).

Myc deregulation may be assessed by molecular analysis. More accessibly, circulating antibodies against c-*myc* protein have been detected in the sera of about 10% of cancer patients, however without any specific mention of lung cancer (Ben-Mahrez et al, 1988).

4.3.2.4. Low Molecular Weight Regulatory Proteins It has become clear that a series of regulatory proteins is modulating the progression through the cell cycle induced by the expression of successive (or simultaneously acting) cyclin-cdk complexes. The role of p21 WAF has been evoked previously in relation with its expression induced by wild-type p53, resulting in the inhibition of the cyclin D1/cdk4, the Cyclin E/Cdk2, and other cyclin cdk complexes. Whereas the inhibitory action of p21 WAF seems to be unspecific, directed against several of the cyclin/cdk complexes, other – more specific – inhibitors have been identified.

p21 WAF1/CIP1/Sdi1 We have already reported the independent discovery of p21CIP1 (for: cdk inhibiting protein) by Harper and Elledge (1993); of p21 WAF1 (for wild-type p53 activated fragment) by B. Vogelstein's team (El-Deiry et al., 1993) and of p21Sdi1 (for senescent cell-derived inhibitor) by Smith's team (Noda et al., 1994), all three proteins having identical structure, and we also have reported the main targets for the action of this inhibitory protein; indeed p21 WAF1/CIP1 seems to abolish the enzymatic kinase activity of all cyclin/cdk complexes; it also prevents the phosphorylation and resulting inactivation of the pRb105 protein; the overexpression of p21 WAF in fibroblasts induces arrest of proliferation. Interestingly p21 also inhibits the PCNA dependent (PCNA: proliferating-cell nuclear antigen, to be considered later) DNA replication (Waga et al., 1994), by a direct p21-PCNA interaction.

p27 Kip 1 The inhibitory protein, p27KIP1 (for cdk inhibiting protein) mediates the antiproliferative actions of TGFβ (Transforming Growth Factor β) (Koff et al., 1993) and of cyclic AMP (Kato et al., 1994), by preventing the activation of the Cyclin D1-cdk4 complex. The cloning of c-DNA of both p21 and p27 has revealed a structural analogy in the N-terminal regions.

p16 INK4 It is a fairly common observation that the short arm of chromosome 9 (in humans) is the seat of alterations – mainly deletions – in several cancers including melanomas, gliomas, lung tumours and leukemia; so it was suspected to harbour a tumour suppressor gene(s), of which the search was then initiated. Simultaneously the teams led by Kamb and Skolnick (Kamb et al., 1994) and by Carson (Nobori et al, 1994) discovered the MTS1 gene (Multiple Tumour Suppressor gene 1), coding for a p16INK4 (for: inhibitor of cdk4) protein that had already been identified (Xiong et al., 1993) and had been shown to specifically inhibit cyclin D-cdk4 and cyclin D-cdk6 complexes (Serrano et al., 1993).

As if it were not enough, a second potential tumour suppressor gene MTS2 has been located in the vicinity of MTS1 (Kamb et al., 1994); it codes for a p15INK4B protein that shows considerable homology with p16INK4 (Hannon and Beach, 1994) and is a mediator of TGF-β action on cyclin D-cdk4 complex. p15INK4 deletions are observed in approximately 20% of all cancers (Cairns et al., 1994) but point mutations are significantly more frequent and underline the importance of this tumour suppressor gene.

Alterations of the MTS 1 gene have been observed *in vivo* in NSCLC (Washimi et al, 1995), in about 30% of cases. The reciprocal behaviour of Rb and p16 has been observed in lung cancer: Rb-positive NSCLC express little or no p16, while Rb-negative NSCLC and SCLC express abundant p16 (Shapiro et al., 1995). These authors propose a model of lung tumourigenesis in which overexpression of Cyclin D1 would be an early event, followed either by Rb loss – a frequent event in SCLC, or by loss of p16 expression – a common event in NSCLC.

The relations between the different agents intervening in the cell cycle and its regulation are schematically represented in Figures 4.4 and 4.5. They have been considered in some extent because the mechanisms driving the cell cycle and consequently proliferation lie at the very base of carcinogenesis and will doubtlessly experience further spectacular developments during coming years. Except direct molecular analysis, the techniques enabling the assessment of these mechanisms are rather scanty; however as we speak, following approaches may be considered:

- c-*fos*, c-*jun*: immunohistocytochemistry
- p53: immunohistochemistry, mutated p53 in fresh serum, detection of mutations using the yeast test, detection of circulating antibodies in serum
- pRb105: molecular analysis
- c-*myc* (L-*myc*, N-*myc*), circulating antibodies (?)
- p21 WAF1/CIP1: immunohistochemistry
- p16 INK4: immunohistochemistry.

Presently the use of a panel of these markers, in association with proliferation markers (see later) enables an accurate evaluation of escapes from the normal and strongly regulated progression through the cell cycle; the quality of this approach will be further enhanced by the assessment of a series of factors that will presently be considered. While some of the assays are performed on serum, in most cases accuracy will depend on obtaining adequate tissue samples.

4.3.3. Growth Factors, Growth Factor Receptors and Signal Transduction Pathways

The activation of the "immediate-early" genes c-*fos* and c-*jun*, mentioned in the previous section, as well as of c-*myc*, occurs after an external mitogenic signal – represented by the presence of a growth factor or substitutes in the extracellular environment – has reached the nucleus after being transmitted through the cellular membrane by a growth factor receptor, and further carried on through the cytoplasm and finally into the nucleus by DNA-binding proteins (Marx, 1993). The different steps of this process will now be considered.

4.3.3.1. Growth Factors and Receptors The effect of GFs is to force resting cells (in G0 phase) to enter the cell cycle and to proceed through it; this is a two-phase process, cells first having to leave the G0 for the G1 phase under the influence of "competence" factors, and afterwards to proceed through the cycle under the influence of "progression" factors. Passage through of the aforementioned restriction point R necessitates the presence of both types of factors, but once past R, only the presence of a progression factor such as insulin-like growth factor 1 (IGF-1) is required (Pardee, 1989). Cytokines such as Transforming Growth Factorβ (TGFβ) and several Interferons can antagonize the proliferative effects of GFs (Aaronson, 1991) and deprivation of GFs can induce apoptosis (Evan et al., 1992). Conversely, in several cell lines, several oncogenes can specifically substitute for the competence factor requirement (Falco et al., 1988; Aaronson et al., 1990).

Insulin-like Growth Factor I and Receptor The importance of the Insulin-like Growth Factor I (IGF-I) has been recently emphasized (Aaronson, 1991; Baserga, 1995), this progression factor being able (as is PDGF) to inhibit *myc*-induced apoptosis, thus fulfilling the requirements for growth factors (Evan et al., 1992).

IGF-I is a single chain polypeptide binding a transmembrane receptor IGFI-R with a very characteristic disulfide-linked $\alpha 2$-$\beta 2$ heterodimeric complex composed of two extracellular α subunits providing the binding sites, and of two transmembrane-intracellular β subunits possessing intrinsic tyrosine-specific protein kinase activity. Ligand binding to the α subunit induces autophosphorylation of the β subunit and triggers the signal transducing pathway carrying the signal to the nucleus and initiating biological responses.

IGFs, also called somatomedins, stimulate the growth of tracheobronchial epithelial cells (Macaulay et al., 1988) and may be produced by fibroblasts and macrophages, stimulating the growth of epithelial cells via a paracrine mechanism (Nathan, 1987; Stiles and Moats-Staats, 1989).

The practical exploitation of this important growth factor has been hampered by the fact that – in extracellular fluids – IGFs circulate in a complexed form with binding proteins, this binding preventing adequate immunological recognition. Nonetheless, elevated levels of IGF-I have been found both in pulmonary tumour tissue (Macaulay et al., 1988) and in cultured cells lines (Favoni et al., 1994), regardless of the histological subtype; this elevation is particularly striking in adenocarcinomas. The serum levels of the binding proteins have been found to be significantly elevated in the lung cancer patients as compared with normal subjects (Reeve et al., 1990).

Epidermal Growth Factor and Receptor family (EGFr, c-*erb*B-2, HER-2/*neu*) The importance of Epidermal Growth Factor (EGF) as a competence factor has been experimentally demonstrated when it was shown that the growth of mouse keratinocytes could be sustained by the complementing action of only two GFs: EGF and IGF-I (Falco et al., 1988). However in practice, the EGFr-receptor has been the subject of more attention: EGFr is a transmembrane protein of mw170 encoded by the c-*erb*B-1 oncogene (a cellular homologue of the viral oncogene inducing avian erythroblastosis, hence the name) and is homologous to the p185 transmembrane receptor protein encoded by the c-*erb*B-2 oncogene – also known as *neu* or HER-2. The intracellular domain of these receptors has a tyrosine protein kinase activity. The extracellular domain can be released into the extracellular environment after proteolytic cleavage, and assessed in the serum or plasma. The c-*erb*B-2 protein product is overexpressed in a wide variety of human cancers (King et al., 1990), including lung cancers in which overexpression is reported in 30 - 64% of cases (Schneider et al., 1989, Weiner et al., 1990; Sozzi et al, 1991; Paako et al., 1992; Shi et al., 1992; Brandt-Rauf et al., 1994; Brandt-Rauf et al., 1995); increased c-*erb*B-2 levels have often been associated with poor prognosis, also in breast cancer (Kandl et al., 1994). The potential importance of this biomarker, that can readily been assessed in serum using the ELISA technique, is further stressed by the observation that high serum levels can be observed in asymptomatic individuals up to five years before the occurrence of overt cancer, making the serum c-*erb*B-2 oncopeptide potentially useful as a marker of early oncogenic change (Luo et al., 1993; Breuer et al., 1993; Brandt-Rauf et al., 1994).

Several studies assert the usefulness of EGFr-ECD and of c-*erb*B-2ECD in clinical settings (ECD = Extracellular Domain).

Using an ELISA (Tenney et al., 1993), the ECD of EGFr has been found to be significantly elevated in asbestosis cases who subsequently developed cancer, when compared to matched asbestosis cases who did not develop cancer, and to non-cancer non-asbestosis controls (Partanen et al., submitted; reported in Brandt-Rauf et al., 1995). The cancer cases had positive serum levels well before the time of disease diagnosis, as concluded from the assessment of banked serum samples, with an average lead time of 51 months (ibid).

Significantly elevated levels of the ECD of the c-*erb*B-2 oncoprotein are reported in several studies, mainly in breast cancer. In a series of pneumoconiosis patients who subsequently developed lung cancer, 64% of the lung cancer cases had elevated levels of the oncoprotein compared to 0 - 5% in two control series; mean levels also were significantly ($P < 0.001$) higher in cases than in controls; in four out of the seven cancer cases, the serum samples were positive well before the time of diagnosis, with an average lead time of 35 months (Brandt-Rauf et al., 1994; Brandt-Rauf et al., 1995).

A recently published study (Rusch et al., 1995) has brought about new and striking information in a search for genetic abnormalities in preneoplastic bronchial lesions –

p53, EGF receptor and Transforming Growth Factor α (TGFα) have been assessed by immunostaining in bronchial lesions associated with invasive carcinomas. The authors conclude that TGFα does not appear a reliable marker of malignant transformation, whereas abnormal p53 expression is almost exclusively observed in preinvasive lesions associated with squamous cell carcinoma. In contrast, aberrant EGFr expression is observed in bronchial lesions associated with all NSCLC histotypes and appears to be an early and more frequent marker of malignant transformation that does p53. Finally, the simultaneous aberrant expression of EGFr and p53 occurs predominantly in SCC and its associated bronchial lesions.

These findings should make the ECD of c-*erb*B-2 and EGF-r exceedingly important biomarkers in individuals at risk of developing lung cancer, as well as other cancers such as breast and ovary; c-*erb*B2-ECD has also been proposed as a base for anti-tumour vaccine and for adoptive immunotherapy (Yoshino et al., 1994).

Transforming Growth Factor α is a mitogenic polypeptide with approximately 30% homology to EGF at the amino acid level; it binds to the EGF receptor and activates it in the same way as EGF.

All the molecules considered in this subsection can be assessed in serum, or by immunohistochemistry.

Platelet-Derived Growth Factor and Receptor (PDGF) Platelet-Derived Growth Factor (PDGF) is a potent mitogen for a variety of cell types; its presence in culture media is essential for growth of cells such as fibroblasts and mesenchyme-derived cells (Ross, 1989). First isolated from blood platelets – hence the name –, this is in fact a misnomer, as PDGF can be synthesized and secreted by many cell types, including transformed and tumour cells, vascular endothelial cells, but also monocyte-derived macrophages and – under certain conditions – fibroblasts (Ross, 1989).

Structurally, PDGF is a $\sim$ 30 KDa dimer consisting of two structurally related polypeptide chains denoted A and B – demonstrating about 60% aminoacid sequence homology – encoded by two different genes located on chromosomes 7 (A-chain) and 22 (B-chain) (Westermark and Heldin, 1993). PDGF exists as homo- (AA and BB) and hetero- (AB) dimers. The B chain has been found to be similar to the protein product of the c-*sis* oncogene, the cellular counterpart of the v-*sis* simian sarcoma virus (Waterfield et al., 1983).

The structural complexity of PDGF is reflected in the structure of its receptor: an α-receptor binds all three isoforms of PDGF, whereas the β-receptor binds only PDGF-BB with high affinity. As with other transmembrane receptors, there is an extracellular ligand-binding domain made up of five immunoglobin domains (a structure to be compared with that of carcino-embryonic antigen – see later), and an intracellular domain with tyrosine kinase activity responsible for the signal transduction (Westermark and Heldin, 1993). The two receptor subunits are encoded by different genes. PDGF receptors are found on all mesenchymal connective-tissue-forming cells, but not on epithelial cells; cells of fibroblastic origin possess both α and β receptors, and mesothelial cells only a receptors. It has recently been reported that lung carcinoma cells may express both α and β receptors, and that malignant cells may produce one or several isoforms of PDGF concomitantly with the cognate receptor type, thus initiating an autocrine loop (Westermark and Heldin, 1993); PDGF is also involved, in a paracrine fashion, in different human fibrotic disorders, e.g. in pulmonary fibrosis after release by alveolar macrophages (Martinet et al., 1987; Gauldie et al., 1993). This process may also be implicated in tumour stroma development (Vignaud et al., 1994).

In the course of several clinical evaluations, elevated PDGF levels have been found to correlate with the presence of cancer (Leitzel et al., 1991), and more precisely with the presence of tumours of mesenchymal origin such as soft tissue sarcomas (Smits et al., 1992; Wang et al., 1994); most often the B-chain has been assessed and found to be elevated also in benign tumours, albeit at lower levels. Interestingly, Wang et al. (1994) have observed that in their series of mesenchymal tumours, PDGF-B expression correlated with increased cell proliferation, as measured by PCNA index (Proliferating Cell Nuclear Antigen, see later); indeed 69% of the PCNA-positive cells immunostained for PDGF-B, and these authors hypothesize that PCNA overexpression may be directly coupled to exogenous growth factor stimulation.

In their already mentioned study, Vignaud et al. (1994) describe that NSCLC tumour cells express PDGF-A and/or PDGF-B chains in about one third of all cases (64 tumours studied) and both α and β receptors in about one sixth of cases, in spite of the fact that normal epithelial cells express none of these genes. Moreover they insist on the production of both growth factors and receptors by tumour-associated macrophages, resulting in their common availability in lung tumours. These observations might well open a pathway to practical implementations, as selective blockers of platelet-derived growth factor tyrosine kinase activity have been developed and seem to reverse *sis*-induced transformation (Kovalenko et al., 1994).

On the other hand, the role of PDGF and PDGF receptors in the development of fibrotic lesions is well documented (Martinet and Crystal, 1987; Antoniades et al., 1990; Vignaud et al., 1991; Shaw et al. , 1991; Vignaud et al., 1994), be it in pulmonary pathologies or in others, e.g. atherosclerosis (Ross, 1993). PDGF levels in BAL (Bronchoalveolar Lavage Fluid) have been found to be significantly elevated in lung transplantation patients who subsequently developed obliterative bronchiolitis (Hertz et al., 1992), as well as in asbestosis and silicosis patients (Brandt-Rauf et al., 1992); in the latter study, elevated serum PDGF levels occurred more frequently in advanced pneumoconiosis cases, and tended to be indicative of progressive disease.

The PDGF-B protein can be assessed in extracellular fluids such as serum or BAL and the receptor by immnunohistochemistry, and of course by molecular analysis. The evaluation of the tyrosine kinase activity will be considered in the subsection on Tyrosine Kinases.

The Fibroblast Growth Factor This growth factor, first isolated from bovine neural tissue (Gospodarowicz, 1975) exists in both an acidic and a basic form showing similar features. Basic FGF exerts a proliferative effect on many cells of mesenchymal origin, especially endothelial cells, making the assessment of this growth factor rewarding when those cellular families are involved in carcinogenesis. Moreover bFGF has been shown to be expressed by other families of malignant cells, such as melanoma cells

(Halaban et al., 1988); and similarly FGF receptors have been identified in carcinoma cell lines (Soman et al., 1991); autocrine loops seem to be common features. The FGF-receptor is a transmembrane tyrosine kinase of which the extracellular domain contains three immunoglobulin-like repeats, thus being structurally related to the PDGF receptor. Functionally, PDGF and FGF appear to be interchangeable as competence factors, but their receptors phosphorylate different substrates belonging to different mitogenic signaling pathways, or inducing other cellular responses (Aaronson, 1991). Recent findings point to a role of FGF-family members in epithelial cell proliferation (Aaronson et al, 1990).

Transforming Growth Factor β TGF-β is a multifunctional peptide Growth Factor (GF) belonging to a family of potent regulators of growth and differentiation (Massagué, 1987). One of the hallmarks of its biological activity is its ability to inhibit the growth of many types of epithelial cells *in vitro* (Moses et al., 1985), while demonstrating a proliferative effect on some others, e.g. fibroblasts (Moses et al., 1990); it also regulates apoptosis. Presently, the central role of TGF-β in proliferation and cell cycle regulation has been recognized; in many cell types, it can antagonize the proliferative effects of growth factors, even when the cytokine is added to cultured cells relatively late in G1 phase, thus preventing the G1-S transition (Moses et al., 1990; Alexandrow and Moses, 1995). Among the targets of the negative signalling pathways induced by TGF-β1 are G1 cyclins, notably cyclins E and A, as well as cyclin-dependent kinases such as cdk4 (Koff et al., 1993; Ewen et al., 1993; Geng and Weinberg, 1993), but also the accumulation of hypophosphorylated pRb (Laiho et al., 1990), the form of the Rb protein preventing overtaking the checkpoint R (see earlier).

The effects of TGF-β treatment on cultured colon carcinoma cells have been described by Chakrabarty et al. (Chakrabarty et al., 1988; Chakrabarty et al., 1990) and may be characterized as follows: growth inhibition; up-modulation of protein expression and secretion; up-modulation of the expression and secretion of Carcino-Embryonic Antigen (CEA) and CEA-related glycoproteins; up-modulation of the expression of the Extra-Cellular Matrix (ECM) glycoproteins fibronectin and laminin and finally down-modulation of the proliferation related nucleolar protein B23. Several of these findings are important and might be relevant to cancer risk assessment. CEA is an accessory adhesion molecule (Benchimol et al., 1989) encoded by a gene on chromosome 19 located in close vicinity to the one encoding TGF-β, and has been proposed as a biomarker of the promotional phase of carcinogenesis (Pluygers et al., 1990). Fibronectin and laminin are implicated in tumourigenesis; these topics will be explicitely considered later, as well as the B23 nucleolar protein.

By contrast, TGF-β stimulates the growth of several cell lines of mesenchymal origin: this has been observed in mouse fibroblasts after down-regulation of the p27 Kip1 inhibitory protein and subsequent activation of the Cyclin E-cdk 2 complex (Ravitz et al., 1995). In humans, TGF-β overexpression has been observed during the early phases of the development of fibrotic lesions in the lung (Limper et al., 1991). In human mesothelial cells, TGF-β induces DNA synthesis, additive to that induced by EGF (Gabrielson et al., 1988).

Interleukins Primarily the term "interleukin" covers a series of soluble factors governing communication among cellular components of the immune system. Some members of the interleukin family exert growth-related effects on other cellular targets, justifying them to be mentioned. For instance Interleukin 6 has been shown to inhibit the growth of breast and colon carcinomas (Revel, 1992). On the other hand the serum level of this cytokine correlates with tumour burden and is an adverse prognostic factor in some patients, particularly with ovarian and renal cell carcinomas (Berek et al., 1991; Blay et al., 1992). Similarly, Interleukin 9 overexpression has been associated with Hodgkin's Disease and some large-cell anaplastic lymphomas (Merz et al., 1991; Gruss et al., 1992).

4.3.3.2. Growth Factor Receptors

Transmembrane Receptors The role of GF receptors has already been mentioned when considering the role of individual GFs; however a few peculiarities deserve further emphasis. The transmembrane GF receptors belong to three major categories: Firstly, the receptors with intrinsic Tyrosine Kinase activity, consisting of an extracellular growth factor binding domain, a transmembrane domain, and finally an intracellular domain possessing the TRK activity; secondly, neurotransmitters composed of seven transmembrane domains, a NH2-terminal extracellular domain and an intracellular COOH-terminal domain containing regulatory serine and threonine residues; these receptors activate the Guanine nucleotide proteins (G proteins); thirdly, the receptors for interleukins and related cytokines, shown to be membrane glycoproteins with one single transmembrane domain, an extra-cellular NH2-terminal domain and an intracellular domain devoid of TRK activity; however, members of the Src tyrosine kinase family might participate in signal transduction by this class of receptors (Aaronson, 1991) (see Figure 4.6).

Receptors with Tyrosine-Kinase activity A majority of the Growth Factor Receptors display intrinsic Tyrosine Kinase activity, i.e. the ability to catalyze the phosphorylation of protein tyrosine. While serine and threonine phosphorylation account for more than 99% of the protein phosphorylated residues present in normal cells, tyrosine phosphorylation is an important property of the molecules involved in the control of cell proliferation (Comoglio et al., 1990). In fact, this unique tyrosine phosphorylation of transmembrane receptors with TRK activity can be evaluated using an "integrated" assessment of the TRK activity of several different receptors belonging to the same family and all expressing TRK acitivity, making this a valuable marker of carcinogenesis (Giordano et al., 1987). On the other hand, the signal transduction process for these receptors involves increased intracellular TRK activity accompanied by the proteolytic cleavage of the extracellular domain (ECD) which then accumulates in the extracellular environment, where it may be quantified (Brandt-Rauf et al., 1995). This approach will yield separate evaluations for each receptor, as opposed to the "integrating" TRK activity assay.

The signal transduction involving G-proteins will be considered in the next section,

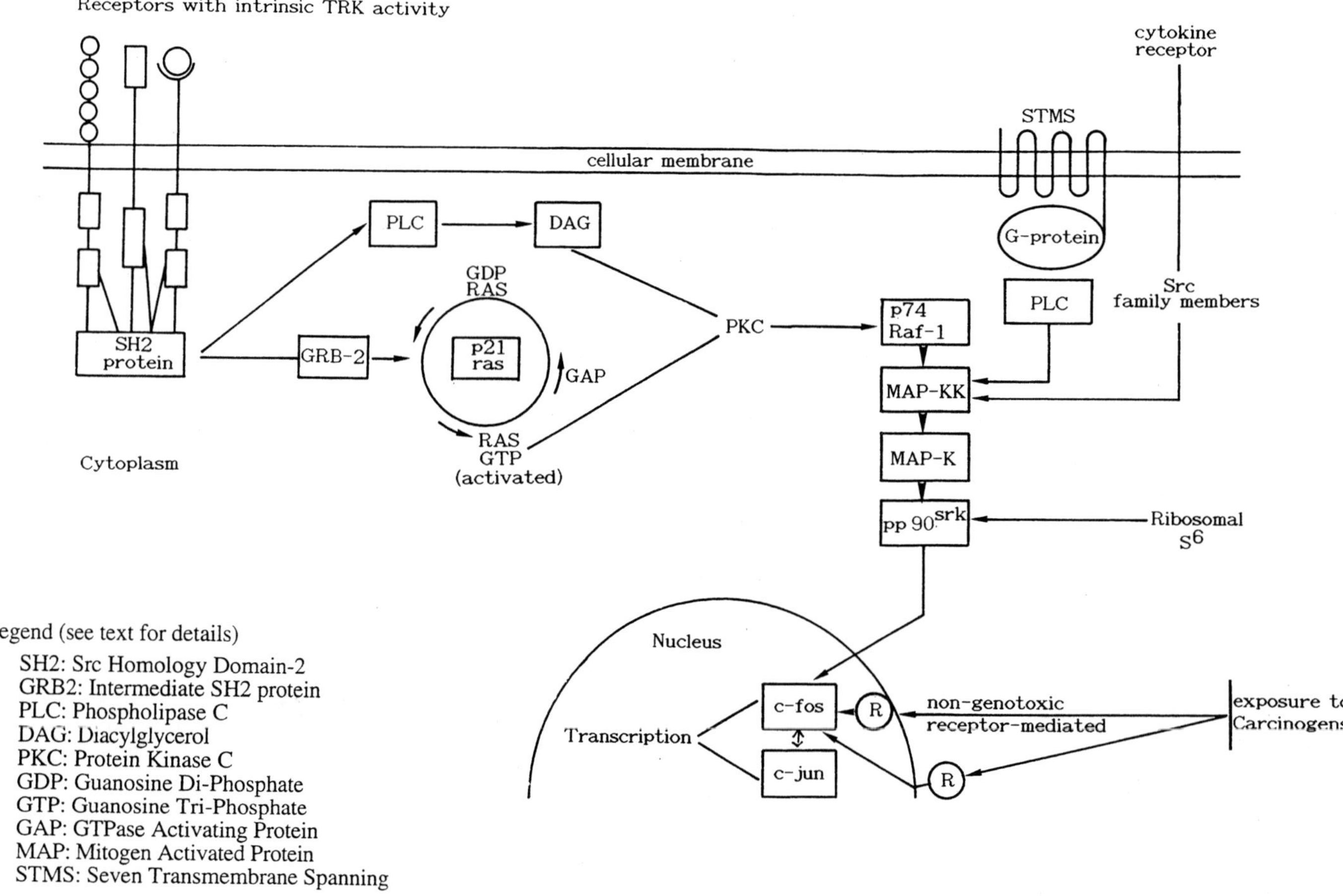

Figure 4.6: *Signal transduction pathways*

together with other signalling pathways.

Cytoplasmic receptors The prototypic example for this family of receptors is the aromatic hydrocarbon receptor AhR, a component of the cytosol responsible, among others, for dioxin toxicity (Okey et al., 1994). For some time considered to be a member of the steroid/thyroid/retinoic acid receptor family (Evans, 1988), some distinctive features have later been identified (Burbach et al., 1992). The cytosolic receptor-mediated mechanism of action can be summarized as follows: a) passive diffusion of the carcinogen into the cells; b) binding to the Ah receptor; c) translocation of the ligand-receptor complex into the nucleus and binding to DNA recognition sites; d) expression of specific genes and translation of their protein products; e) expression of the effects of these protein products (Landers and Bunce, 1991). Compared to the transmembrane-related signal transduction pathways (to be considered hereafter), this mechanism represents a short cut permitting the escape from several control steps or rate-limiting factors. In the case of 2,3,7,8-tetrachlorodibenzo-p-dioxin (TCDD), binding to the AhR requires the association with a 90 KDa heat shock protein (Perdew, 1988), an association also found for the glucocorticoid receptor (Denis et al., 1988). The ligand-receptor-Hsp 90-complex is translocated into the nucleus at the intervention of the Ah-receptor nuclear translocator protein (Arnt protein) after release of the HSP (Reyes et al., 1992). After binding to specific DNA regions, the Ah responsive elements, a series of genes is induced, including CYP1A1, CYP1A2, TGF-α, TGF-β2, EGF-receptor and others (Okey et al., 1994; Sutter and Greenlee, 1992). As mentioned in the section on cancer susceptibility, genetic polymorphism in Ah responsiveness has been reported and may be a determinant of susceptibility to lung cancer in smokers, mediated by CYP1A1 inducibility (Nebert et al., 1991). A similar polymorphism for the Arnt protein production has been demonstrated by Hayashi et al. (1994). The potential role of the AhR is further emphasized by the observation that ultraviolet photoproducts of tryptophan are binding the receptor with high affinity (Helferich and Denison, 1991).

Nuclear receptors Evidence is presently available showing the nuclear localization of a series of receptors including the steroid hormone receptors (estrogen, progesterone and androgen), the vitamin D and retinoic acid receptors and the glycocorticoid and mineralocorticoid receptors.

As an example we shall consider the mechanism of action of the estrogen receptor (ER) in influencing breast and liver cancer, although many other cancer sites are the seat of estrogen-induced cancers (Henderson et al., 1988), ERs having been detected in most tissues of the body (Lucier, 1992). It has long been admitted that unoccupied estrogen-receptors were located in the cytoplasm, to be translocated to the nucleus after binding to their ligand; presently it is known that both the unoccupied and bound forms have a nuclear localization (King and Greene, 1984; Welshons et al., 1984). The cloning of the human ER cDNA has demonstrated that the receptor consists of at least two major functional domains: an evolutionary highly conserved DNA binding domain called Region C, binding to a DNA Responsive Element (RE) and a slightly less strongly conserved carboxy terminal, representing the hormone binding domain HBD (Dreicer and Wilding, 1992); this is called region E. The HBD contains an inducible transcription activation function (Webster et al., 1988), as do the progesterone and glycocorticoid receptors, implicating that when this domain is unoccupied, this prevents the activating function. Also, a deletion of the HBD abolishes the capacity of the receptor to bind the hormone and to activate transcription. A significant homology has been demonstrated between several steroid hormone receptors and the V-*erb*-A oncogene product, whereas the cellular gene c-*erb*-A has been found to code for the thyroid hormone receptor (Weinberger et al., 1986).

The ER-mediated effects of estrogens include the induction of large numbers of enzymes and of growth factors among which EGF, TGFα, IGFs, PDGF, TGF-β and FGFs (Dreicer and Wilding, 1992). To trigger these effects and to induce DNA synthesis in target cells, a sustained occupancy of the nuclear ER seems to be required (Korach et al., 1985); however, this may be at a low level, as Campen et al. (1990) have demonstrated. A receptor occupancy of approximately 15% was sufficient to cause increased cell proliferation in the liver. As mentioned in the consensus report published by the IARC Working Group on the use of data on mechanisms of carcinogenesis in risk identification (IARC, 1992), receptor-mediated stimulation of mitogenesis may occur at low concentrations of ligand and, because a proportional relationship between receptor occupancy and biochemical biological responses exists for some receptor-mediated processes, "one ligand-receptor molecule could theoretically produce a change (although indetectable) in gene expression". This observation is of considerable interest owing to the worldwide dispersion of enormous amounts of chemicals (chlorinated biphenyls, some pesticides, alkyl-substituted phenols present in detergents, etc.) exhibiting estrogen-like activities. In spite of their low binding affinity, these chemicals may lead to sustained estrogen exposure as the result of massive introduction into the environment (several hundred thousand tons a year), persistence and additive effects of different compounds binding the same receptor.

The literature pertaining to the clinical effects of exposure to estrogens is extremely bulky and could not possibly be reviewed here; presently there is however pertinent evidence that exposure to increased levels of estrogens (endogenous, exogenous e.g. after prolonged hormonal replacement therapy, environmental xenoestrogens) encompasses an enhanced cancer risk in target organs, as underscored for instance for breast cancer (et al., 1995) and fatal ovarian cancer (Rodriguez et al., 1995).

4.3.4. Signal Transduction Pathways

In the case of the aforementioned cytoplasmic and nuclear receptors, ilustrated respectively by the Ah and the estrogen receptors, the ligand binds to the receptor after passively passing through the cell membrane and is immediately (or after translocation into the nucleus) bound to a DNA Responsive Element to trigger transcription. When transmembrane receptors are involved, the mechanism is quite different. The ligand binds to the extracellular domain of the receptor, resulting in activation of the intrinsic tyrosine kinase (TRK) activity. This information will then be transduced to Responsive DNA Elements in the nucleus through a wide array of extremely complex signal transduction pathways, of which the major steps have been elucidated and will presently be schematically considered, as they represent valuable intermediate endpoints contributing important information for the evaluation of cellular proliferation. Three major signal transduction pathways have been identified; some of their pecularities have already been evoked (see Figure 4.6).

4.3.4.1. Transmembrane Receptors with Intrinsic TRK Activity After activation of the receptor TRK activity, the information is transmitted to the interior of the cell through non-receptor tyrosine kinases and other signal transduction proteins possessing SH2 (Src homology region 2) domains (Fawson and Gish, 1992), to finally activate the proto-oncogene product p21 *ras* and phospholipase C. This latter induces the production of Diacylglycerol (DAG), a second messenger activating the serine/threonine specific Protein Kinase C, which plays a central role in this signal transduction pathway (Weinstein, 1987, O'Brian and Ward, 1989). Down-stream from *ras* the signals flow through *raf*-1 kinase, thence to MAP (Mitogen Activated Protein) kinases, the ribosomal S6 (pp90rsk) kinase and finally to the nucleus and the proto-oncogene products (Kahn, 1992; Roberts, 1992). Several steps in this process can be readily assessed.

Tyrosine Kinase Activity We have previously mentioned that, in normal cells, phosphorylation on tyrosine residues is a property practically restricted to molecules involved in the control of cell proliferation (Comoglio et al., 1990), in such a way that the assessment of TRK activity represents an integrated evaluation of the activation induced by several different GFs proceeding through the same mechanism. Proteins phosphorylated on tyrosine can be detected by immunological methods (Di Renzo et al., 1986) and commercial reagents are available. P-tyr antibodies have been used to screen a panel of human tumour cell lines (Giordano et al., 1987); proteins phosphorylated on tyrosine have been detected in a bladder carcinoma, a colon carcinoma, a fibrosarcoma, an epidermoid carcinoma; untransformed human cells lines or normal human tissue were constantly negative (id). Excessive levels of tyrosine phosphorylation have been observed in each of 19 human cell lines derived from head-and-neck malignancies, with respect to normal human keratinocytes; in 14 of the cell lines, enhanced EGF-R activity was detected (Cardinali et al., 1995). In node-positive breast cancer, high levels of TRK activity have been associated with poor prognosis (Romain et al., 1994) and, in leukemic cell lines, with aggressiveness (together with high PKC levels) (Aflalo, 1992). Elevated levels of TRK activity have also been observed in the histologically normal-appearing thyroid tissue of patients with thyroid cancer (Hatada et al., 1994); the authors interpret this finding as a potential increased risk of developing cancer in the apparently normal thyroid tissue.

p21*ras* The *ras* gene family includes at least three members: Harvey-*ras* (H-*ras*), Kirsten-*ras* (K-*ras*) identified as being the cellular counterparts of Harvey and Kirsten murine sarcoma viruses and N-*ras*, identified in a neuroblastoma cell line. These oncogenes code for three closely related 21-KDa proteins, such as GRB-2, that appear to be guanosine-binding G proteins. The intermediate SH2 proteins mediate the receptor-generated signal and transduce it towards *ras*-GDP (Guanosine Diphosphate), activating it to *ras*-GTP (G-Triphosphate). This moves along the inner side of the cytoplasmic membrane towards an effector which is then activated, while simultaneously *ras*-GTP is deactivated to *ras*-GDP by p120 GAP. This means that p21*ras* can be switched on or off; when *ras* is mutated, it cannot be switched off, resulting in continuous activation of the effector and continuous transmission of proliferation-stimulating signals.

Ras mutations are frequently observed in human tumours; they typically consist in point mutations at one of the critical positions 12, 13 and 61; often the mutations are specific for a given carcinogen. (Bos, 1989). The percentage of tumours displaying *ras* mutations is quite variable from one tumour type to another; it is very high in pancreatic adenocarcinomas – around 80 - 90% (Almoquera et al., 1988); in colon adenocarcinomas – 40 to 50% (Vogelstein et al., 1988); in adenocarcinomas of the lung – about 30%, exclusively K-*ras* mutations at colon 12 (Rodenhuis and Slebos, 1990), however a recent study (Mills et al., 1995) shows that these codon 12 mutations might be definitely more frequent, exceeding the 50% range; in follicular and undifferentiated carcinomas of the thyroid (Lemoine et al., 1989), in myeloid disorders (Hirai et al., 1987; and many others). On the contrary, *ras* mutations are not frequent in breast, ovary, cervix and stomach tumours (Bos, 1989); these results have however been challenged. Indeed, increased levels of p21*ras* have been detected in breast cancer tissues compared with normal counterparts or fibro-adenomas (De Biasi et al., 1989). Moderate levels of p21*ras* have been detected in benign colonic conditions, the levels of the oncoprotein being predictive of evolution towards malignancy (Michelassi et al., 1987). For several tumour sites, elevated p21*ras* levels have been detected during the early stages of carcinogenesis and in occupational settings, the finding of elevated levels of p21*ras* oncoprotein in the serum of workers exposed to diverse chemicals has been interpreted as corresponding to an increase in cancer risk (Brandt-Rauf, 1988; Brandt-Rauf and Niman, 1988). Similarly, an overexpression of the p21*ras* oncoprotein has been detected twice as frequently in the serum of residents in a heavily polluted area in Poland as in the controls (Perera et al., 1992).

Protein Kinase C (PKC) PKC is an ubiquitously expressed enzyme transducing multifarious signals, hence playing a critical role in phenomena as diverse as platelet activation, neurotransmission, muscle contraction, hormonal responses, growth factor action and tumour promotion (Nishizuka, 1986). The hydrolysis of membrane phospholipids, including phosphatidylinositol, catalyzed by phospholipase C, produces the second messenger diacylglycerol that activates PKC (Weinstein, 1987, O'Brian and Ward, 1989). PKC can also be activated by the potent tumour promoter 12-O-tetradecanoylphorbol-13-acetate, TPA (Castagna et al., 1982), confirming the critical role of PKC in promotion and in carcinogenesis, as its stimulation elevates the activity of the immediate early genes c-*fos* and c-*jun*, after transmission of the signals further down the cascade. Activated PKC is translocated from the cytosolic to the particulate cell fraction and the activation may be enhanced by the production of reactive oxygen mediated by lipid peroxidation, emphasizing the importance of the lipid background within the cell (O'Brian et al., 1987).

Depending on the cellular system studied, PKC activation can either stimulate or inhibit proliferation. In colon carcinomas, a reduced expression is observed as compared to adjacent mucosal tissue and mucosa in control subjects (Kopp et al., 1991). Moreover, in patients with colorectal carcinoma, the PKC activity of the normal colonic mucosa was only a third or one half of levels in individuals without cancer (Sakanoue et al., 1991); these authors suggest that PKC activity may be used as a biological marker of risk of developing colorectal cancer or risk of bearing an asymptomatic tumour. According to Hirai et al. (1989), PKC activity is often elevated in lung cancer cell lines (various types), while it was reduced in squamous cell carcinomas of the tongue and vulva. In breast cancer specimens, PKC activity was strongly increased in comparison with normal breast tissue from the same patients, to such an extent that this might be a potential marker for malignant disease in the breast (O'Brian et al., 1989).

Mediators of Signal Transduction Pathways as Targets for Cancer Prevention and Treatment In the endeavours to control carcinogenesis, treatment strategies have been developed that rely on the functional impairment of several key mediators of the signal transduction pathways. For instance, compounds called tyrphostins have been synthetized and shown to be inhibitors of the EGF-receptor tyrosine kinase; they inhibit EGF-R autophosphorylation, EGF-dependent tyrosine phosphorylation of endogenous substrates such as the SH2 domain carriers, and the EGF induced breakdown of the phosphoinositides and subsequent production of diacylglycerol; these effects are correlated with inhibition of cell proliferation. Tyrphostins containing an indole moiety are potent blockers of PDGF (AB and BB) related mitogenesis and tyrosine phosphorylation in fibroblasts (Bryckaert et al, 1992).

The effect of *ras* impairment is often consequence of a single point mutation. It seems tempting to replace a misfunctioning *ras* gene with a wild-type functionally normal one. J. Roth and his team have brought evidence that the introduction of an antisense k-*ras* fragment was able to specifically inhibit the expression of a mutant k-*ras* protein in human non-small cell lung cancer cells (Mukhopadhyay et al, 1991). In order to overcome the difficulty of transfering this gene construct into the tumour cells, a retroviral expression vector has been developed by these authors; this effectively prevents the growth of human lung cancer cells in *nu/nu* mice (Georges et al., 1993).

The inhibition of PKC activity is believed to be at least partially responsible for the antitumour effects of several classes of drugs, including the antiestrogen tamoxifen and related triphenylethylenes (O'Brian et al., 1986) – of which the role in the treatment of breast cancer is well established –, glycyrrhetic acid, dequalinium and several others; the inhibitory action may exert itself either on the catalytic or on the regulatory domain of the enzyme (for a review see Gescher, 1992). The practical implications of these findings still remain somewhat confused, as subtle differences in PKC modulation seem to exist between different cell types, whereas PKC isozymes appear to be functionally cell type-specific.

4.3.4.2. Receptors with Seven Transmembrane-spanning Domains Fundamentally, this signal transduction pathway follows the same mechanisms as the preceding one: the receptor contains seven transmembrane domains and its intracellular part reacts with an hetero-trimeric G protein of which the α subunit activates the effector enzyme adenylate cyclase; the latter transforms ATP into the second messenger cyclic AMP which in turn activates Protein Kinase A. One of the most extensively studied systems is the Gs/Gi system, coupling adrenaline to its receptor, transducing the signal to the effector by a stimulated Gs protein, leading to production of cAMP, which is interrupted by switching back the G protein to its inhibiting form Gi (Bourne et al., 1990). This signal transduction pathway, frequently involved in neurotransmitter action, is less frequently observed in carcinogenesis and will not be further considered.

4.3.4.3. Cytoskeletal Signal Transduction Pathways It has been demonstrated that cytoskeletal elements participate in signal transduction; however as yet their precise role is not clearly understood. Proteins possessing SH3 domains (similar to the above-mentioned SH2 proteins) could regulate interactions between enzymes such as phospholipase C – whose key role has been previously underlined – and cytoskeletal elements (Koch et al., 1991). It has been hypothesized that the cytoskeleton acts as a coordinator by providing a matrix on which the many enzymes implicated in signal transduction are associated in a highly efficient way, to facilitate the enzymatic cascade (Payrastre et al., 1991). The cytoskeletal protein vinculin is a substrate of PKC.

Tubulin and microtubules have been shown to associate in complexes with signal transducing G proteins (Wang et al., 1990), and with the transactivation domain of the c-*myc* oncoprotein (Alexandrova et al., 1995). Considering the central role of these proteins in the control of cell proliferation, the importance of these cytoskeletal pathways may be presumed. Interesting, the proliferation biomarker TPA that will be later considered and discussed is recognized by monoclonal antibodies to cytokeratins 8, 18 and 19.

4.3.5. The Outcome: The Clonal Expansion of the Initiated Cells

As a result of the multiple processes that have been described, the initiated cells acquire a proliferative advantage leading to their clonal expansion. If the proliferation rate exceeds the spontaneous cellular death rate (apoptosis) in a tumour, this will grow. Thus the growth of a tumour represents an unbalance between proliferation and apoptosis; both may be evaluated by appropriate biomarkers.

4.3.5.1. Proliferation Several methods are available to assess proliferation and are in regular, although not really common, use; they have been reviewed (Quinn and Wright, 1990).

Mitotic count This is defined as the number of mitoses per ten high-power fields, and has for instance been applied in distinguishing leiomyomas from leiomyosarcomas. However the method is burdened with many shortcomings, the lesser being that it does not account for differences in cell size; obviously a large-cell tumour will contain fewer cells than a small cell tumour within the same number of high-power fields. Hence the development of a "mitotic index", representing the fraction of mitoses expressed as a percentage. Unfortunately, this assessment is extremely timeconsuming.

Thymidine Labelling Index This is a S-phase marker, measuring the incorporation of tritiated thymidine into DNA; the method necessitates the preparation of autoradiographs, in which the labelled cells are counted and their frequency compared with the labelling index of cells in the interphase. This technique is not readily available and is also very timeconsuming.

Bromodeoxyuridine (BrdUr) Bromodeoxyuridine is a thymidine analog which is readily incorporated into cells during S-phase and can be detected using specific monoclonal antibodies, making this technique much more accessible than the radioactive thymidine incorporation; it can be applied in routine clinical practice as well as in experimental systems. The results are expressed as a labelling index. The labelling index has been found to be statistically lower in low grade tumour compared to high-grade tumours. Moreover, as BrdUr is a therapeutic agent, it may be administered *in vivo*, allowing to carry out kinetic studies, including estimation of the S-phase and calculation of the potential doubling time of the tumour (Wilson et al., 1988).

Flow Cytometry This automated technique enables the quantification of the cellular DNA content, as well as its distribution along the cell cycle, known as its ploidy status. Normal resting cells are diploid, corresponding to a "DNA-index" of 1 (ratio of the G0/G1 cells in the cell population being studied to that of a standard diploid cell population). A DNA-index of 2 corresponds to tetraploid cells, higher indexes to aneuploidly or polyploidy. Aneuploidy is frequent in tumour cells and has been reported in up to 90% of breast carcinomas; it has been correlated with poor prognosis (McGuire et al., 1985) and inversely correlated with oestrogen receptor positivity. Similar observations are reported for ovarian cancer, colorectal carcinomas and preneoplastic conditions such as ulcerative colitis (Hammarberg et al, 1984), bladder cancer, lymphoproliferative diseases.

The proliferation-associated Ki-67 protein In the search for antibodies reactive with nuclear antigens specific for proliferating cells, Gerdes et al. (1983) have developed a mouse monoclonal antibody designated Ki-67 that recognizes a nuclear antigen associated with cell proliferation. Since this initial research a panel of Ki-67 antibodies have been prepared of which one precisely reflects the growth fraction (McCormick et al., 1993) of a given human cell population, allowing for its rather easy determination using routine immunocytochemical methods. The Ki-67 protein has been shown to be a strictly nuclear protein present in steadily increasing quantities from G1 to G2 + M phase and seeming to be an absolute requirement for cell proliferation (for details on these and other characteristics, see Duchrow et al., 1994); quiescent G0 cells are not recognized by the antibody.

Several studies have evaluated the significance of Ki-67 immunostaining in human tumours. In breast cancer the Ki-67 score (proportion of Ki-67-positive cells) was significantly higher in aneuploid than euploid cells; it correlated significantly with the S-phase fraction and the mitotic count (Isola et al., 1990). The advantages of Ki-67 immunostaining over other proliferation indexes in colorectal tumours are underscored by Porschen et al. (1991); these authors observed a significant increase of the Ki-67 score in relapsing carcinomas. In ovarian carcinomas, high Ki-67 activity has been correlated with the occurrence of distant metastases (Wong and Tattersall, 1989; Henzen-Logmans et al., 1994).

Due to the extreme lability of the epitope labelled by the Ki-67 antibody, this technique can be used only on frozen tissue. A novel antibody, called Ki-S1, overcomes this difficulty and labels a very stable epitope; it correlates positively with S-phase fraction and might be a valuable alternative to Ki-67 (Camplejohn et al, 1993). On the other hand, antibodies have been raised to a recombinant Ki-67 motif-containing sequence and may be used on formalin-fixed paraffin-embedded tissues, making the technique more readily available.

The Proliferating Cell Nuclear Antigen, PCNA Proliferating Cell Nuclear Antigen is a 36KDa nuclear protein functioning as the auxiliary protein of DNA-polymerase delta, hence is an absolute requirement for adequate leading strand synthesis (Bravo et al., 1987; Prelich et al., 1987). Several antibodies against this antigen have been developed; the PC10 antibody has been shown to be an excellent S-phase marker, displaying better accurracy than DNA histograms (Landberg and Roos, 1991). Practically undetected in non-cycling cells, PCNA can be detected – sometimes at high levels – in seemingly normal tissues surrounding malignant tumours; it can also be induced in these normal tissues after administration of growth factors (Hall et al., 1994). PCNA participates in DNA repair processes and is required for DNA nucleotid excision repair (Shivji et al., 1992); it may be expressed in non-cycling cells *in vivo* when they undergo DNA repair (Hall et al., 1993), as has been demonstrated in UV-treated human epidermal keratinocytes. However, in normal tissue PCNA staining usually remains confined to proliferating cells and can be used as an index of cell proliferation; in malignant tissue, higher levels of immunostaining correspond to more aggressive tumours. In clinical settings, PCNA immunostaining is inversely correlated with survival in ovarian cancer (Thomas et al., 1995) and has proven useful in identifying tumours with high growth potential in prostatic adenocarcinomas; in these tumours treatment should not be delayed (Vesalainen et al, 1994). Relapsing colon cancer also shows higher PCNA indices both in malignant and normal cells. In mesothelioma PCNA immunoreactivity may be helpful in discriminating between malignant and benign mesothelial cells, and it also may have a prognostic value (Ramael et al., 1994).

Nucleolar Antigens Nucleolar organizer regions (NORs) are loops of DNA which transcribe to ribosomal RNA; they are associated with certain proteins, including e.g. RNA polymerase 1 and B23, characterized by argyrophilia, an affinity for silver staining. Hence their common denomination of AgNOR proteins. The AgNOR technique has been standardized and an AgNOR index has been developed (Ploton et al., 1986); it has been applied to a series of clinical studies and higher counts have been correlated to conditions of increased malignancy (e.g. Crocker and Skilbeck, 1987). AgNOR staining parallels the percentage of cells in the S-phase and is indicative of a high proliferation rate; the proliferation index determined by this method is comparable to PCNA and Ki-67 indexes (Egan and Crocker, 1992). During mitosis, NOR proteins are associated with ribosomal genes and the AgNOR staining represents a good marker to predict active and repressed genes (Roussel and Hernandez-Verdun, 1994).

A p120 antigen has been identified in nucleoli during G1 phase; decreased levels of the protein are detected during differentiation, whereas phytohaemagglutinin stimulation in peripheral blood mononuclear cells leads to increased p120 mRNA expression, paralleling that of c-*myc* mRNA (Jhiang et al., 1990).

Tissue Polypeptide Antigen (TPA), Tissue-Specific Polypeptide Antigen (TPS) Whereas the hitherto considered proliferation markers necessitate intact cellular material (tissue specimens, eventually cytological specimens) to be assessed, the common characteristic of TPA and TPS is that the proliferation index is based on the assessment of the soluble fractions in the extracellular fluids, mostly serum, making this assay completely non-invasive.

TPA is a tumour-related antigen originally isolated from the cytosolic fraction of pooled tumours (Bjorklund et al., 1958); it is released from the cells during and immediately after the completion of mitosis and may then be detected and assessed in extracellular fluids, in which its levels are believed to parallel mitotic frequency, making it a proliferation marker. Indeed elevated serum levels have been observed in many malignant conditions and the biomarker is currently used for the monitoring of cancer patients whose tumours express the marker. The precise nature of the TPA antigen has yet to be determined; it is identified in serum by antibodies to cytokeratins 8, 18 and 19. Cytokeratins are constituents of the intermediate filaments building up the cytoskeleton, whose potential role in signal transduction has already been evoked. The antibody identifying TPA would then recognize solubilized breakdown products released from intermediate filaments during mitosis (Bjorklund, 1992). However, breakdown products are similarly released from dying cells – be it through apoptosis or infectious (predominantly viral) cytolysis. TPA could then express either cell proliferation or cell destruction, both processes being involved in carcinogenesis. An antibody has been developed, called TPS for Tissue Polypeptide Specific Antigen, supposed to recognize an epitope present only on proliferating cells, making this a "true" proliferation marker. However in cytosols prepared from breast cancer cells, the levels of TPA and TPS are strongly correlated and both tend to show an inverse association with the Thymidine Labelling Index (Gion et al., 1994). Whatever the involved mechanisms, TPA serum levels have been correlated e.g. with exposure to asbestos and a dose-response relationship has been established (Pluygers et al., 1991/1992; Pluygers and Baldewyns, 1993). The hypothesis has been formulated that serum TPA levels might be indicative of free-radical-induced damage, as these levels tend to decrease after the administration of anti-oxidants (Pluygers and Sadowska, unpublished data). Significant elevations in serum TPA levels have also been demonstrated in populations residing in the vicinity of waste disposal sites, the levels being inversely correlated with distance from the waste site (Pluygers et al., 1993).

4.3.5.2. Apoptosis Homeostasis in normal tissues is a result from the balance of cell proliferation and programmed cell death or apoptosis. This also occurs in tumour tissues, in which the rate of cell loss may be inferred by comparing the doubling time of the tumour cells and the doubling time of the tumour mass. High rates of cell loss, exceeding 70%, have been detected in several human tumours (Arends and Wyllie, 1991). Cell loss may result from necrosis or apoptosis, two completely distinct mechanisms, the latter being characterized by typical morphologic changes (Kerr et al., 1991). Nuclear DNA undergoes unique changes, consisting in double-strand cleavage in the linker regions between nucleosomes, resulting in the formation of fragments comprising 180 - 200 base pairs; these assume a typical "ladder" appearance on agarose gel electrophoresis. Mitochondrial DNA is not affected. Cytoskeletal elements participate in the process.

One of the most intriguing features of apoptosis is its dependency on genetic control; several of the regulatory genes appear to be oncogenes or tumour suppressor genes, bringing additional evidence of the relation between apoptosis and oncogenesis.

Regulatory genes Among the sofar identified regulatory genes, a conspicuous role is devoted to c-*myc*, its overexpression leading to proliferation or apoptosis depending on the availability of mitogenic signals (Evan et al., 1992). In the presence of growth factors (IGF-1 being the most relevant for fibroblasts), c-*myc* overexpression leads to proliferation; however after complete withdrawal of the GFs, a similar overexpression will induce apoptosis. With Willie (1993) three extreme cells states may be identified: growth arrest (c-*myc* off, growth factors absent); population expansion (c-*myc* on , GFs present) and apoptosis (c-*myc* on, GFs off). As previously mentioned, cells undergoing apoptosis under these conditions may be rescued by overexpression of the *bcl*-2 proto-oncogene product (Hockenbery et al, 1990; Bissonnette et al., 1992). The *bcl*-2 proto-oncogene, first identified in human B-cell lymphomas, opened the way for a new type of proto-oncogenes, of which the product does not stimulate proliferation, but inhibits apoptosis (Korsmeyer, 1992). Its mechanism of action is not fully elucidated; it does not inhibit apoptosis in all circumstances; for instance it does not block the apoptosis induced by cytotoxic T-lymphocytes. An interesting working hypothesis emphasizes the protective role of *bcl*-2 against the lipid peroxidation induced by reactive oxygen species, themselves potent inducers of apoptosis (Hockenbery et al, 1993).

Overexpression of *ras* has been shown to induce apoptosis and – in experimental settings – wild-type p53 has induced extensive apoptosis and is involved in triggering the deletion – through apoptosis – of cells whose DNA has been damaged. Mutated p53 is unable to induce the apoptosis of the damaged cells. From these observations, a cooperation between c-*myc* and p53 appears to be likely.

Identification of apoptosis The distinctive morphologic patterns of apoptosis and the striking differences between apoptosis and necrosis have been described (Kerr et al., 1994). However, identification of apoptotic bodies by light microscopy is uneasy and requires practice; on the other hand the characteristic features of each process are clearly demonstrated by electron microscopy.

The endonuclease-mediated DNA fragmentation that occurs in apoptotic cells leads to the formation of numerous fragments of about 180 - 200 base pairs, resulting in the above mentioned "DNA laddering" in standard agarose gels of DNA extracted from apoptotic cells. This fragmentation generates a multitude of 3'OH-DNA ends, in contrast to normal or proliferating nuclei in which these ends are few. The 3'OH ends can be specifically labelled and stained, making their identification both on cryosections and paraffin-embedded tissues much easier; presently several techniques are available (e.g. Gavrieli et al., 1992).

Appealing new developments proceed from the finding that apoptosis may be induced by activation of a transmembrane receptor belonging to the TNF-Receptor (Tumour Necrosis Factor) and NGF-R (Nerve Growth Factor Receptor) families. The Fas/APO-1 antigen is a transmembrane receptor identified in haematopoietic cell lines, of which the binding to a specific anti-Fas monoclonal antibody induces apoptosis, independently of any complementary activation (Trauth et al., 1989; Itoh et al., 1991). This finding may bring forth far-reaching consequences.

4.4. ADJUVANT DETERMINANTS OF THE CLONAL EXPANSION

In the previous section we have considered what we believe to be the basic mechanims of carcinogenesis. Obviously, other mechanisms also do participate in this complex process and some of these "adjuvant determinants" may correspond to important, frequent – and indeed decisive – steps in the carcinogenic process. Adjuvant therefore should not be confounded with unimportant. These determinants will be briefly considered.

4.4.1. Oxidative Damage and its Repair

The detailed description of the mechanisms of carcinogenesis induced by free radicals (FR) and reactive oxygen species (ROS) would lead well beyond the scope of this analysis, the more since excellent reviews have been published (Cerutti, 1985; Meneghini, 1988; Halliwell and Aruoma, 1992); we ourselves have considered the topic in our study on the mechanisms and prevention of asbestos carcinogenesis (Pluygers et al., 1991-1992). Indeed, a variety of agents and mechanisms can induce the pro-oxidant states that will trigger or contribute to carcinogenesis. Among them, as enumerated by Cerutti (1985): hyperbaric oxygen, radiation, xenobiotic metabolism and Fenton-type reactions, peroxisome proliferators, agents interacting with membrane functions, lipid peroxidation of the polyunsaturated fatty acid side chains of membrane lipids. The effects elicited by such diverse inducers of course demonstrate considerable diversity but are consistent with the concept of pro-oxidant states exerting a promotional activity; they include an increase in intracellular free Ca^{2+} that activates a Ca^{2+}/calmodulin dependent kinase and, as a consequence, a ribosomal S6 kinase; the oxidation of critical sulfhydryl groups in the regulatory lipid binding domain of Protein Kinase C (PKC) (Cerutti, 1989); the activation – presumably by PKC – of the phosphorylating capacity toward ADP-ribosyl-transferase (ADPRT).-Poly-ADP-ribosylation of chromosomal proteins represents an epigenetic consequence of DNA breakage induced by oxidants (Cerutti, 1989) and reflects the intensity of DNA repair activity (Pero et al., 1990).

This mechanism has been further elucidated by the observation that oxidants not only increase the cellular content of Nicotinamide Adenine Dinucleotide (NAD) which serves as a substrate for ADPRT, but also – being clastogens – that they induce the DNA strand breaks acting as a co-factor of ADPRT, a combination finally stimulating poly-ADP-ribosylation of chromosomal proteins and, consequently, resulting in the modulation of gene expression. Interestingly, this poly-AD-ribosylation involves topoisomerase I and c-*fos* protein, product of the "immediate early" c-*fos* oncogene.

Several of the above mentioned mechanisms are modulated by endogenous anti-oxidant defence mechanisms (catalase, Super-Oxide Dismutases – SOD, Glutathione transferases) as well as by exogenous supplies of anti-oxidants, thus providing additional evidence of the role of pro-oxidant states in carcinogenesis. However these observations also bring further support to the complexity of the processes, as these are modulated not only by the type of involved ROS (displaying different levels of potency), but also by the efficiency of the endogenous defence systems and by the abundance of the exogenous supplies of anti-oxidants. Numerous experimental and clinical (case-control and epidemiological) studies bring evidence of the delaying action of anti-oxidant administration on carcinogenesis.

Contrarily to the direct induction of DNA damage by electrophilic metabolites of carcinogens, an indirect mechanism has been identified that is responsible for the DNA-damage elicited by ROS, by lipid hydroperoxides and their radical and aldehydic degradation products and others (Cerutti, 1985). These indirect mechanisms may induce single- and double-strand breaks, but also characteristic mutations such as a tandem CC to TT double substitution (Tkeshelashvili et al., 1991), that may be considered as a marker of free radical mutagenesis (Feig et al., 1994) and serve as an indicator for evaluating the oxidative DNA damage contributing to the clonal expansion. DNA polymerases αa and η play an important role in determining the different sites and types of mutations produced as a result of ROS-induced DNA damage; the occurrence of specific mutations has been discussed for human hepatocellular carcinomas, lung and prostate cancer (Feig et al., 1994).

4.4.1.1. Identification of Oxidative Damage The direct *in vivo* measurement of free radicals is extremely difficult if not impossible because of the low concentrations and very short half-lives of these reactive compounds. Indirect methods assess DNA-damage products appearing in urine after having been excised in the course of the repair process.

4.4.1.2. Thymine Glycol and Thymidine Glycol These products appear *in vitro* as a consequence of chemical oxidation (or ionizing radiation – similarly oxidative), are excised by DNA repair systems and are excreted in urine where their assessment has been proposed as a monitor for oxidative DNA damage (Cathcart et al., 1984). Unfortunately the assay, though non-invasive, is extremely cumbersome and time-consuming.

Alternative techniques using a monoclonal antibody against thymine glycol have been developed.

4.4.1.3. 8-Hydroxydeoxyguanosine (8OHdG) A conceptually similar approach assesses the 8-hydroxylation of the guanine base as evidence of oxidative DNA damage; this technique – consisting in the detection of 8-hydroxyguanine in DNA – is successfully applied to the measurement of oxidative DNA damage *in vitro* (Kasai et al., 1986). *In vivo*, DNA excision repair results in the production of water-soluble free 80HdG, which is excreted into the urine without being further metabolized (Shigenaga et al., 1989). As exogenous DNA – e.g. of dietary origin – does not contribute to the excretion, the urinary measurement of 80HdG will reflect the extent of oxidative DNA damage. The urinary excretion of 8-OHdG has been correlated with smoking, gender and body mass index (Loft et al., 1992), and has been proposed as an effective tool for measuring the effects of oxidative damage on ageing, carcinogenesis and other chronic health impairments (See also subsection 4.2.1).

4.4.1.4. ADPRT The role of ADP-ribosyl-transferase in the excision repair of oxidative DNA damage has been aforementioned; its assessment – in human mononuclear leukocytes in pheripheral blood – has been used to evaluate the levels of DNA damage induced by different pro-oxidant generating systems (Pero et al., 1990). According to Pero et al. (1990) pro-oxidant sensitive ADPRT activity is associated with some of the most common dominantly inherited cancers, such as breast, colon and lung. About a tenfold variation in constitutive ADPRT levels is observed in a randomly selected human population, and these variations are significantly correlated to the levels observed after exposure to different activating pro-oxidant systems. It is proposed that constitutive (basic) ADPRT levels are under a genetic control involving a host factor affecting all pro-oxidant systems, such as cellular redox cycling.

4.4.1.5. Others Fluorometric techniques are available to visualize oxidative processes at the cellular level. The assessment of several DNA repair enzymes in human peripheral blood leukocytes has been mentioned in Section 4.2.3 (Hall et al., 1993).

4.4.2. Intercellular Communication

The harmonious development of multicellular organisms requires a constant equilibrium between three major cellular functions, i.e. cellular proliferation and its control, ordered differentiation of stem and progenitor cells and finally adaptive control of differentiated functions (Trosko and Chang, 1989). The homeostatic control of these functions is mediated by signals that may be transmitted to distant cells (e.g. hormones, peptide growth regulators, neurotransmitters), or from cell to cell by intercellular communication, or within the cell ("second messengers") (Trosko and Chang, 1989).

The role of cell-to-cell communication in carcinogenesis has emerged from a series of observations. Intercellular communication is provided by Gap Junctions (GJs), specialized intercellular channels between contiguous plasma membranes. The structure of the GJs has been unraveled, both of the adjacent cells each contributing one half structure or connexon, itself composed of six proteins called connexins (Cxs) (Loewenstein 1981; Holder et al., 1993). Several structurally related connexins with different molecular weights have been identified, such as e.g Cx 32 and Cx 43. Many GJ can be clustered and form a "plaque", facilitating bulk exchange between cells of small molecular weight ions and molecules; this seems indispensable to ensure homeostasis. Cellular Adhesion Molecules (CAMs) (to be considered in next subsection) can facilitate gap junctional intercellular communication, at least in epidermal cells, demonstrating the importance of cooperation between these mechanisms.

Tumour promoters of the phorbol ester class inhibit gap junctional cell communication (Yotti et al., 1979) and this property has been found to be shared by other tumour promoters (Kanno, 1985; Holder et al., 1993). It is proposed that the chronic inhibition of GJ intercellular communication in carcinogen-initiated tissues brings about the promotional stage of carcinogenesis (Yamasaki, 1990). An inverse correlation between cell growth and GJ intercellular communication has been demonstrated; for instance enhanced cell-to-cell communication inhibits proliferation, a mechanism shown to be inherent to several cancer preventive agents, and representing a novel pathway for chemoprevention of cancer (Zhang et al., 1992), through the up-regulation of connexin mRNA and protein. Conversely, agents inhibiting GJ intercellular communication should be considered as good candidates for tumour promoters; this has for instance been proven for airborne particulate matter (APM) (Heussen, 1991).

Several oncogene products tend to disrupt intercellular communications; among them the pp^{60} product of the src oncogene, *ras*, *mos* and *neu*.

Impairments in GJ intercellular communication can be evaluated through a series of *in vitro* assays, such as metabolic cooperation, fluorescent dye transfer and electrical coupling. None of them is fully satisfactory due to the organ specificity of many tumour promoters, making extrapolations from one cellular system to another somewhat hazardous.

4.4.3. Intercellular Adhesion

The necessary cooperation between adhesion molecules and molecules involved in cell-to-cell communication has been mentioned in the previous subsection. Indeed several types of adhesion molecules participate in the regulation of cellular differentiation and the maintenance of tissue integrity, and the down-regulation of these molecules has been implicated in the neoplastic process, although rather in its later stages.

Four main groups of adhesion molecules have been identified: integrins, cadherins, selectins and the immunoglobulin superfamily (Hynes and Lander, 1992); they mediate adhesion not only from cell to cell, but also with extracellular matrix macromolecules to which they act as receptors. *Integrins* are heterodimers composed of α subunits (at least 14 types) and β subunits (at least 8 types) resulting in at least 20 identified combinations (Hynes, 1992) acting as receptors for fibronectin, vitronectin, fibrinogen, laminin and collagen (Hynes, 1992); they also mediate signalling events. *Cadherins* are calcium-dependent transmembrane adhesion molecules representing the major mediators of intercellular interaction; several subclasses have been described: E-cadherin, uvomorulin, L-CAM. Increased invasive and metastatic potential has been reported upon loss of E-cadherin expression (Vleminckx et al., 1991).

The *immunoglobulin superfamily* of adhesion molecules includes at least thirty identified members, of which the most intensively studied are the neural cell adhesion molecule, N-CAM, and carcino-embryonic antigen CEA.

The members of this superfamily are characterized by the presence of several extracellular domains corresponding to the immunoglobulin constant domains: five for N-CAM, seven for CEA; the variable domains of the immunoglobulins are lacking in the adhesion molecules clearly illustrating fundamental differences in function.

The *neural cell adhesion molecule* corresponds to a family of closely related sialoglycoproteins, involved in cell-cell interactions through homotypic binding. This binding occurs through the outer three of the five immunoglobin domains in adult tissues, mainly brain and muscle; in these tissues only the fifth IG domain closest to the cell membrane, is moderately sialylated. In embryonic tissues, but also in tumours with neuroendocrine differentiation such as small-cell lung cancer (SCLC), the sialylation is much heavier – up to three times more sialic acid being bound: this induces a bending in the extracellular domain of NCAM that reduces its adhesion properties (Thiery and Boyer, 1992; Michalides et al., 1994). Soluble forms of NCAM do exist and allow for its detection not only in culture media, but also in serum. Serum levels have been found to be significantly higher in patients with extensive disease than in those with limited disease, and in those with active vs quiescent disease (Ledermann et al., 1994). The highest specificity seems to be obtained when using an antibody directed against the α-(2,8) polysialylated side chain of NCAM, as this polysialylation occurs rarely in healthy subjects (Jaques et al., 1993).

We may infer from this observation that NCAM alterations are rather late events in carcinogenesis and that characteristic patterns rather are related to well-established tumours.

While *carcino-embryonic antigen* (CEA) has been first described in relation with digestive cancers (Gold and Freedman, 1965; Thomson et al., 1969) and is widely used as a "tumour marker" in clinical oncology to monitor treatment results and disease evolution, it has soon been recognized that this membrane glycoprotein also occurs in non-malignant conditions (Herbeth and Bagrel, 1980), and that its serum levels tend to be more elevated in conditions carrying a higher risk of developing cancer, such as smoking, ageing and some chronic inflammatory diseases. Higher CEA serum levels have been positively correlated with residence in industrial areas (Schlipköter et al., 1978) or with diverse occupational settings (Pluygers et al., 1992). Follow-up studies of a large asymptomatic population have brought striking evidence that higher CEA levels correlated with the risk of subsequent cancer development, above-threshold levels corresponding to a tenfold increase in risk (Pluygers et al., 1986) and making CEA a marker of the promotional phase of carcinogenesis (Pluygers et al., 1990). The exact mode of action of CEA has remained unresolved; its structural relationship to the immunoglobulin superfamily has made it to be considered as an accessory adhesion molecule (Benchimol et al., 1989). Very recently, the finding has been published that changes in the expression of CEA can lead to alterations in the expression of other – unrelated – adhesion molecules and contribute to the general deregulation of adhesion interactions that is frequently observed in tumour cells (Grimm and Johnson, 1995) and possibly also in premalignant conditions. It is therefore possible that progressive alterations in adhesion molecules as well as in intercellular communication structures contribute to the transformation of the initiated cells.

4.4.4. Cell-Surface Structures

Cell surface carbohydrates undergo remarkable alterations during differentiation, development and carcinogenesis (Muramatsu, 1988; Itzkowitz and Kim, 1986). Blood group antigens participate in this process and have been the focus of considerable interest, mainly directed to the epitopes characteristic of the Lewis (Le) antigens. The blood group determinants are carried on the terminal carbohydrate chains of the core glycolipids and glycoproteins; two basic structures – called type 1 and type 2 – have been identified for these carbohydrate chains. Fucosylation of the type 1 structure leads to the expression of Le^a and Le^b antigens, while fucosylation of the type 2 structure leads to the expression of Le^x and Le^y antigens (see Figures 4.7 and 4.8).

These different antigens are recognized by specific monoclonal antibodies, and so are related structures of increasing complexity. For instance, 2-6 sialylated Le^a is identified by the MoAb FH-7; 2-3 sialyl Le^a by the MoAb CA19-9 (a widely used clinical tumour marker); dimeric sialyl Le^{x-i} (also called SLX) by MoAb FH-6; dimeric and trimeric forms of Le^x and extended forms of Le^y can also be identified (Kawai et al., 1993). It is important to identify the extended forms of the Lewis antigens (sialylated Le^a and Le^x, extended Le^y), as these are preferentially synthesized by malignant cells, but also by premalignant dysplastic cells, making them good candidates not only for cancer – but also for carcinogenesis markers (Hakomori et al., 1984; Kim et al., 1988). High levels of CA19-9, SLX and extended Le^y have been repeatedly reported in malignant and premalignant tissues, as well as in serum, in relation, with the development of several cancer types: colon (Waldock et al., 1989); stomach (Sakamoto et al., 1989); pancreas (Kim et al., 1988); pulmonary adenocarcinoma (Kawai et al., 1993); adenocarcinoma generally (Singhal et al., 1990).

The relevance of polysialylation to carcinogenesis has been mentioned in the previous subsection. On the other hand, as sialic acid (N-acetylneuraminic acid) usually occurs as a terminal component of the carbohydrate chains of glycolipids and glycoproteins, it can be shed or secreted form the cell surface and assessed in blood. Several studies have demonstrated elevated levels in malignant conditions (Musset, 1985; Shamberger, 1986); acute phase reactions also increase the levels of sialic acid, mainly in inflammatory and rheumatoid diseases. In cancer-bearing subjects, the highest specificity is observed for Lipid-Associated Sialic Acid (LASA) (Katopodis et al., 1982).

Anomalous expression of blood group antigens (A in A-negative subjects, B in B-subjects) is occasionally observed, due to aberrant fucosylation or sialylation leading to aberrant oligosaccharide expression in neoplastic cells.

Worthy to be mentioned is the membrane glycoprotein called CD 44, that functions

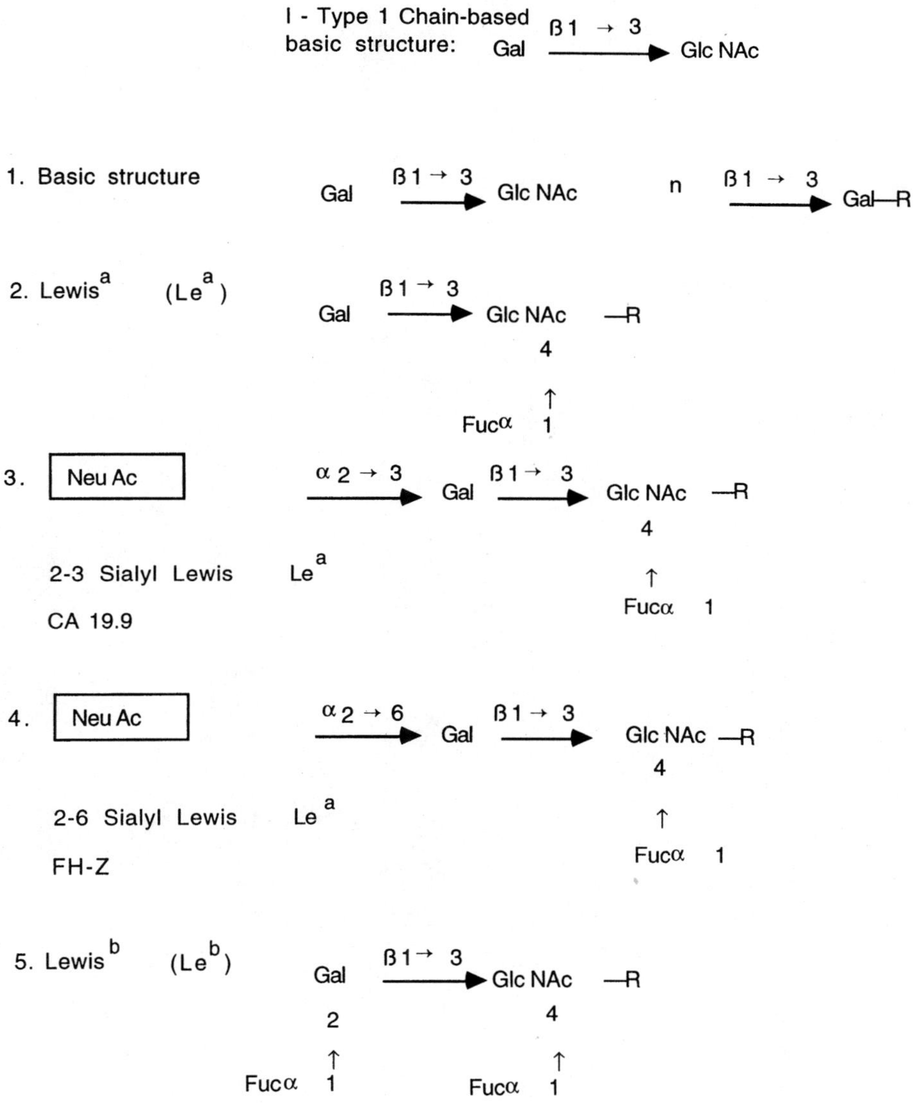

I - Type 1 Chain-based basic structure: Gal $\xrightarrow{\beta 1 \rightarrow 3}$ Glc NAc

1. Basic structure
Gal $\xrightarrow{\beta 1 \rightarrow 3}$ Glc NAc n $\xrightarrow{\beta 1 \rightarrow 3}$ Gal—R

2. Lewis^a (Le^a)
Gal $\xrightarrow{\beta 1 \rightarrow 3}$ Glc NAc —R
4
↑
Fucα 1

3. Neu Ac $\xrightarrow{\alpha 2 \rightarrow 3}$ Gal $\xrightarrow{\beta 1 \rightarrow 3}$ Glc NAc —R
4
↑
Fucα 1

2-3 Sialyl Lewis Le^a

CA 19.9

4. Neu Ac $\xrightarrow{\alpha 2 \rightarrow 6}$ Gal $\xrightarrow{\beta 1 \rightarrow 3}$ Glc NAc —R
4
↑
Fucα 1

2-6 Sialyl Lewis Le^a

FH-Z

5. Lewis^b (Le^b)
Gal $\xrightarrow{\beta 1 \rightarrow 3}$ Glc NAc —R
2 4
↑ ↑
Fucα 1 Fucα 1

Gal: Galactose; Glc Nac: N-acetylglucosamine

Tuc: Tucota; Neu Ac: N-acetylneuraminic (Sialic acid)

R: core glycolipid or glycoprotein

In the boxes: sialic acid

The identifying monoclonal antibodies are mentioned under the antigen and underlined with a dobled line (CA 19.9, FH-7, etc.)

Figure 4.7: *Structures of blood group related antigens I*

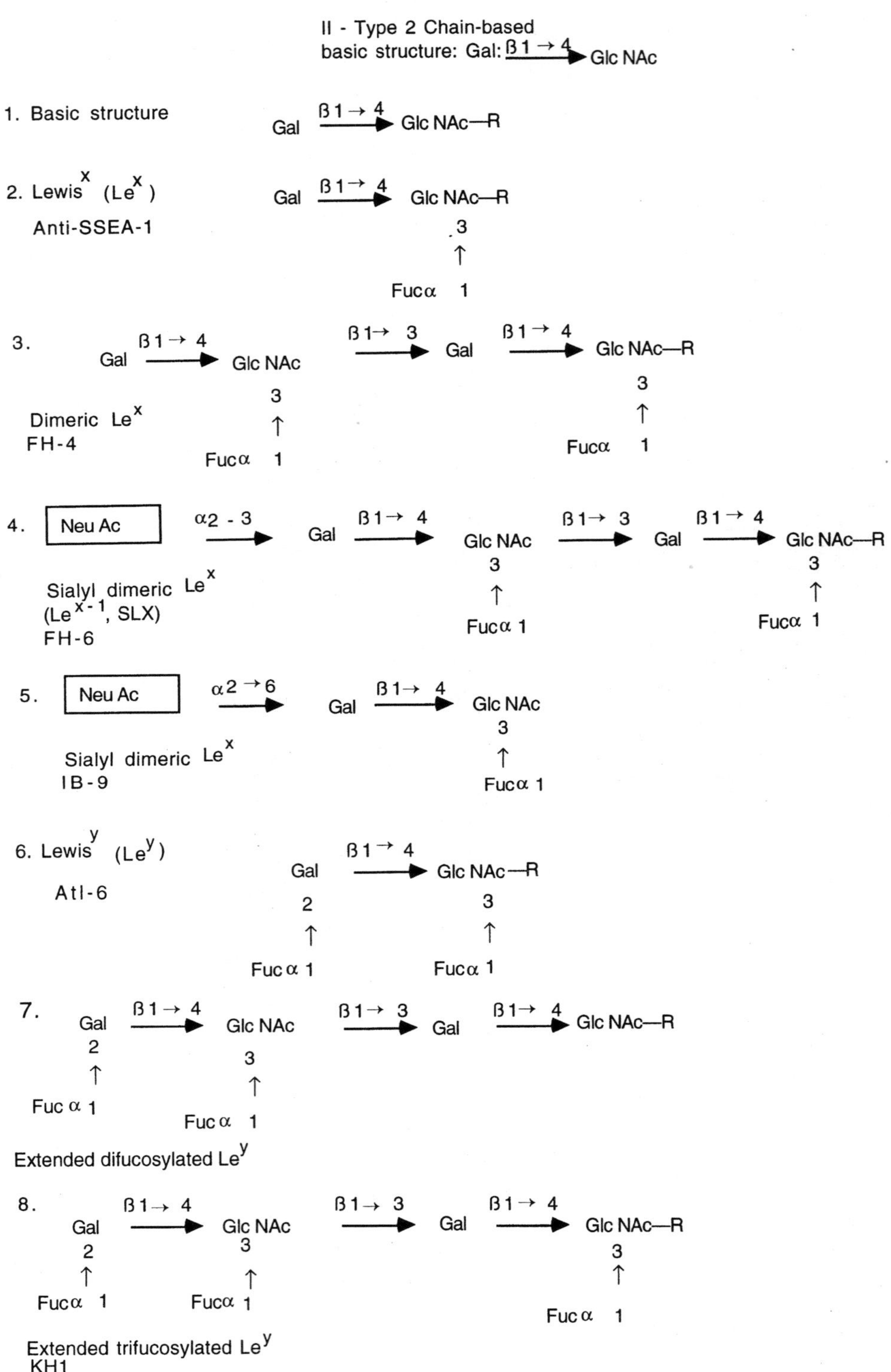

Figure 4.8: *Structures of blood group related antigens II*

as a receptor for the extracellular matrix glycan, hyaluronan (Aruffo et al., 1990). CD 44 exists under two major isoforms: a protein product with a molecular weight of $\pm$ 90,000, present in normal serum, and an alternately spliced variant (CD44v) of higher molecular weight; 130,000 - 160,000. This latter variant is predominantly expressed in tumour cells, in which standard CD 44 expression is lost or reduced (Birch et al., 1991; Shtivelman and Bishop, 1991). Hyaluronan (hyaluronic acid) is a polysaccharid consisting of repeating disaccharide units of N-acetyl-D-glucosamine and D-glucuronic acid; it is a major constituent of the extracellular matrix, believed to create a low resistance matrix that facilitates cell motility. Elevated serum CD 44 levels have been reported in gastric and colon cancer cases (Guo et al., 1994), as well as Non-Small-Cell-Lung-Cancers (NSCLC) (Penno et al., 1994); this elevation could be mediated by *ras* and *myc* overexpression (Penno et al., 1994); a functional link between p21*ras* and a cell surface hyaluronan binding protein has been suggested (Turley and Auersperg, 1989). It has been shown that the invasion of normal tissues by glioma cells is mediated by CD 44, as well as adhesion to the extracellular matrix proteins fibronectin, vitronectin, laminin and collagen I (Merzak et al., 1994).

High levels of Hyaluronan in serum or in pleural effusions have been associated with malignant disease and – in the latter case – specifically with mesothelioma for which it has been considered to be diagnostic (Frebourg et al., 1987). This finding has however been challenged (Hillerdal et al., 1991), and it seems that high serum values are in fact correlated with rather advanced malignant disease of any origin, as well as with some benign conditions. It does not allow the differential diagnosis between malignant mesothelioma and other malignant pulmonary conditions (Pluygers et al., 1991-1992). The potential role of hyaluronan in carcinogenesis is illustrated by the finding that its synthesis is enhanced by several growth factors such as IGF-I, EGF and PDGF, and inhibited by the tyrosine kinase inhibitor genistein (Honda et al., 1991; Heldin et al., 1992). Interestingly, it has been demonstrated that specific hyaluronan binding sites (including CD 44) are present on human malignant mesothelioma, cells but absent on normal human mesothelial cells (Asplund and Heldin, 1994).

4.4.5. Miscellaneous Determinants

The topics mentioned in this subsection will not be given full discussion in spite of their relevance to the carcinogenic process generally; it has been considered, however, that they do not directly participate in the basic mechanisms of carcinogenesis. On the other hand, expert up-to-date reviews are available.

4.4.5.1. Immune Status The concept of immunosurveillance has been developed by Burnet (1965) and postulates that tumour cells, being antigenically different, are identified by a healthy immune system and eliminated by it. Immunodysfunction or suppression, acquired or constitutional, will deteriorate this function and allow the proliferation of the malignant cells. Abundant evidence has proceeded from the observation of transplant recipients, especially renal transplant recipients, in whom the incidence of several cancers shows a considerable increase, a relatively short time after transplantion

(2 - 3 years). For instance lip cancers show a 29fold increase in incidence, Non-Hodgkins Lymphomas a 28-49-fold, hepatobiliary carcinomas a 30fold, vulvar and anal carcinomas a 100fold and Kaposi Sarcoma (KS) a 400-500-fold increase (Penn 1988). Similar results are observed in patients receiving immunosuppressive theraphy for reasons other than organ transplantation (Kinlen, 1992). The extending AIDS epidemic has brougth further evidence of the cancer-enhancing effects of immunodeficiency: in AIDS patients the incidence of Kaposi's sarcoma has been estimated to be at least 20.000 times greater than in the general population (Beral et al, 1990); strong increases in high-grade B-cell lymphomas are also observed.

Presently, the better understanding of the mechanisms of the immune system, the identification of subsets of lymphocytes possessing specific functions, as well as of the cell surface structures and of the cytokines governing their interactions, have opened new avenues in our knowledge of the immunological control of tumour development (and in the development of immunotherapy).

4.4.5.2. Nutritional Status Undoubtedly carcinogenesis is influenced by numerous nutritional factors, both at the level of macro and micronutrients. The literature covering this topic is extremely bulky and only a few major points will be mentioned, among them are those that may have a broader influence on the carcinogenic process.

Macronutrients The influence of caloric uptake on carcinogenesis has been suspected ever since dietary restriction had been show to inhibit tumour growth in mice (Moreschi, 1909; Rous, 1914) and confirmed in the fourties by the pioneering studies of Tannenbaum on mamary tumour incidence in mice: in the underfed group, 2% develop tumours versus 40% in the controls (Tannenbaum, 1940; Tannenbaum, 1942). These preliminary experimental data have triggered a vast amount of observations and research and relevant human data have become available. For instance in a huge prospective study, Lew and Garfinkel (1979) compared the relative risks – after accounting for potential biases – of dying from several cancers in average-weight men and women (risk = 100%) and overweight men (i.e. at least 40% heavier than average): colon/rectum 173%; prostate 129%; pancreas 162%; stomach 188%; all cancers 133%; - or women: endometrium 542%; uterine cervix 239%; gall bladder 358%; kidney 203%; colon/rectum 122%; breast 153%; any cancer 155%. Men and women with less than 85% of the average weight had significantly lower risks. These findings have been confirmed later by a series of organ-targeted studies, e.g. those of Snowdon et al. (1984) demonstrating a relative risk of 2.5 for prostate cancer in overweight men, and of Phillips and Snowdon (1985) showing a RR of 2.8 for rectal cancer in both sexes combined and of 3.3 for colon cancer in overweight (percent of desirable weight $\geq$ 125) males among Californian Seventh-Day Adventists. Body weight has been shown to correlate with breast cancer risk, mainly in postmenopausal women (London et al., 1989; Tretli, 1989) and so does – even more strongly – body height (Baanders and de Waard, 1992). While a general consensus prevails about the positive correlation between bodyweight and cancer risk, the importance of the energy source still is a matter of controversy, although there are indications that lipid-derived calories play a major role (for discussion: Prentice et al., 1989). A recent experimental study on skin tumourigenesis in SENCAR mice, after initiation by DMBA and promotion by TPA, has compared the effects of fat calories restriction and carbohydrate calories restriction. Both protocols resulted in comparable inhibition of skin carcinomas, but fat restriction more strongly inhibited papillomas; caloric restriction reduced protein kinase C activity, possibly through reduced phosphotidylinositol turnover (Birt et al., 1992). There is also accumulating evidence of the importance of the types of fatty acids consumed in the form of triglycerides. For instance Alaska and Greenland Eskimos, as well as Cretans (Creta island) have a rather low cancer incidence in spite of a very high percentage of calories derived from dietary fat. The former consume large quantities of n-3 highly polyunsaturated fatty acids such as eicosapentaenoic acid (c 20:5, n-3) and docosahexaenoic acid (c 22:6, n-3) and the latter the mono-unsaturated monoenoic fatty acids such as oleic acid found in olive oil. This is in confirmation of numerous experimental data showing the promotion-inhibitory effects of the aforementioned fatty acids, whereas on the contrary n-6, polyunsaturated fatty acids such as linoleic acid (C 18:2) enhanced tumour (notably mammary) development (for discussion, see Welsch, 1992). An optimal amount of about 4.4% of linoleic acid in diet is required to ensure maximum mammary tumour development in the rat (Ip et al., 1985), and there are reasons to believe that similar considerations might apply to humans. Indeed, the role of n-6 polyunsaturated fatty acids in carcinogenesis is supported by a line of evidence, since many years (see e.g. Kort et al., 1987).

These findings raise the questions of mechanisms underlying the relationship between caloric intake, source of the calories, and carcinogenesis. An array of theories have been proposed and recently discussed by Roe et al. (1995), in relation with the Biosure Study. As repeatedly emphasized in this review, the clonal expansion, i.e. the proliferation, of the initiated cells represents a major event in carcinogenesis (Cohen and Ellwein, 1990). Increased cell proliferation substantially increases the risk that DNA damage will be transmitted unrepaired to daughter cells, for lack of time to ensure adequate repair, and induce fixed mutations of which the rate will consequently be increased. Much of the endogenous damage inflicted to DNA is oxidative and is estimated to occur at an average of 10^4 times a day per cell in humans (Ames, 1989); other mechanisms include demethylation, deamination and depurination.

Methods for identifying oxidative DNA damage have been mentioned in an earlier section; these urinary biomarkers of oxidative DNA base damage (UBODBD) have been shown to correlate strongly with the amount of caloric intake, in such a way that caloric restriction in human results in the supression of UBODBD excretion, reflecting a reduction in levels of oxidative DNA damage (Simic and Bergtold, 1991). Cell proliferation has been found to be reduced by food restriction in several experimental systems (Heller et al., 1990; Lok et al., 1990) as well in humans. The particular relevance of n-6 polyunsaturated fatty acids to carcinogenesis results from their potency to induce peroxidation of inner cell membrane lipids, with subsequent free radical generation.

These studies indicate that caloric restriction down-modulates both cell proliferation and oxidative DNA damage – two major determinants of carcinogenesis –, hence reducing tumourigenesis. The available human data are in perfect agreement with those of two huge experimental studies: the already reported Biosure study (Roe et al., 1995) on 1200 animals, and the MRL study – on 1400 rats – reported by Keenan and Soper (1995). Based on the estimation by Doll and Peto (1981) that diet is responsible for approximately 35% of all cancers deaths, and that cancer itself accounts for 20 - 25% of all deaths, Lutz and Schlatter (1992) have calculated that in westernized countries, over-nutrition could be responsible, by its effects on cancer alone, for 60,000 out of every million deaths.

In some instances, restrictions in protinaceous components of the diet also have been related to reduced cancer risk. Of particular interest are the dietary sources of the methylated amino-acid methionine, and its precursor choline. There is abundant evidence that DNA methylation (i.e. its contents of 5-methylcytosine [5 MeC]) plays a variety of roles in carcinogenesis (Laird et al., 1995; Counts and Goodman, 1995). In rats, a methyl-deficient diet causes the depletion of S-adenosylmethionine pools, followed by DNA hypomethylation, itself inducing altered gene expression yielding patterns closely resembling those occurring in the livers of animals exposed to cancer promoting chemicals (Wainfan and Poirier, 1992). Increased levels of expression of c-*myc*, c-*fos* and C-Ha-*ras* genes are indicative of greater proneness to cancer. Global DNA hypomethylation and site-specific gene hypomethylation are reported in several human neoplasia (Goelz and Vogelstein, 1985). In humans as well as in rodents, gene hypomethylation seems to enhance transcription (Baylin et al., 1992). Increased hypomethylation is reported with increasing grade of cervical neoplasia, suggesting that global hypomethylation may serve as a biochemical marker of cervical neoplasia (Kim et al., 1994). It is suggested that choline deficiency – leading to methionine deficiency – might induce increased cancer risk, although DNA hypermethylation is reported in some human cancers; thus regional chromosome hypermethylation is believed to inactivate tumour supressor genes (reported in Wainfan and Poirier, 1992).

Micronutrients The influence of micronutrients, on the other hand, has long been suspected (Wattenberg, 1983 and subsequent publications) and has received a decisive impetus after the publication of Peto's history-making paper (Peto et al., 1981) about the anti-carcinogenic effects of *β-carotene*. For several of the micronutrients considered to potentially mediate carcinogenesis, this activity is related to their anti-oxidant properties.

β-carotene and *carotenoids* rank among the most extensively studied anti-oxidants. *β-carotene* is a non-stoichiometric scavenger for singlet oxygen, a common reactive oxygen species (ROS); together with related carotenoids such as lycopene and canthaxanthin, it has been shown to lower the risk for several cancers, confirming Peto's report; this effect seems to be unrelated to provitamin A activity (Micozzi et al., 1990). Carotene and carotenoids are abundant in yellow-green vegetables and in some fruits, of wich the consumption has been associated with reduced cancer risks, especially for lung cancer (Connett et al., 1989; Ziegler, 1991, Stähelin et al., 1991), but also for other cancers; in specific cancers, carotenoids other than β-carotene may prove most effective (Ziegler et al., 1992). Remission of precancerous lesions has also been evidenced. Among the invoked mechanisms, enhancement of immunocompetence should be considered in addition to ROS scavenging. An inverse correlation has been demonstrated between serum β-carotene and Tissue Polypeptide Antigen (TPA) levels (Pluygers and Sadowska, unpublished results). β-carotene reduces Ornithine Decarboxylase (ODC) activity, known to be associated with cell proliferation and tumour promotion (Bukin et al., 1993).

Tocopherols (α-Tocopherol, vitamin E) are stoichiometric liposoluble ·OH radical scavengers exerting their effects mainly in relation with lipid peroxidation of polyunsaturated fatty acids in cell membranes, often in combination with selenium. α-Tocopherol is regenerated by ascorbic acid (vitamin C). From the numerous studies that have been published, showing an inverse relationship between serum vitamin E levels and cancer incidence, we shall recall the large prospective finnish study involving 36265 individuals followed for 8 years, and demonstrating a protective effect, at least for some cancer sites (Knekt et al., 1991), including pancreas, urinary organs and nervous system in men, and breast, ovary and stomach in women.

The water-soluble *thiols* are acting both as free radical scavengers and as constituents of enzymatic systems. Glutathione (GSH) is the most important cellular thiol, being a substrate for several enzymes (peroxidases, transferases) involved in cellular anti-oxidant defence systems (De Flora and Ramel, 1988); GSH raises the threshold of susceptibility of the organism to several toxic and carcinogenic xenobiotics ("the glutathione threshold"). Intracellular GSH levels can be increased by the administration of precursors such as N-acetylcysteine (De Flora and Ramel, 1988), and its conjugation with a variety of electrophiles – resulting in their inactivation – is catalyzed by glutathione-transferases (GSTs), themselves inducible by a series of non-nutrient dietary constituents, including phenols, indoles, aromatic isothiocyanates, coumarins, diterpenes, nonpolar flavones, dithiolthiones and thiols (De Flora and Ramel, 1988; Wattenberg, 1992). Most of these are naturally occurring in "green-and-yellow" vegetables and some fruits, of which higher-than-usual consumption is advocated in several cancer-preventing diets (in association with the mono-unsaturated fatty acid present in olive oil) (Hill and Giacosa, 1992).

The inhibitory effect of *selenium* on carcinogenesis in experimental animals is well documented; reviewing 35 studies, Ip (1986) mentions decreased incidences in 31 among them. Being an absolute requirement for the normal functional activity of the seleno-enzyme glutathione-peroxidase, adequate nutritional supplies of selenium are crucial to ensure proper destruction of peroxides (Hochstein and Atallah, 1988). In humans, inverse associations between serum selenium levels and cancer incidence have been suggested by several studies (Shamberger et al., 1973; Salonen et al., 1984). More recent studies confirm these findings: in US rural counties forage selenium status is inversely (and significantly) related to cancers of the lung, rectum, bladder, esophagus and cervix (Clark et al., 1991), whereas selenium contents of nail clippings are inversely related to the incidence of oral cancer in men (Rogers et al, 1991). In a prospective study involving nearly 26,000 persons followed for 12 years, those who developed bladder cancer had significantly lower selenium serum levels (Helzlsouer et al., 1989). Some studies stress the enhanced efficacy when combining several anti-oxidants; selenium and vitamin E display a truly complementary action, as demonstrated by the large-scale Linxian County, China, nutrition intervention trial (Blot et al., 1993). In this study, involving 29584 adults, those receiving a daily supplementation with *β-carotene*, vitamin E and selenium for five years showed a significantly lower total mortality, mainly due to a reduction in cancer rates, especially stomach cancer (RR 0.79; 95% CI = 0.64 - 0.99).

Many *other micronutrients* are known to influence carcinogenesis – hence cancer incidence – through a variety of mechanisms, interfering with basic steps in carcinogenesis, with immune function, etc. To be mentioned: ascorbic acid, riboflavin, zinc, manganese, calcium. Transition metals such as iron, copper, cobalt, are of special interest because of their capacity to enhance ROS formation by catalyzing Fenton-type reactions. *Iron* will be briefly considered.

Indeed, whereas most of the oxygen consumed in biological systems is reduced to water, a small fraction escapes this pathway and is transformed in hydrogen peroxide (H_2O_2) which undergoes metal-catalyzed decomposition to yield the extremely reactive hydroxyl radical (·OH). This reaction – the socalled Fenton reaction – requires the indispensable presence of a transition metal, most often *iron* (Gutteridge and Halliwell, 1989). As a consequence, the presence of an excess of iron enhances the production of ·OH radicals, and might increase the incidence of cancer. Actually, this assumption is supported by a line of evidence. A relation between high iron stores and overall cancer risk has been reported (Stevens et al., 1988) as well as for some specific sites: colon (Stevens et al., 1988), rectum (Freudenheim et al., 1990; Knekt et al., 1994) and lung. Asbestos-related cancers occur in individuals exposed to fibres with high iron contents, the amphiboles, rather than to the iron-poor chrysotile; serum levels of ferritin, the iron storage protein, and also a Fenton reactant, often are extremely high in mesothelioma patients (Pluygers et al., 1991-1992). High ferritin levels are also observed in chronic inflammatory diseases, considered to increase the risk of neoplastic development.

Assessment of anti-oxidants in humans In addition to the few anti-oxidant components that have been considered, numerous exogenous – but also endogenous – anti-oxidants are present in human plasma, also including vitamin C, uric acid, bilirubin, albumin and others. All these anti-oxidants may be assessed separately, but this represents a considerable amount of labour and skill and does not account for any synergistic effects. Therefore methods to measure the total cumulative anti-oxidant capacity of the serum (Cao et al., 1993) or – better – of the plasma (Ghiselli et al., 1993) represent important contributions by providing a simple and single parameter. The Total Radical-trapping Anti-oxidant Parameter (TRAP) defined by Ghiselli et al. (1993) appears to be a useful biomarker in human carcinogenesis studies.

4.5. CONCLUSION

The spectacular developments that have occurred over the last few years in biochemical and biological research (especially at the molecular level), provide us with tools capable of analyzing and quantitating many intricate mechanisms of carcinogenesis, as well as variations in interindividual susceptibility to carcinogens, differences in DNA repair capacity and influences of concomitant endogenous or exogenous carcinogens. It is presently perfectly clear that biomarkers are able to identify not only the very initial, exposure-related steps of carcinogenesis in humans, or the very late alterations characteristic of overt cancer but also – and more importantly – the relevant intermediate steps indicative of physiological alterations occurring prior to truly pathological effects, and hence predictive for increased risk of the development of cancer (Depledge et al., 1993). These alterations may be monitired over time, making *molecular epidemiology* a major component of cancer prevention studies, allowing for the evaluation of their effectiveness as well as for primary prevention.

The biochemical and cellular responses that may be identified directly in humans through the use of biomarkers preclude – to a large extent – the uncertainty proceeding from animal-to- human extrapolations as well as from other factors related with uncertainty (Amaral-Mendes, 1992). They also enable to monitor – directly in humans – the effects of exposures to low levels of complex carcinogen mixtures, frequently prevailing under real conditions, and very alien to experimental settings. Relevant biomarkers in humans yield data that may be directly incorporated into risk assessment models.

One of the difficulties resulting from the multitude of the present available human biomarkers is the inevitable selection. This selection should not be carried out randomly, but it should be based on the precise mechanistic knowledge of the carcinogenesis pathway, that is often differing from one carcinogen (or group of carcinogenic agents) to another. For instance, in nuclear receptor-mediated carcinogenesis, it will be useless to assess cytoplasmic signal transduction pathways. So the concept of "biomarker spectra" emerges, comparable to that of "mutational spectra" characteristic of exposures to specific carcinogens. It will generally be advisable to have recourse to a tiered approach, a set of "general" non-specific biomarkers being assessed in a first phase approach, to be eventually completed by a second – or a third – tier of more specific biomarkers, if necessary (Depledge et al., 1993; Pluygers, 1995). In any case, an accurate evaluation will depend on the use of a broad set of biomarkers, addressing different aspects of the carcinogenic process.

In human medicine generally, there exists a long tradition of the use of biomarkers in assessing multiple escapes from the homeostatic health status (Amaral Mendes et al., 1995). Presently, molecular biology and chemistry provide accurate approaches for assessing carcinogenesis and monitoring its evolution in humans.

4.6. ACKNOWLEDGMENTS

The authors want to express their sincere appreciation to Professor Georg Luebeck from the Fred Hutchinson Cancer Research Center in Seattle, WA, for reading the manuscript and providing valuable advice. They also appreciate the important contribution of Werner Wosniok from the Statistics Institute, Bremen University, Bremen, FRG, for his helpful contribution to the final layout of the chapter.

4.7. REFERENCES

Aaltonen LA, Peltomaki P, Leach FS, Sistonen P, Pylkkänen L, Mecklin JP, Järvinen H, Powell SM, Jen J, Hamilton SR, Petersen GM, Kinzler KW, Vogelstein B and de la Chapelle A. "Clues to the pathogenesis of familial colorectal cancer". Science 1993; 260: 812-816.

Aaronson SA, Rubin JS, Finch PW, Wong J, Marchese C, Falco J, Taylor WG and Kraus MH "Growth factor-regulated pathways in epithelial cell proliferation". Am. Rev. Respir. Dis. 1990; 142:S7-S10.

Aaronson SA. "Growth Factors and Cancer". Science, 1991; 254:1146-1153.

Abate C, Patel L, Rauscher FJ III and Curran T. "Redox regulation of *fos* and *jun* DNA-binding activity *in vitro*. Science 1990; 249:1157-1161.

Aflalo E, Wolfson M, Ofir R and Weinstein Y. "Elevated Activities of Protein Kinase C and Tyrosine Kinase correlate to leukemic cell aggressiveness". Int. Jl. Cancer 1992; 50: 136-141.

Aitio A, Aitio M-L, Camus A-M, Cardis E and Bartsch H. "Cytochrome P-450 isozyme pattern is related to individual susceptibility to Diethylnitrosamine-induced liver cancer in rats". Japn. J. Cancer Res. 1991; 82:146-156.

Albertini RJ, O'Neill JP, Heintz NH and Kelleher P. "Alterations in the hprt gene in human *in vivo* derived 6-thioguanine resistant T-lymphocytes". Nature 1985; 316:369-371.

Alexandrova N, Niklĭnki J, Bliskovsky V, Otterson GA, Blake M, Kaye FJ and Zajac-Kaye M. "The N-terminal domain of c-Myc associates with α-tubulin and microtubules *in vivo* and *in vitro*". Molcular and Cellular Biology 1995; 15: 5188-5195.

Alexandrow MG and Moses HL. "Transforming Growth Factor β and Cell Cycle Regulation". Cancer Research 1995; 55: 1452-1457.

Almoquera C, Shibata D, Forrester K, Martin J, Arnheim N and Perucho M. "Most human carcinomas of the exocrine pancreas contain mutant c-K-*ras* genes". Cell 1988; 53: 549-554.

Amaral-Mendes JJ, Pluygers E and Fariña J. "Environmental health and ecotoxicology: an indispensable link". In: D.J. Rapport, C.L. Gaudet and P. Calow (Eds). "Evaluating and monitoring the health of large-scale ecosystems". Springer-Verlag, Berlin. NATO ASI Series, Vol. I28; 1995; pp 77-93.

Amaral-Mendes JJ. "Biological monitoring-based biomarkers in cancer risk assessment". Arq. Patol., 1992; 24:51-67.

Ambrosone CB, Freudenheim JL, Graham S, Marshall JR, Vena JE, Brasure JR, Laughlin R, Nemoto T, Michalek AM, Harrington A, Ford TD and Shields PG. "Cytochrome P450 1A1 and Glutathione S-Transferase (M1) genetic polymorphisms and post-menopausal breast cancer risks". Cancer Research 1995; 55:3483-3485.

Ames BN, Durston We, Yamasaki E and Lee FD."Carcinogens are mutagens: a simple test system combining liver homogenates for activation and bacteria for detection" – Proc. Nat. Acad. Sci US, 1973; 70:2281-2285.

Ames BN, Mc Cann J and Yamasaki E. "Methods for detecting carcinogens and mutagens with the Salmonellal mammalian-microsome mutagenicity test" – Mutation Research 1975; 31: 347-364.

Ames BN. "Mutagenesis and carcinogenesis: endogenous and exogenous factors". Environmental and Molecular Mutagenesis, 1989; 14 (Suppl 16): 66-77.

Angelopoulou K, Diamandis EP, Sutherland D, Kellen JA and Bunting PS. "Prevalence of serum antibodies against the p53 tumour suppressor gene protein in various cancers". Int J Cancer 1994; 58:480-487.

Antoniades HN, Bravo MA, Avila RE, Galanopoulos T, Neville-Golden T, Maxwell M and Sehman M. "Platelet-derived growth factor in idiopathic pulmonary fibrosis". J. Clin. Invest 1990; 86:1055-1064.

Arends MJ and Wyllie AH. "Apoptosis: mechanisms and roles in pathology". Int. Rev. Exp. Pathol. 1991; 32:223-254.

Aruffo A, Stamenkovic I, Melnick M, Underhill CB and Seed B. "CD44 is the principal cell surface receptor for hyaluronate". Cell 1990; 61:1303-1313.

Ashby J. "The value and limitation of short-term genotoxicity assays and the inadequacy of current cancer bioassay chemical selection criteria" In: C. Maltoni and IJ Selikoff (eds) "Living in a chemical world – Occupational and environmental significance of industrial carcinogens" pp. 133-138. Annals of the New York Academy of Science, Vol 534. The New York Academy of Sciences, New York 1988.

Asplund T and Heldin P. "Hyaluronan receptors are expressed on human malignant mesothelioma cells but not on normal mesothelial cells". Cancer Research, 1994; 54:4516-4523.

Athas WF, Hedayati MA, Matanoski GM, Farmer ER and Grossman L. "Development and Field-Test Validation of an Assay for DNA Repair in Circulating Human Lympocytes". Cancer Res. 1991; 51:5786-5793.

Autrup H. "Human exposure to genotoxic carcinogens: methods and their limitations" – J. Cancer Res. Clin. Oncol. 1991; 117: 6-12.

Autrup H; Seremet T; Wakhisi J and Wasunna A. "Aflatoxin exposure measured by urinary excretion of aflatoxin B1-guanine adduct and hepatitis B virus infection in areas with different liver cancer incidence in Kenya". Cancer Res. 1987; 47:3430-3433.

Ayer DE, Kretzner L and Eisenman RN. "Mad: a heterodlimeric partner for Max that antagonizes Myc transcriptional activity". Cell 1993; 72:1-20.

Ayesh R, Idle JR, Ritchie JC, Crothers MJ and Hetzel MR. "Metabolic oxidation phenotypes as markers for susceptibility to lung cancer". Nature, 1984; 312:169-170.

Baanders An and de Waard F. "Breast Cancer in Europe: the importance of factors operating at an early age". Europ. Jl. Cancer Rev. 1992; 1: 285-291.

Bartek J, Iggo R, Gannon JV and Lane DP. "Genetic and immunochemical analysis of mutant p53 in human breast cancer cell lines". Oncogene 1990; 5:893-899.

Bartkova J, Lukas J, Strauss M and Bartek J. "Cell Cycle-related variation and tissue restricted expression of human Cyclin D1 protein". Jl. Pathology 1994; 172:237-245.

Bartsch H, Malaveille C, Camus A-M, Martel-Planche G, Brun G, Hautefeuille A, Sabadie N, Barbin A, Kuroki T, Drevon C, Piccoli C and Montesano R. "Validation and comparative studies on 180 chemicals with S. typhimurium strains and V79 Chinese hamster cells in the presence of various metabolizing systems" Mutation Research 1980; 76:1-50.

Baserga R, "The insulin-like growth factor I receptor: a key to tumour growth". Cancer Research 1995; 55:249-252.

Baylin SB, Makos M, Wu J, Yen R-WC, de Bustros A, Vertino P, et al. "Abnormal patterns of DNA methylation in human neoplasia: potential consequences for tumour progression". Cancer Cells 1992; 3:383-390

Bell DA, Taylor JA, Paulson DF, Robertson CN, Mohler JL and Lucier GW. "Genetic Risk and carcinogen exposure: a common inherited defect of the carcinogen-metabolism gene Glutathione S-Transferase M1 (GSTM1) that increases susceptibility to bladder cancer". Jl. Natl. Cancer Inst. 1993; 85: 1159-1164.

Bello-Fernandez C, Packham G and Cleveland JL. "The ornithine decarboxylase gene is a transcriptional target of c-Myc". Proc. Natl. Acad. Sci., USA, 1993, 90:7804-7808.

Ben-Mahrez K, Thierry D, Sorokine I, Danna-Muller A and Kohiyama M. "Detection of circulating antibodies against c-*myc* protein in cancer patient sera". Brit J. Cancer 1988; 57:529-534.

Benchimol S, Fuks A, Jothy S, Beauchemin N, Shirota K and Stanners CP. "Carcinoembryonic antigen, a human tumour marker, functions as an intercellular adhesion molecule". Cell 1989; 57:327-334.

Benner S, Lippman S, Wargovich M, Lee J, Velasco M, Martin J, Toth B and Hong WK. "Micronuclei as a biomarker for chemoprevention trials: results in a randomized study in oral pre-malignancy". Int. J. Cancer 1994; 59:457-459.

Beral V, Peterman TA, Berkelman RL and Jaffe HW. "Kaposi's sarcoma among persons with AIDS: a sexually transmitted infection?". Lancet 1990; 335:123-128.

Berek JS, Chung S, Kaldi K, Watson JM, Knox RM, Martinez-Maza O. "Serum interleukin-6 levels correlate with disease status in patients with epithelial ovarian cancer". Am. J. Obstet. Gynecol. 1991; 164:1038-1042.

Berenson JR, Koga H, Yang et al. "Frequent amplification of the *bcl*-1 locus in poorly differentiated squamous cell carcinoma of the lung". Oncogene 1990; 5:1343-1348.

Bergh JC. "Gene amplification in human lung cancer. The *myc* family genes and other proto-oncogenes and growth factor genes". Am. Rev. Respir. Dis 1990; 142:S20-S26.

Berhane K, Widersten M, Engström Å, Kozarich JW and Mannervik B. "Detoxification of base propenals and other, $\alpha\beta$-unsaturated aldehyde products of radical reactions and lipid peroxidation by human glutathione transferases. Proc. Natl. Acad. Sci., USA, 1994; 91:1480-1484.

Berlin A, Yodaiken RE and Henman BA (eds). "Assessment of toxic agents at the workplace"; Martinus Nyhoff Publishers, 1984.

Birch M, Mitchell S and Hart IR "Isolation and Charaterization of human melanoma cell variants expressing high and low levels of CD44". Cancer Research 1991; 51:6660- 6667.

Birrer MJ and Minna JD. "Genetic changes in the pathogenesis of lung cancer". Ann Rev. Med. 1989; 2:461-9.

Birt DF, Kris ES, Choe M and Pelling JC. "Dietary Energy and Fat effects on tumour promotion". Cancer Research (Suppl.) 1992; 52:2035s-2039s.

Bissonnette RP, Echeverri F, Mahboubi A and Green DR. "Apoptotic cell death induced by c-*myc* is inhibited by *bcl*-2". Nature 1992; 359:552-554.

Björklund B, Lundblad G and Björklund V. "Antigenicity of pooled human malignant and normal tissue by cyto-immunological techniques II. Nature of tumour antigen". Int. Archs. Allergy appl. Immunol. 1958; 12:241-261.

Björklund B. "Tumour markers TPA, TPA-S and Cytokeratins. A working hypothesis". Tumordiagnostik U. Ther. 1992; 13:78-80.

Blay JY, Negriez S, Combaret V, Attali S, Goillot E, Merrouche Y, Mercatello A, Ravault A, Tourani JM and Moskovtchenko JF. "Serum level of interleukin 6 as a prognosis factor in metastatic renal cell carcinoma". Cancer Res 1992; 52:3317-3322.

Blot WJ and17 others. "Nutrition intervention trials in Linxian, China: supllementation with specific vitamin/mineral combinations, cancer incidence and disease-specific mortality in the general population". Jl. Natl. Cancer Inst., 1993; 85:1483-1492.

Blum M, Demierre A, Grant D, Heim M and Meyer UA. "Molecular mechanism of slow acetylation of drugs and carcinogens". Proc. Natl. Acad. Sci. USA, 1991; 88:5237-5241.

Bonassi S. "Italian Study on the long-term effect of chromosome damage: Preliminary results of the Chromosome Aberration Cohort". Presented at the Nordtox 1994 Conference Interphase between Human Toxicology and Ecotoxicology", Skyping. Denmark, May 20-23, 1994 – Published as abstract in Pharmacol. Toxicol. 1994; 74 Suppl II: 15.

Boobis AR, Lynch AM, Murray S, de la Torre R, Solans A, Farré M, Segura J, Gooderham NJ and Davies DS. "CYP1A2-catalyzed conversion of dietary heterocyclic amines to their proximate carcinogens is their major route of metabolism in humans". Cancer Res., 1994; 54:89-94.

Boothman DA; Schlegel R and Pardee AB. "Anticarcinogenic potential of DNA-repair modulators". Mutation Research 1988, 202:393-411.

Bos JL. "*Ras* Oncogenes in Human Cancer: a Review. Cancer Research 1989; 49:4682-4689.

Bourne HR, Sanders Da and Mc Cormick F "The GTPase Superfamily: a conserved switch for diverse cell functions", Nature 1990; 348:125-132.

Brandt-Rauf PW, De Vivo I, Marion M-J and Hemminki K. "The molecular epidemiology of growth signal transduction proteins". J. Occup. Envir. Med. 1995; 37:77-83.

Brandt-Rauf PW and Niman HL. "Serum screening for oncogene protein in workers exposed to PCB's". Brit. Jl. Industr. Med. 1988; 45: 689-693.

Brandt-Rauf PW, Luo J-C, Carney WP, Smith S, De Vivo I, Milling C, Hemminki K, Koskinen H, Vainio H and Neugnut AI. "Detection of increased amounts of the extracellular domain of the c-*erb*B-2 oncoprotein in serum during pulmonary carcinogenesis in humans". Int. J. Cancer 1994; 56:383-386.

Brandt-Rauf PW, Smith S, Hemminki K, Koskinen H, Vainio H, Niman H and Ford J. "Serum oncoproteins and growth factors in asbestosis and silicosis patients". Int. J. Cancer 1992; 50:881-885.

Brandt-Rauf PW. "New Markers for Monitoring Occupational Cancer: the example of oncogene proteins". Jl. Occup. Med. 1988; 30:399-404.

Bravo R, Frank R, Blundell PA and Macdonald-Bravo H. "Cyclin-PCNA is the auxiliary protein of DNA polymerase delta". Nature (London) 1987; 326:515-517.

Brenner D, Jeffrey A, Latriano L, Wazneh L, Warburton D, Toor M, Pero R, Andrews L, Walles S and Perera F. "Biomarkers in styrene-exposed boat builders". Mutation Research 1991; 261:225-236.

Breuer B, Luo J-C, De Vivo I, Pincus M, Tatum AH, Daucher J, Minick R, Osborne M, Miller D, Nowak E, Cody H, Carney WP and Brandt-Rauf PW. "Detection of elevated c-*erb*B-2 oncopeptide in the serum and tissue in breast cancer". Med. Sci. Res. 1993; 21:383-384.

Bridges BA, Cole J, Arlett CF, Green MHL, Waugh APW, Beare D, Henshaw DL and Last RD. "Possible association between mutant frequency in peripheral lymphocytes and domestic radon concentrations": Lancet 1991; 237:1187-1189.

Brockmöller J, Kerb R, Drakoulis N, Staffeldt B and Roots I. "Glutathione S-transferase M1 and its variants A and B as host factors of bladder cancer susceptibility: a case-control study". Cancer Research 1994; 54: 4103-4111.

Bronner CE and 17 others, including Fishel R and Kolodner R. "Mutation in the DNA mismatch repair gene homolog hMLH1 is associated with hereditary non-polyposis cancer". Nature 1994; 368; 258-261.

Bryckaert MC, Eldor A, Fontenay M, Gazit A, Osherov N, Gilon C, Levitzki A and Tobelem G. "Inhibition of Plateled-derived growth factor-induced mitogenesis and tyrosine kinase activity in cultured bone marrow fibroblasts by Tyrphostins". Exper Cell Res. 1992; 199:255-261.

Bukin YV, Zaridze DG, Draudin-Kaylenko VA, Orlov EN, Sigacheva NA, Dawei F, Kurtzman MY, Schlenskaya IN, Gorbacheva ON, Nechipai AM, Kuvschinov YP, Poddubny BK and Maximovitch DM "Effect of *β-carotene* supplementation on the acitivity of ornithine decarboxylase (ODC) in stomach mucosa of patients with chronic gastritis". Europ. Jl. Cancer Prev., 1993; 2:61-68.

Burbach KM, Poland A and Bradfield CA. "Cloning of the Ah-receptor cDNA reveals a distinct ligand-activated transcription factor". Proc. Natl. Acad. Sci., USA, 1992; 89:8185-8189.

Burnet, FM. "Somatic mutation and chronic disease". Brit. Med. Jl. 1965; I:338-342. Butterworth BE and Slaga TJ (eds). "Non-genotoxic mechanisms in carcinogenesis" (Banbury Report 25) Cold Spring Harbor Laboratory, Cold Spring Harbor, 1987.

Butterworth BE. "Consideration of both genotoxic and non-genotoxic mechanisms in predicting carcinogenic potential" Mutation Research 1990; 239:117-132.

Cairns P, Mao L, Merlo A, Lee DJ, Schwab D, Eby Y, Tokino K, Van der Riet P, Blaugrund JE and Sidransky D. "Rates of p16 (MTS) mutations in primary tumours with 9p loss". Science 1994; 265:415-416.

Calleman CJ, Ehrenberg L; Jansson B; Osterman-Golkar S; Segerback D; Svensson K and Watchtmeister CA. "Monitoring and risk assessment by means of alkyl groups in hemoglobin in persons occupationally exposed to ethylene oxide". J. Environ. Pathol. Toxicol., 1978; 2:427-442

Camoglio PM, Di Renzo MF, Gaudino G, Ponzetto C and Prat M. "Tyrosine Kinase and control of cell proliferation". Am. Rev. Respi. Dis., 1990; 142:S16-S19.

Campen D, Maronpot R and Lucier G. "Dose-response relationships in promotion of rat hepatocarcinogenesis by 17-α ethinyl estradiol". J. Toxicol. Environ. Health 1990; 29:257-268.

Camplejohn RS, Brock A, Barnes DM, Gillett C, Raikundalia B, Kreipe H and Parwaresch MR. "Ki-S1, a novel proliferative marker: flow cytometric assessment of staining in human breast carcinoma cells". Brit Jl. Cancer 1993; 67:657-662.

Cao G, Alessio HM and Cutler RG. "Oxygen-Radical Absorbance Capacity (ORAC) assay for antioxidants". Free Radical Biol. Med., 1993; 14.303-311.

Caporaso NE, Hayes RB, Dosemeci M, Hoover RN, Idle J and Ayesh R. "Debrisoquine metabolic phenotype (MP), asbestos exposure and lung cancer". Proc. Ann. Meeting Am. Soc. Clin. Oncol., 1988; 6:229 (abstract 904).

Caporaso NE, Tucker MA, Hoover RN, Hayes RB, Pickle LW, Issaq HJ, Muschik GM, Green-Gallo L, Buivys D, Aisner S, Reseau JH, Trump BF, Tollerud D, Weston A and Harris CC. "Lung cancer and the debrisoquine metabolic phenotype". Jl. Natl. Cancer Inst., 1990; 82: 1264-1272.

Caporaso NE. "Study design and genetic susceptibility factors in the risk assessment of chemical carcinogens". Ann. Ist. Super. Sanità, 1991; 27:621-630.

Cardinali M, Pietraszkiewicz H, Ensley JF and Robbins KC "Tyrosine-phosphorylation as a marker for aberrantly regulated growth-promoting pathways in cell lines derived from head-and-neck malignancies". Int Jl.Cancer 1995; 61:98-103.

Caron de Fromentel C, May-Levin F, Mouriesse H, Lemerle J, Chandrasekaran K and May P. "Presence of circulating antibodies against cellular protein p53 in a notable proportion of children with B-cell lymphoma". Int J Cancer 1987; 39:185-189.

Carrano A and Moore D. "The rationale and methodology for quantifying sister chromatid exchange in humans". In: Heddle J (ed) Mutagenicity: New Horizons in Genetic Toxicology. Academic Press, New York, 1982, pp. 307-316.

Castagna M and Martely, I. "Overview of promotion as a mechanism in carcinogenesis" In: CC Travis (Ed) Biologically Based Methods for Cancer Risk Assessment, pp. 144-153 - Plenum Press, New York, 1989.

Castagna M. Takai Y, Kaibuchi K, Sano K, Kikkawa U and Nishizuka Y. "Direct activation of calcium-activated Phospholipid-dependent protein kinase by tumour-promoting phorbol esters". Jl. Biol. Chem. 1982; 257:7847-7851.

Cathcart R, Schweirs E, Saul RL and Ames BN. "Thymine glycol and thymidine glycol in human and rat urine: a possible assay for oxidative DNA damage". Proc. Nat. Acad. Sci. US, 1984; 81:5633-5637.

Cathcart R, Schwiers E, Saul RL and Ames BN "Thymine glycol and thymidine glycol in human and rat urine: a possible assay for oxidative DNA damage" Proc. Natl. Acad. Sci. USA, 1984; 81:5633-5637.

Cerutti PA "Mechanisms of action of oxidant carcinogens". Cancer Det. and Prev. 1989; 14:281-284.

Cerutti PA "Pro-oxidant states and tumour promotion". Science, 1985; 227:375-381 Chakrabarty S, Fan D and Varani J. "Modulation of differentiation and proliferation in human colon carcinoma cells by transforming growth factor-β1 and β2". Int. J. Cancer. 1990; 46: 493-499.

Chakrabarty S, Tobon A, Varani J and Brattain MG. "Induction of carcinoembryonic antigen secretion and modulation of protein secretion/expression and fibronectin/laminin expression in human colon carcinoma cells by transforming growth factor-β". Cancer Research 1988; 48: 4059-4064.

Clark LC, Cantor KP and Allayway WH. "Selenium in Forage Crops and cancer mortality in US counties". Archives Environm. Health, 1991; 46:37-42.

Cleaver JE. "Defective repair replication of DNA in xeroderma pigmentosum". Nature 1968; 218: 652-656.

Cohen SM and Ellwein LB. "Biological theory of carcinogenesis: implications for risk assessment". In: S Olin, W Farland, C Park, L Rhomberg, R Schenplein, T Starr and J Wilson (Eds). "Low-dose extrapolation of cancer risks: issues and perspectives". ILSI Press, Washington DC, 1995. Pp. 145-161.

Cohen SM and Ellwein LB. "Cell proliferation in carcinogenesis" – Science 1990; 249:1007-1011.

Cole J. Green MHL, James SE, Henderson L and Cole H. "A further assessment of factors influencing measurements of thioguanine resistant mutant frequency in circulating T- lymphocytes". Mutation Research, 1988; 204:493-507.

Connett JE, Kuller LH, Kjelsberg MO, Polk BF, Collins G, Rider A, and Hulley SB. "Relationship between carotenoids and Cancer. Cancer 1989; 64:126-134.

Cosma GN, Crofts F, Currie D, Wirgin I, Toniolo P and Garte Sj. "Racial differences in restriction fragment lenght polymorphism and mRNA inducibility of the human CYP1A1 gene". Cancer Epidem., Biomarkers, Prev., 1993; 2:53-57.

Counts JL and Goodman JI. "Alterations in DNA methylation may play a variety of roles in carcinogenesis". Cell 1995; 83:13-15.

Cox R, Debenham PG, Masson WK and Webb MBT. "Ataxia-telangiectasia: a human mutation giving high frequency misrepair of DNA double stranded scissions". Mol. Biol. Med. 1986; 3:229-244.

Crawford LV, Pim DC and Bulbrook RD. "Detection of antibodies against the cellular protein p53 in sera from patients with breast cancer". Int J Cancer 1982; 30:403-408.

Crocker J and Skilbeck N. "nucleolar organiser region associated protein in cutaneous melanocytic lesions: a quantitative study". Jl. Clin. Pathol. 1987; 40: 885-889.

Curran T and Franza BR, Jr. "Fos and Jun: the AP-1 connection" – Cell, 1988; 55:395-397.

Cuzick J, Routledge MN, Jenkins D and Garner C. "DNA adducts in different tissues of smokers and non-smokers". Inst. J. Cancer 1990; 45:673-678.

Davidoff AM, Iglehart JD and Marks JR. "Immune response to p53 is dependent upon p53/HSP 70 complexes in breast cancers". Proc. Natl. Acad. Sci. US, 1992; 89:3439-3442.

Daya-Grosjean L, Robert C, Drougard C, Suarez HG and Sarasin A. "High Mutation frequency in *ras* gene of skin tumours isolated from DNA-repair deficent xeroderma pigmentosum patients". Cancer Research 1993; 53:1629-1629.

De Biasi F, Del Sal G and Horan Hand P. "Evidence of enhancement of the *ras* oncogene protein product (p21) in a spectrum of human tumours". Int. Jl. Cancer 1989; 43:431-435.

De Ferrari M, Artuso M, Bonassi S, Bonatti S, Cavalieri Z, Pescatore D, Marchini E, Pisano V and Abbondandolo A. "Cytogenetic biomonitoring of an Italian population exposed to pesticides: chromosome aberration and sister-chromatid exchange analysis in pheripheral blood lymphocytes". Mutation Research 1991; 260:105-113.

De Flora S and Ramel C. "Mechanism of inhibitors of mutagenesis and carcinogenesis - Classification and overview". Mutation Research 1988; 202:285-306.

Denis M, Cuthill S, Wikstrom AC, Poellinger L and Gustafsson JA. "Association of the dioxin receptor with the M 90.000 heat shock protein: a structural kinship with the the gluco-corticoid receptor". Biochem Biophys. Res. Comm. 1988; 155:801-807.

Depledge MH, Amaral-Mendes JJ, Daniel B, Halbrook RS, Kloepper-Sams P, Moore MN and Peakall DB. "The conceptual basis of the biomarker approach". In DB Peakall and LR Shugart (Eds)

"Biomarkers: research and application in the assessment of environmental health". Springer Verlag, Berlin, NATO ASI series, Vol H68: 1993, pp 15-30.

Dewailly E; Dodin S; Verreault R; Ayotte P; Sauvé L; Morin J and Brisson J. "High organochlorine body burden in women with Estrogen-Receptor positive breast cancer" Jl. Nat. Cancer Inst. 1994; 86:232-237.

Di Renzo MF, Ferracini R, Naldini L, Giordano S and Comoglio PM. "Immunological detection of proteins phospohrylated at tyrosine in cells stimulated by growth factors or transformed by retroviral-oncogene-encoded proteins". Eur. Jl. Biochem. 1986; 158:383-391.

Digweed M. "Human genetic instability syndromes. Single gene defects with increased risk of cancer". Toxicology Letters, 1993; 67:259-281.

Doll R and Peto R. "The cause of cancer: quantitative estimates of avoidable risks of cancer in the US today" Jl. Natl. Cancer Inst. 1981; 66: 1191-1308.

Dreicer R and Wilding G. "Steroid Hormone Agonists and Antagonists in the treatment of Cancer". Cancer Investigation 1992; 10:27-41.

Duchrow M, Gerdes J and Schlüter C. "The proliferation associated Ki-67 protein: definition in molecular terms". Cell Prolif., 1994; 27:235-242.

Dumaz N, Drougard C, Sarasin A and Daya-Grosjean L. "Specific U-V-induced mutation spectrum in the p53 gene of skin tumours from DNA repair deficient xeroderma pigmentatosa patients". Proc. Natl. Acad. Sci., USA, 1993; 90:10529-10533.

Dunn BP; Vedal S; San RHC; Kwan WF; Nelems B; Enarson DA and Stich HF. "DNA adducts in bronchial biopsies". Int J. Cancer 1991; 48:485-492. Egan MJ and Crocker J. "Nucleolar organiser regions in pathology". Brit. Jl. Cancer 1992; 65:1-7.

Ehrenberg L. "Introduction to Molecular Dosimetry" In : CC Travis (Ed). "Use of Biomarkers in Assessing Health and Environmental Impacts of Chemical Pollutants" – NATO ASI Series, volume 250. Plenum Press, New York, 1993, pp 1-7.

El-Deiry WS, Tokino T, Velculescu VE, Levy DB, Parsons R, Trent JM, Lin D, Mercer WE, Kinzler KW and Vogelstein B. "WAF1, a potential mediator of p53 tumour suppression". Cell 1993; 75:817-825.

Essigmann JM and Wood L. "The relationship between the chemical structures and mutagenic specificities of the DNA lesions formed by chemical and physical mutagens". Toxicology Letters 1993; 67:29-39.

Evan GI, Wyllie AH, Gilbert CS, Littlewood TD, Land H, Brooks M, Waters CM, Penn LZ and Hancock DC. "Induction of apoptosis in fibroblasts by c-*myc* protein". Cell 1992; 69:119-128.

Evans HJ, Buckton KE, Hamilton GE and Carothers A. "Radiation induced chromosome aberrations in nuclear docky hard workers" – Nature 1979; 271:531-534. Evans RM. "The steroid and thyroid hormone receptor superfamily". Science 1988; 240:889- 895.

Ewen ME, Sluss HK, Whitehouse LL and Livingston DM. "TGF β inhibition of Cdk 4 synthesis in linked to cell cycle arrest". Cell 1993; 74: 1009-1020.

Falco JP, Taylor WG, Di Fiore PP, Weissman BE and Aaronson SA. "Interactions of growth factors and retroviral oncogenes with mitogenic signal transduction pathways of Batb/MK keratinocytes". Oncogene 1988; 2:573-578.

Favoni RE, de Cupis A, Ravera F, Cantoni C, Pirani P, Ardizzoni A, Noonan D and Biassoni R. "Expression and function of the insulin-like growth factor I system in human non- small-cell lung cancer and normal lung cell lines". Int. J. Cancer 1994; 56:858-866.

Fawson T and Gish GD. "SH2 and SH3 domains: from structure to function". Cell 1992; 71:359-362.

Feig DI, Reid TM and Loeb LA "Reactive Oxygen Species in Tumourigenesis" Cancer Research (Suppl) 1994; 54:1890S-1894S.

Fishel R, Lescoe MK, Rao MRS, Copeland NG, Jenkins NA, Garber J, Kane M and Kolodner R. "The human mutator gene homolog MSH2 and its association with hereditary non- polyposis colon cancer". Cell 1993; 75:1027-1038.

Flesch-Janys D, Berger J, Manz A, Nagel S and Ollroge L."Exposure to Polychlorinated Dibenzo-p-dioxins and furans and breast cancer mortality in a cohort of female workers of a herbicide producing plant in Hamburg, FRG" – Hutzinger and Batik (eds.). Proceedings of the 13th International Symposium on Chlorinated Dioxins and Related Compounds", Vienna 1993. Vol. 13: pp.381-384.

Fontham E, Correa P. Rodriguez E and Lin Y. "Validation of smoking history with the micronuclei test". In: D. Hoffman and C. Harris (Eds): Mechanisms in tobacco carcinogenesis – Cold Spring Harbor Laboratory, New York, 1986, pp. 113-119.

Fraga CG, Shigenaga MK, Park J-W, Degan P and Ames BN. "Oxidative damage to DNA during aging : 8-hydroxy-2-deoxyguanosine in rat organ DNA and urine". Proc. Nat. Acad. Sci. US, 1990; 87:4533-37.

Frebourg T, Lerebourg G, Delpech B, Benhamou D, Bertrand P, Maingonnat C, Boutin C and Nouvet G. "Serum hyaluronate in malignant pleural mesothelioma". Cancer 1987; 59:2104-2107.

Freudenheim Jl. Graham S, Marshall JR, Haughey BP and Wilkinson G. "A case-control study of diet and rectal cancer in Western New York". Am Jl. Epidemiol. 1990; 131:612-624.

Fry MJ. "Structure, regulation and function of phosphoinositide 3-kinases". Biochem. Byophys. Acta 1994; 1226:237-268.

Gabrielson EW, Gerwin BI, Harris CC, Roberts AB, Sporn MB and Lechner JF. "Stimulation of DNA synthesis in cultured primary human mesothelial cells by specific growth factors". FASEB J 1988; 2:2717-2721.

Gallagher EP, Wienkers LC, Stapleton PL, Kunze KL and Eaton DL. "Role of human microsomal and human complementary DNA-expressed Cytochromes P4501A2 and P450 3A4 in the bioactivation of Aflatoxin B1" Cancer Res. 1994; 54:101-108.

Galloway S, Berry P, Nichols W, Wolman S. Soper K, Stolley P and Archer P. "Chromosome aberrations in individuals occupationally exposed to ethylene oxide, and in a large control population". Mutation Research 1986; 170:55-74.

Gannon JV, Greaves R, Iggo R and Lane DP. "Activating mutations in p53 produce a common conformational effect – a monoclonal antibody specific for the mutant form". EMBO Jl 1990; 9:1595-1602.

Garabrant DH; Held J; Langholz B; Peters JM and Mack TM. "DDT and related compounds and risk of pancreatic cancer". Jl Nat. Cancer Inst. 1992; 84:764-771.

Garner C. "Molecular Potential" – Nature (London) 1992; 360:207-208.

Garry VF, Hozier J, Jacobs D, Wade RL and Gray DG. "Ethylene Oxide: evidence of human chromosomal effects". Environm. Mutag., 1979; 1:375-382.

Gatti RA and McConville CM. "Meeting Report. Sixth International Workshop on Ataxia- Telangiectasia". Cancer Research 1994; 54:6007-6010.

Gauldie J, Jordana M and Cox G. "Cytokines and pulmonary fibrosis" – Thorax 1993; 48:931-935.

Gavrieli Y, Sherman Y and Ben-Sasson SA. "Identification of programmed cell death *in situ* via specific labelling of nuclear DNA fragmentation" Jl Cell Biol 1992; 119:493-501.

Gazzeri S, Brambilla E, Caron de Fromentel C, Gouyer V, Moro D, Perron P, Berger F and Brambilla C. "p53 genetic abnormalities and *myc* activation in human lung carcinoma". Int J Cancer 1994; 58:24-32.

Gazzeri S, Brambilla E, Jacrot M, Chauvin C, Benabid AL and Brambilla B. "Activation of *myc* gene family in human lung carcinomas during heterotransplantation into nude mice". Cancer Research 1991; 51:2566-2571.

Geng Y and Weinberg RA. "Transforming growth factor β effects on expression of G1 cyclins and cyclin-dependent protein kinases". Proc Natl. Acad. Sci. USA, 1993;90: 10315-10319.

Georges RN, Mukhopadhyay T, Zhang Y, Yen N and Roth JA "Prevention of orthotopic human lung cancer growth by intratracheal instilattion of retrovitral antisense K-*ras* construct". Cancer Research 1993; 53:1743-1746.

Gerdes J, Schwab U, Lemke H and Stein H. "Production of a mouse monoclonal antibody reactive with a nuclear antigen associated with cell proliferation". Int. Jl. Cancer 1983; 31: 13-20.

Gescher A. "Towards selective pharmacological modulation of protein kinase C - opportunities for the development of novel antineoplastic agents". Brit. Jl. Cancer 1992; 66:10-19.

Ghiselli A, Serafini M, Azzini M and Ferro-Luzzi A. "A fluorescence-based method for measurig total plasma antioxidant capability". Submitted for publication in Free Rad. Biol. Med. 1995.

Gillett C, Fantl V, Smith R, Fisher C, Bartek J, Dickson C, Barnes D and Peters G. "Amplification and overexpression of Cyclin D1 in breast cancer detected by immunohistochemical staining". Cancer Research 1994; 54:1812-1817.

Gion M, Mione R, Becciolini A, Balzi M , Correale M, Piffanelli A, Giovannini G, Saccani Jotti G and Fontanesi M. "Relationship between cytosol TPS, TPA and cell proliferation". Intl. Jl. Biol. Markers 1994: 9:109-114.

Giordano S, Di Renzo MF, Cirillo D, Naldini L, Chiado 'Piat L and Comoglio PM. "Proteins phosphorylated on tyrosine as markers of human tumour cell lines". "Int. J. Cancer 1987; 39:482-487.

Goelz SE and Vogelstein B "Hypomethylation of DNA from benign and malignant human colon neoplasms" Science 1985; 228:187-190.

Gold P and Freedman S. "Specific carcino-embryonic antigens of the human digestive system". Jl. Exper. Med. 1965; 122:467-481.

Grafstrom RC, Pegg AE, Trump BF and Harris CC. "O^6-Alkylguanine-DNA alkyltransferase activity in normal human tissues and cells". Cancer Research 1984; 44:2855-2857.

Grant DM, Tang BK and Kalow W. "A simple test for acetylator phenotype using caffeine". Brit. Jl. Clin. Pharmacol., 1984; 17: 459-464.

Greenblatt MS, Benett WP, Hollstein M and Harris CC. "Mutations in the p53 tumour suppressor gene: clues to cancer etiology and molecular pathogenesis". Cancer Research 1994, 54:4855-4878.

Greenwald P, Witkin KM, Malone WF, Byar DP, Freedman LS and Stern HR. "The study of markers of biological effect in cancer prevention research trials". Int J. Cancer 1992, 52: 189-196.

Grimm T and Johnson JP. "Ectopic Expression of carcino-embryonic antigen by a melanoma cell leads to changes in the transcription of two additional cell adhesion molecules" Cancer Research 1995; 55:3254-3257.

Groopman JD, Trudel LJ, Donahue PR, Marshak-Rothstein A and Wogan GN. "High affinity monoclonal antibodies for aflatoxins and their application to solid phase immunoassays". Proc. Nat. Acad. Sci. US, 1984; 81:7728-7731.

Groopman JD; Donahue PR; Zhu J; Chen J and Wogan GN. "Aflatoxin metabolism in humans: detection of metabolites and nucleic acid adducts in urine by affinity chromatography" – Proc. Nat. Acad. Sci. US, 1985; 82:6492-6496.

Groopman JD; Wogan GN, Roebuck BD and Kensler TW. "Molecular biomarkers for aflatoxins and their application to human cancer prevention". Cancer Res (suppl) 1994; 54s:1907s-1911s.

Gruss HJ, Brach MA, Drexler HG, Bross KJ and Herrmann F. "Interleukin-9 is expressed by primary and cultured Hodgkin and Reed-Sternberg cells". Cancer Res., 1992; 52:1026-1031.

Guo Y-J, Wang X, Jim D, Wu M, Ma J and Sy M-S. "Potential use of soluble CD-44 in serum as indicator of tumour burden and metastasis in patients with gastric or colon cancer". Cancer Research 1994; 54:422-426.

Gutterridge JMC and Halliwell B. "Iron toxicity and oxygen radicals". Bailliere's Clinical Hematology, 1989; 2:195-256.

Hakoda M, Akiyama M,Kyoizumi S, Awa AA, Yamakido M and Otake M. "Increased somatic cell mutant frequency in atomic bomb survivors". Mutation Research, 1988; 201:39-48.

Hakomori S, Nudelman E, Levery SB and Kannagi R. "Novel fucolipids accumulating in human adenocarcinoma. I. Glycolipids with di-or-tri-fucosylated type 2 chain". Jl. Biol. Chem. 1984; 259:4672-4680.

Hall J, Brésil H, Donato F, Wild CP, Loktionova NA, Kazanova OI, Komyakov IP, Lemekhov VG, Likhachev AJ, and Montesano R. "Alkylation and oxidative DNA damage repair activity in blood leukocytes of smokers and non-smokers". Int. Jl. Cancer 1993; 54:728-733.

Hall PA, Coates PJ, Goodlad RA, Hart IR and Lane DP. "Proliferating cell nuclear expression in non-cycling cells may be induced by growth factors *in vivo*". Brit. Jl. Cancer 1994; 70:244-247.

Hall PA, McKee PM, Ménage H du P, Dover R and Lane DP "High levels of p53 protein in UV irradiated normal human epidermal keratinocytes". Oncogene 1993; 8:203-207.

Hall PA, Ray A, Lemoine NR, Midgley CA, Krausz T and Lane DP. "p53 immunostaining as a marker of malignant disease in diagnostic cytopathology". Lancet 1991; 338: 513.

Halliwell B and Aruoma OI (Editors) "DNA and Free Radicals". Ellis Harwood, New York, 1992.

Hammarberg C, Slezak P and Tribukait B "Early detection of malignancy in ulcerative colitis". Cancer 1984; 53:291-295.

Hanawalt PC and Sarasin A. "Cancer-prone hereditary discases with DNA processing abnormalities". Trends Genet., 1986; 2:124-129.

Hannon GJ and Beach D. "p15INK4B is a potential effector of TGFβ-induced cell cycle arrest". Nature 1994; 371:257-261.

Harbour JW, Lai SL, Whang-Peng J, Gazdar AF and Minna J. "Abnormalities in structure and expression of the human retinoblastoma gene in small-cell lung cancer". Science (Washington DC) 1988; 241:353-357.

Harper JW, Adami GR, Wei N, Keyormarsi K and Elledge SJ. "The p21 cdk-interacting protein Cip1 is a potent inhibitor of G1 cyclin-dependent kinases". Cell 1993; 75:805–816.

Harris CC, Vähäkangas K, Newman MJ, Trivers GE, Shamsuddin A, Sinopoli N, Mann DL and Wright WE. "Detection of benzo[a] pyrene diolepoxide. DNA adducts in peripheral blood lymphocytes and antibodies to the adducts in serum from coke oven workers". Proc Nat. Acad. Sci. (US) 1985; 82:6672-6676.

Harris CC. "Chemical and physical carcinogenesis: advances and perspectives for the 1990's". Cancer Res. suppl 1991; 51 suppl: 5023s-5044s.

Hatada T, Sakanoue Y, Kusunoki M, Kobayashi A and Utsunomiya J. "Variable activity of protein Tyrosine Kinase in apparently normal thyroid glands". Cancer Investigation 1994; 12:26-32.

Hatton DH, Mitchell DL, Strickland PT and Johnson RT. "Enhanced photoproduct repair: its role in the DNA Damage-resistance phenotype of human malignant melanoma cells". Cancer Research, 1995; 55:181-189.

Hayashi S-i, Watanabe J and Kawajiri K. "High susceptibility to lung cancer analysed in terms of combined genotypes pf P450 IAI and Mu-class glutathione S-Transferase genes". Japn Jl. Cancer Res., 1992; 83:866-870.

Hayashi S-i, Watanabe J, Nakachi K and Kawajiri K. "Genetic linkage of lung cancer Msp I polymorphisms with amino acid replacement in the heme binding region of the human Cytochrome P450IAI gene". Jl. Biochem. 1991; 110:407-411.

Hayashi S-i, Watanabe J, Nakachi K, Eguchi H, Gotoh O and Kawajizi K. "Interindividual difference in expression of human Ah receptor and related P450 genes". Carcinogenesis, 1994; 15:801-806.

Hecht SS, Camella SG, Foiles PG and Murphy SE. "Biomarkers for Human Uptake and Metabolic Activation of Tobacco-Specific Nitrosamines". Cancer Res. (suppl) 1994; 54: 1912s-1917s.

Heim S, Johansson B and Mertens F. "Constitutional chromosome instability and cancer risk". Mutation Research 1989; 221:39-51.

Hein DW. Acetylator genotype and arylamine-induced carcinogenesis". Biochem. Biophys Acta 1988; 948: 37-66.

Heintz NH, Janssen Y and Mossman BT. "Persistent induction of c-*fos* and c-*jun* proto oncogene expression by asbestos" – Proc. Natl. Acad. Sci. USA 1993; 90:3299-3303.

Heldin P, Asplund T, Ytterberg D, Thelin S and Laurent TC. "Characterization of the molecular mechanism involved in the activation of hyaluronan synthetase by platelet-derived growth factor in human mesothelial cells". Biochem. Jl. 1992; 283:165-170.

Helferich WG and Denison MS. "Ultraviolet photoproducts of tryptophan can act as dioxin agonists". Mol. Pharmacol. 1991; 40:674-678.

Heller TD, Holt PR and Richardson A. "Food restriction retards age-related histological changes in rat small instestine". Gastroenterology 1990; 98:387-391.

Helzlsouer KJ, Comstock GW and Morris JS. "Selenium, lycopene, α-tocopherol, β-carotene, retinol and subsequent bladder cancer". Cancer Research 1989; 49:6144-6148.

Hemminki K. "Use of chemical, biochemical and genetic markers in cancer epidemiology and risk assessment". Amer. Jl. Industr. Med. 1992; 21:65-76.

Henderson BE, Ross R and Bernstein L. "Estrogens as a cause of human cancer: the Richard and Hinda Rosenthal Foundation Award Lecture". Cancer Research 1988; 48: 246-253.

Henzen-Logmans SC, Fieret E, Berns E, van der Burg M, Klijn J and Foekens JA. "Ki-67 staining in benign, border-line, malignant primary and metastatic ovarian tumours: correlatio with steroid receptors, epidermal-growth-factor receptor and cathepsin-D". Int. Jl. Cancer 1994; 57:468-472.

Herbeth B and Bagrel A. "A study of factors influencing plasma CEA levels in an unselected population". Oncodevelopmental Biol. Med. 1980; 1:191-198.

Hertz MI, Henke CA, Nakhleh RE, Harmon KR, Marinelli WA, Fox JMK, Kubo SH, Shumway SJ, Bolman III RM and Bitterman PB. "Obliterative bronchiolitis after lung transplantation: a fibroproliferative disorder associated with platelet-derived growth factor". Proc. Nat. Acad. Sci. USA 1992; 89:10385-10389.

Heussen GAH. "Inhibition of intercellular communication by airborne particulate matter". Arch. Toxicol. 1991; 65:252-256.

Hill M and Giacosa A. "The mediterranean diet-Editorial". Europ. Jl. Cancer Rev. 1992; 1:339-340.

Hillerdal G, Lindqvist U and Engström-Laurent A. "Hyaluronan in pleural effusions and in serum". Cancer 1991; 67:2410-2414.

Hirai H, Kobayashi Y, Mano H, Hagiwara K, Maru Y, Omine M, Mizoguchi H, Nishida J and Takaku F. "A point mutation at codon 13 of the N-*ras* oncogene in myelodysplastic syndrome". Nature (London) 1987; 330:186-188.

Hirai M, Gamon S, Kobayashi M and Shimizu N. "Lung Cancer Cells often express high levels of protein kinase C activity". Japan Jl. Cancer Res. 1989; 80:204-208.

Hirvonen A, Husgafvel-Pursiainen K, Anttila S and Vainio H. "The GSTM1-null genotype as a potential risk modifier for squamous cell carcinoma of the lung". Carcinogenesis (London) 1993; 14:1479-1481.

Hochstein P and Atallah AS. "The nature of oxidants and anti-oxidant systems in the inhibition of mutation and cancer". Mutation Research 1988; 202:363-375.

Hockenbery D, Nunez G, Milliman C, Schreiber RD and Korsmeyer SJ. "Bcl-2 is an inner mitochrondrial membrane protein that blocks programmed cell death". Nature 1990; 348:334-336.

Hockenbery DM, Oltvai ZN, Yin X-M, Milliman CM and Korsmeyer SJ. "Bcl-2 functions in an antioxidant pathway to prevent apoptosis". Cell 1993; 75:241-251.

Hogstedt B. "Micronuclei in lymphocytes with preserved cytoplasm: A method for assessment of cytogenetic damage in man". Mutation Research 1984; 69:357-368.

Hogstedt C; Aringer and Gustavsson A. "Epidemiologic support for ethylene-oxide as a cancer-causing agent". JAMA 1986; 255:1575-1578.

Holder JW, Elmore E and Barrett JC. "Gap Junction function and cancer": Cancer Research 1993; 53:3475-3480.

Hollstein M and Mc Cann J. "Short-term tests for carcinogens and mutagens" Mutation Research 1979; 65:133-226.

Hollstein M, Sidransky D, Vogelstein B and Harris CC. "p53 mutations in human cancers". Science (Washington DC) 1991; 253:49-53.

Honda A, Noguchi N, Takehara H, Ohashi Y, Asuwa N and Mori Y. "Cooperative enhancement of hyaluronic acid synthesis by combined use of IGF-I and EGF and inhibition by tyrosine kinase inhibitor genistein in cultured mesothelial cells from rabbit pericardial cavity". Jl Cell. Sci. 1991; 98:91-98.

Hunter T and Pines J. "Cyclins and Cancer". Cell 1991; 66:1071-1074.

Husgafvel-Pursiainen K. "Sister chromatid exchange and cell proliferation in cultured lymphocytes of passively and actively smoking restaurant personnel". Mutation Research 1987; 190:211-215.

Husgafvel-Pursiainen K, Sorsa M, Engström K and Einistö P. "Passive smoking at work: biochemical and biological measures of exposure to environmental tobacco smoke". Int. Arch. Occup. Environ Health, 1987; 59:337-345.

Hynes RO and Lander AD. "Contact and adhesive specificities in the associations, migrations and targeting of cells and axons". Cell 1992; 68: 303-322.

Hynes RO, "Integrins versatility, modulation and signalling in cell adhesion" Cell 1992; 69: 11-25.

IARC, Scientific Publications no 116. "Mechanisms of Carcinogenesis in Risk Identification". H. Vainio, PN Magee, DB Mc Gregor and AJ Mc Michael (Eds.). International Agency for Research on Cancer, Lyon, 1992; 615 pp.

Ide F, Ishikawa T, Takagi M, Umemura S and Takayama S. "Unscheduled DNA synthesis in human oral mucosa treated with chemical carcinogens in short-term organ culture" Jl. Natl. Cancer Inst. 1982; 69:557-563.

Idle J. "Cytochrome P450 2D phenotypes and human cancer risk". Cancer Det. Prev., 1989; 14:275-280.

Idle JR, Mahgoub A, Sloan TP, Smith RL, Mbanefo CO and Bababunmi EA. "Some observations on the oxidation phenotype status of Nigerian patients presenting with cancer". Cancer Letters, 1981; 11:331-338.

Ionov Y, Peinado MA, Malkhosyar S, Shibata D and Perucho M. "Ubiquitous somatic mutations in simple repeated sequences reveal a new mechanism for colonic carcinogenesis". Nature 1993; 363:558-561.

Ip C, Carter CM and Ip MM. "Requirement of essential fatty acid of mammary tumourigenesis in the rat". Cancer Res. 1985; 45:1997-2001.

Ip C. "The chemopreventive role of selenium in carcinogenesis". Jl. Am. Coll. Toxicol. 1986; 5:7-20.

Ishioka C, Freburg T, Yan Y, Vidal M, Friend SH, Schmidt S and Iggo R. "Screening patients for heterozygotous p53 mutations using a functional assay in yeast" Nature Genet. 1993; 5:124-129.

Islas AL, Vos J-M and Hanawalt PC "Differential introduction and repair of psoralen photoadducts to DNA in specific human genes". Cancer Research 1991; 51:2867-2873.

Isola JJ, Helin HJ, Helle MJ and Kallioniemi O-P. "Evaluation of cell proliferation in breast carcinoma. Comparison of Ki-67 immunohistochemical study, DNA flow cytometric analysis and mitotic count". Cancer 1990; 65:1180-1184.

Itoh N, Yonehara S, Ishii A, Yonehara M, Mizushima SI, Sameshima M, Hase A, Seto Y and Nagata S. "The polypeptide encoded by the cDNA for human cell surface antigen Fas can mediate apoptosis" Cell 1991; 66:233-243.

Itzkowitz SH and Kim Y. "New carbohydrate tumour markers". Gastroenterology 1986; 90:491-494.

Jaques G, Auerbach B, Pritsch M, Wolf M, Madry N and Havemann K. "Evaluation of serum neural cell adhesion molecule as a new tumour marker in small-cell lung cancer". Cancer 1993; 72:418-425.

Jhiang SM, Yaneva M and Busch H. "Expression of human proliferation-associated nucleolar antigen p120". Cell Growth and Differentiation. 1990; 1:319-324.

Jones PA, Buchley JD, Henderson BE, Ross RK and Pike MC. "From gene to carcinogen: a rapidly Evolving Field in Molecular Epidemiology" - Cancer Research 1991; 51:3617-3620.

Kadlubar FF. "Detection of human DNA-carcinogen adducts" - Nature 1992; 360:189.

Kahn A. "La transmission du signal en amont et en aval de *Ras*". Médecine/Sciences 1992; 8:1097-1099. (In French).

Kamb A, Gruis NA, Weaver-Feldhaus J, Lin Q, Harshman K, Tavtigian SV, Stockert E, Day III RS, Johnson BE and Skolnick MH. "A cell cycle regulator potentially involved in genesis of many tumour types". Science 1994; 264: 436:440.

Kandl H, Seymour L, and Bezwoda WR. "Soluble c-*erb*B-2 fragment in serum correlates with disease stage and predicts for shortened survival in patients with early-stage and advanced breast cancer". Brit. J. Cancer 1994; 70:739-742.

Kanno Y "Modulation of cell communication and carcinogenesis". Japan Jl. Physiol. 1985; 35: 693-707.

Kao-Shan CS, Fine RL, Whang-Peng J, Lee EC and Chabner BA. "Increased Fragile Sites and Sister Chromatid Exchanges in Bone Marrow and Peripheral Bloood of Young Cigarrette Smokers". Cancer Research 1987; 47:6278-6282.

Kasai H, Crain PF, Kuchino Y, Nishimura S, Ootsuyama A and Tanooka H. "Formation of 8- hydroxyguanine moiety in cellular DNA by agents producing oxygen radicals and evidence for its repair" Carcinogenesis (London) 1986; 7:1849-51.

Kastan MB, Zhan Q, El-Deiry WS, Carrier F, Jacks T, Walsh WV, Plunkett BS, Vogelstein B and Fornace JA, Jr. "A mammalian cell cycle checkpoint pathway utilizing p53 and GADD45 is defective in ataxia-telangiectasia". Cell 1992; 71:587-597.

Kato GJ and Dang CV. "Function of the c-*myc* oncoprotein" FASEB J 1992; 6:3065-3072.

Kato JY, Matsuoka M, Polyak K, Massagué J and Sherr CJ. "Cyclic AMP-induced G1 phase arrest mediated by an inhibitor (p27KIP1) of cyclin-dependent kinase 4 activation". Cell 1994; 79:487-496.

Kato JY, Matsushiue H, Hiebert SW, Ewen ME and Sherr CJ. "Direct binding of cyclin D to the retinoblastoma gene product (pRb) and pRb phosphorylation by the cyclin d- dependent kinase CDK4". Genes Dev. 1993; 7:331-342.

Katopodis N, Hirshaut Y, Geller N and Stock CC. "Lipid-associated sialic acid test for the detection of human cancer". Cancer Research 1982; 42:5270-5275.

Kawai T, Suzuki M, Kase K and Ozeki Y "Expression of carbohydrate antigens in human pulmonary adenocarcinoma". Cancer 1993; 72:1581-1587.

Kawajiri K, Nakachi K , Imai K, Yoshii A, Shinoda M and Watanabe J. "Identification of genetically high risk individuals to lung cancer by DNA polymorphisms of the cytochrome P4501A1gene". Febs Letters 1990; 263:131-133.

Kaye FJ, Kratzke RA, Gerster JL and Lin PS. "Recessive oncogenes in lung cancer". Am. Rev. Respir. Dis. 1990; 142:S44-S47.

Keenan KP and Soper KA. "The effects of overfeeding and moderate dietary restriction on Sprague-Dawley rat survival Spontaneous Carcinogenesis, chronic disease and the toxicological response to pharmaceuticals". In: "Dietary restriction: implications for design and interpretation of Toxicity and Carcinogenicity Studies". R. Hart, DA Neuann and R. Roberston (Eds.). ILSI Press, Washington DC, 1995.

Kellermann G, Shaw CR and Luyten-Kellermann M "Aryl hydrocarbon hydroxylase inducibility and bronchogenic carcinoma". New Engl. Jl. Med. 1973; 289:934-937.

Kelsey K, Wiencke J, Eisen E, Lynch D, Lewis T and Little J. "Persistently elevated sister chromatid exchanges in ethylene oxide-exposed primates: the role of a subpopulation of high frequency cells". Cancer Research 1988; 48:5045-5050.

Kerr JFR, Winterford CM and Harmon BV. "Apoptosis. Its significance in cancer and cancer therapy". Cancer 1994; 73:2013-2026.

Kim Y, Itzkowitz SH, Yuan M, Chung Y-S, Satake K, Umeyama K and Hakomori S-i "Le^x and Le^y antigen expression in human pancreatic cancer". Cancer Research, 1988; 48:475-482.

Kim Y-I, Giuliano A, Hatch KD, Schneider A, Nour MA, Dallal GE, Selhub J and Mason JB "Global DNA hypomethylation progressively in cervical: dysplasia and carcinoma". Cancer 1994; 74:893-899.

King CR, Krauss MH , Di Fiore PP, Paik S and Kasprzyk PG. "Implications of *erb*B-2 overexpression for basic science and clinical medicine". Sem. Cancer Biol. 1990; 1:329-337.

King WJ and Greene GL. "Monoclonal antibodies localize estrogen receptor in the nuclei target cells". Nature, 1984; 307:745-747.

Kinlen LJ. "Immunosuppression and cancer" In "Mechanisms of Carcinogenesis in Risk Identification". Eds: H. Vainio, PN Magee, DB McGregor and AJMc Michael. Lyon, International Agency for Research on Cancer, pp. 237-253. IARC, 1992.

Klein N, Vignaud JM, Sadmi M, Plenat F, Borelly J, Duprez A, Martinet Y and Martinet N. "Squamous metaplasia expression of protooncogenes and p53 in lung cancer patients". Lab. Invest 1993; 68:26-32.

Knekt P, Aromaa A, Maatela J. Aaran RK, Nikkari T, Hakama M, Hakulinen T, Peto R and Teppo L. "Vitamin E and cancer prevention". Am. J. Clin. Nutr. 1991; 53:283s-286s.

Knekt P, Reunanen A, Takkunen H, Aromaa A, Heliövaara M and Hakulinen T. "Body iron stores and risk of cancer". Int. Jl. Cancer, 1994; 56:379-382.

Knudsen L, Boisen T, Christensen J, Jelnes J, Jensen G, Jensen J, Lundgren K, Lundsteen C, Pedersen B, Wassermman K, Wilhardt P, Wulf H and Zebitz U. "Biomonitoring of genotoxic exposure among stainless steel welders". Mutation Research 1992; 279:129- 143.

Knudsen LE, Sorsa M and the Nordic Study Group on the Health Risk of Chromosome Damage. "An increased level of chromosomal aberrations in lymphocytes appears to be a relevant biomarker of future cancer risk". Presented at the Nordtox 1994 Conference. "Interphase between Human Toxicology and Ecotoxicology". Skyping, Denmark, May 20-23, 1994. Published as abstract in Pharmacol. Toxicol., 1994; Suppl. II 74:25.

Knudson AG, Jr. "Hereditary cancer, oncogenes and anti-oncogenes". Cancer Research 1985; 45:1437-1443

Koch AC, Anderson D, Moran MF, Ellis C and Dawson T "SH2 and SH3 domains: elements that control interaction of cytoplasmic signalling proteins". Science 1991; 252:668-674.

Koff A, Ohtsuki M, Polyak K, Roberts JM and Massagué J. "Negative Regulation of G1 in mammalian cells: inhibition of cyclin E-dependent kinase by TGF β". Science 1993; 260: 536-539.

Kopp R, Noelke B, Sauter G, Shildberg FW, Baumgartner G and Pfeiffer A. "Altered protein kinase C activity in biopsies of human colonic adenomas and carcinomas". Cancer Research 1991; 51:4271-4278.

Korach KS, Levy LA and Sarver PJ. "Stereochemical analysis of stilbene estrogens: receptor binding and hormone responsiveness". In: JA. McLachlan (Ed.) "Estrogens in the Environment. Vol. II. Influences on Development". New York, Elsevier 1985; pp43-68.

Korsmeyer SJ. "Bcl-2 initiates a new category of oncogenes: regulators of cell death". Blood 1992; 80:879-886.

Kort WJ, Weijma IM, Bijma AM, van Schalkwijk WP, Vergroesen AJ and Westbrock DL. "Omega-3 fatty acids inhibiting the growth of a transplantable rat mammary adenocarcinoma". Jl. Natl. Cancer Inst. 1987; 79:593-599.

Kouri RE, McKinney CE, Slomiany DJ, Snodgrass DR, Wray NP and McLemore TL. "Positive correlation between high aryl hydroxylase activity and primary lung cancer as analyzed in cryopreserved lymphocytes". Cancer Research 1982; 42:5030-5037.

Kovalenko M, Gazit A, Böhmer A, Rorsman C, Rönnstrand L, Heldin C-H, Waltenberger J, Böhmer F-D and Levitzki A. "Selective platelet-derived growth factor receptor kinase blockers reverse *sis*-transformation". Cancer Research, 1994; 54:6106-6114.

Krokan HE. "Variation in DNA repair". Pharmacol. Toxicol., 1994; 74 suppl. II, p. 12 (Abstract).

Kubota M, Sogawa K, Kaizu Y, Sawaya T, Watanabe J, Kawajiri K, Gotoh O and Fujii- Kuriyama Y. "Xenobiotic responsive element in the 5'-upstream region of the human P450 c gene". Jl. Biochem., 1991; 110:232-236.

Ladero JM, Gonzalez FJ, Benitez JB, Vargas E, Fernandez MJ, Baki W and Diaz-Rubio M. "Acetylator polymorphism in human colorectal carcinoma". Cancer Research, 1991; 51: 2098-2100.

Lahue RS, Au KG and Modrich P. "DNA mismatch correction in a defined system". Science (Washington DC) 1989; 245:160-164.

Laiho M, De Caprio JA, Ludlow JW, Livingston DM and Massagué J. "Growth inhibition by TGF-β linked to suppression of retinoblastoma protein phosphorylation". Cell 1990; 62:175-185.

Laird PW, Jackson-Grusby L, Fazeli A, Dicinson SL, Jung WE, Li E, Weinberg RA and Jaenisch R. Cell 1995; 81:197-205.

Lake RS, Kropko ML, McLachlan S, Pezzutti MR, Shoemaker RH and Igel HJ. "Chemical carcinogen induction of DNA-repair synthesis in human peripheral blood monocytes". Mutation Research 1980; 74:357-377.

Lambert B. "Biological markers in exposed humans: gene mutation". In: Vainio H, Magee PN, McGregor DB and McMichael AJ (eds) "Mechanisms of Carcinogenesis in Risk Identification". IARC 1992; Lyon, pp. 535-542.

Lammie GA and Peters G. "Chromosome 11q13 abnormalities in human cancer". Cancer Cells (Cold Spring Harbor) 1991; 3:413-420.

Landberg G and Roos G. "Antibodies to Proliferating Cell Nuclear Antigen as S-Phase Probes in Flow Cytometric Cell Cycle Analysis". Cancer Research 1991; 51:4570-4574.

Landers JP and Bunce NJ. "The Ah receptor and the mechanism of dioxin toxicity". Biochem. Jl., 1991; 276:273-287.

Lane DP. "Cancer. A death in the life of p53", Nature (London) 1993; 362: 786-787.

Lane DP. "p53, guardian of the genome", Nature (London) 1992; 358:15-16.

Langlois RG, Bigbee WL and Jensen RH. "Measurements of the frequency of human erythrocytes with gene expression loss phenotypes of the glycophorin A locus". Human Genet., 1986; 74:353-362.

Langlois RG, Bigbee WL, Kyoizumi S, Nakamura N, Bean MA, Akiyama M and Jensen RH. "Evidence for increased somatic mutations at the glycophorin A locus in atomic bomb survivors". Science 1987; 236:445-448.

Leach FS and 34 others, including Lynch HT, de la Chapelle A and Vogelstein B. "Mutations of a *mut*S homologue in hereditary non-polyposis colorectal cancer". Cell 1993; 75:1215-1226.

Ledermann JA, Pasini F, Olabiran Y and Pelosi G "Detection of the Neural Cell Adhesion Molecule (NCAM) in serum of patients with small-cell lung cancer (SCLC) with "Limited" or "Extensive" disease and bone marrow infiltration" Inter. Jl. Cancer 1994; Suppl. 8:49-52.

Leitzel K, Bryce W, Tomita J, Manderino G, Tribby I, Thomason A, Billingsley M, Podczaski E, Harvey H, Bartholomew M and Lipton A. "Elevated plasma platelet- derived growth factor B-chain levels in cancer patients" Cancer Res. 1991; 51:4149- 4154.

Lemoine NR, Mayall ES, Wyllie FW, Williams ED, Goyns M, Stringer B and Wynford Thomas D. "High frequency of *ras* oncogene activation in all stages of human thyroid tumourigenesis". Oncogene 1989; 4:159-164.

Lew EA and Garfinkel L. "Variations in mortality by weight among 750.00 men and women". Jl Chronic Dis. 1979; 32:563-567.

Limper AH, Broekelmann TJ, Colby TV, Malizia G and McDonald JA. "Analysis of local mRNA expression for extracellular matrix proteins and growth factors using *in situ* hybridization in fibroproliferative lung disorders". Chest 1991; 99: 555-565.

Lipkin M. "Biomarkers of increased susceptibility to gastrointestinal cancer: new applications to studies of cancer prevention in human subjects". Cancer Res. 1988; 48:235-245.

Lippman S, Lee J, Lotan R. Hittelman W, Wargovich M and Hong WK. "Biomarkers as intermediate end points in chemoprevention trials". J. Natl. Cancer Inst. 1990b; 82:555-560.

Lippman S, Peters E, Wargovich M, Stadnyk A, Dixon D, Dekmezian R, Loewy J, Morice R, Cunningham J and Hong W. "Bronchial micronuclei as a marker of an early carcinogenesis in the human tracheobronchial epithelium" Int. J. Cancer 1990a; 45:811- 815.

Loeb LA. "Microsatellite Instability: Marker of a Mutator Phenotype in Cancer". Cancer Res, 1994; 54:5059-5063.

Loewenstein W. "Junctional intercellular communication: the cell-to-cell membrane channel". Physiol. Rev. 1981; 61: 829-913.

Loft S, Vistisen K, Ewertz M, Tjønneland A, Overvad K and Poulsen HE. "Oxidative DNA damage estimated by 8-hydroxydeoxyguanosine excretion in humans: influence of smoking, gender and body mass index". Carcinogenesis (London) 1992; 13:2241-2247.

Lok E, Scott FW, Mongeau R, Nera EA, Malcolm S and Clayson DB. "Caloric restriction and cellular proliferation in various tissues of the female Swiss Webster mouse". Cancer Letters 1990; 51:67-73.

London SJ, Colditz GA, Stampfer MJ, Willett WC, Rosner B and Speizer FE. "Prospective Study of relative weight, height and risk breast cancer". JAMA 1989; 262:2853-2858.

Lubin R, Schlichtholz B, Bengoufa D, 16 others and Soussi T. "Analysis of p53 antibodies in patients with various cancers define B-cell epitopes of human p53: distribution on primary structure and exposure on protein surface". Cancer Research 1993; 53:5872- 5876.

Lucier GW. "Receptor-mediated carcinogenesis". In H. Vainio, PN Magee, DB McGregor and AJ McMichael (Eds.). "Mechanisms of Carcinogenesis in Risk Identification", Lyon, International Agency for Research on Cancer, pp. 87-112.IARC 1992.

Lukas J, Pagano M, Staskovic Z, Draetta G and Bartek J. "Cyclin D1 protein oscillates and is essential for cell cycle progression in human tumour cell lines". Oncogene 1994; 9:707- 718.

Luo J-C, Yu MW, Chen CJ, Santella RM, Carney WP and Brandt-Rauf PW. "Serum c-*erb*B-2 oncopeptide in hepatocellular carcinogenesis". Med. Sci. Res. 1993; 21:305-307.

Lutz WK and Schlatter J. "Chemical carcinogenesis and overnutrition in diet-related cancer". Carcinogenesis 1992; 13:2211-2216.

Lynch HT, Smyrk TC, Watson P, Lanepa SJ, Lynch JF, Lynch PM, Cavalieri RJ and Boland CR. "Genetics, natural history, tumour spectrum and pathology of hereditary non-polyposis colorectal cancer: an updated review". Gastroenterology, 1993; 104:1535–1549.

Macaulay VM, Teale JD, Everard MJ, Joshi GP, Smith IE and Millar JL. "Somatomedin- C/insulin-like growth factor I is a mitogen for human small-cell lung cancer". Brit. J. Cancer, 1988, 57:91-93.

Maki-Paakkanen J. "Chromosome aberrations, micronuclei and sister chromatide exchanges in blood lymphocytes after occupational exposure to low levels of styrene". Mutation Research 1987; 189:399-406.

Mannervik B, Alin P, Guthenberg C, Jensson H, Kalim TH, Warholm J and Jornvall H. "Identification of three classes of cytosolic glutathione transferase common to several mammalian species: correlation between structural data and enzymatic properties.". Proc. Natl. Acad. Sci. USA, 1985; 82:7202-7206.

Martinet Y and Crystal RG. "Pathogenesis of tissue fibrosis: inflammatory cell modulation of mesenchymal cell accumulation". In: J.P. Revillard and N. Wierzbicki (eds.) "Tissue Fibrosis: Immune cells and mediators". Published by Foundation Franco-Allemande, Suresnes, France, 1987, pp. 13-31.

Martinet Y, Rom W, Grotendorst GR, Martin GR and Crystal RG "Exaggerated spontaneous release of platelet-derived growth factor by alveolar macrophages of patients with idiopathic pulmonary fibrosis". New Engl. J. Med. 1987;317:202-209.

Marx J. "Forging a path to the nucleus". Science; 1993; 260:1588-1590.

Marzin D. "Utilisation des tests de genotoxicité pour la surveillance biologique du personnel exposé". Jl. de Toxicologie Clinique et Expérimentale, 1989; 53-71. (in French).

Massagué J. The TGF-β family of growth and differentiation factors". Cell 1987; 49:437-438.

Matsumura Y and Tarin D. "DNA figer printing survey of various human tumours and their metastases". Cancer Research, 1992; 52:2174-2179.

Matter B and Schmid W. "Trenimon-induced chromosomal damage in bone marrow of six mammalian species evaluated by the micronucleus test". Mutation Research 1971; 12: 417-425.

Maximovitch DM. Effect of β-carotene supplementation on the activity of ornithine decarboxylase (ODC) in stomach mucosa of patients with chronic atrophic gastritis". Europ. Jl. Cancer Prev. 1993; 2:61-68.

Maxwell SA, Ames SK, Sawai ET, Decker GL, Cook RG and Butel JS "Simian virus 40 large T antigen and p53 are microtubule-associated proteins in transformed cells". Cell Growth Differ, 1991; 2:115-127.

Mayer J, Warburton D, Jeffrey AM, Pero R, Walles S, Andrews L, Toor M, Latriano L, Wazneh L, Tang D, Tsai W-Y, Kuroda M and Perera F. "Biologic markers in ethylene exposed workers and controls". Mutation Research 1991; 248:163-176.

Mc Cann J,Coi E, Yamasaki E and Ames BN. "Detection of carcinogens as mutagens in the *Salmonella* / microsome test: assay of 300 chemicals" – Proc. Nat. Acad. Sci US, 1975; 72 : 5135-5139.

Mc Guire WL, Meyer JS, Barlogie B and Kute TE "Impact of flow cytometry on predicting recurrence and survive in breast cancer patients". Breast Cancer Res. Treat. 1985; 5:117-128.

McCormick D, Yu C, Hobbs C and Hall PA. "The relevance of antibody concentration to the immunohistological quantification of cell proliferation associated antigens". Histopathology 1993; 22:543.

Mendelsohn ML. "Can chemical carcinogenicity be predicted by short-term tests?" In: C. Maltoni and IJ Selikoff (eds) "Living in a chemical world – Occupational and environmental significance of industrial carcinogens" pp: 115-126. Annals of the New York Academy of Science, Vol 534. The New York Academy of Sciences, New York 1988.

Meneghini R. "Genotoxicity of active oxygen species in mammalian cells" Mutation Research 1988, 195:215-230.

Merz H, Houssiau FA, Orschescheck K, Renauld JC, Fliedner A, Herin M, Noel H, Kadin M, Mueller-Hermelink HK, Van Snick J and Feller AC. "Interleukin-9, expression in human malignant lymphomas: Unique association with Hodgkin disease and large cell anaplastic lymphoma". Blood 1991; 78:1311-1317.

Merzak A, Koochechkpour S and Pilkington GJ. "CD44 mediates human glioma cell adhesion and invasion *in vitro*" Cancer Research 1994; 54:3988-3992.

Mezzina M, Nardelli J, Nocentini S, Renault G and Sarasin A. "DNA ligase activity in human cell lines from normal donors and Bloom's syndrome patients". Nucleic Acids Research 1989; 17:3091-3106.

Michalides R, Kwa B, Springall D, Van Zandwyk N, Koopman J, Hilkens J and Mooi W. "NCAM and lung cancer". Intern. Jl. Cancer, 1994; Suppl. 8:34-37.

Michelassi F, Leuthner S, Lubienski M, Bostwick D, Rodgers J, Handcock M and Block GE. Ras oncogene p21 levels parallel malignant potential of different human colonic benign conditions". Arch. Surg. 1987; 122:1414-1416.

Michnovicz JJ and Bradlow HL. "Induction of estradiol metabolism by dietary indole-3-carbinol in humans". Jl. Natl. Cancer Inst. 1990; 82:947-949.

Micozzi MS, Beecher GR, Taylor PR and Khachik F. "Carotenoid analyses of selected raw and cooked foods associated with a lower risk for cancer". Jl Natl. Cancer Inst. 1990; 82:282-285.

Mills NE, Fishman CL, Rom WN, Dubin N and Jacobson DR. "Increased prevalence of K-*ras* oncogene mutations in lung adenocarcinoma". Cancer Research 1995; 55: 1444-1447.

Mitelman F. "Catalog of chromosome aberrations in cancer" 3rd Edn – Alan R. Liss, New York, 1988.

Modrich P. "Mechanism and biological effects of mismatch repair". Ann. Rev. Genet., 1991; 25; 229-253.

Moore D and Carrano A. "Statistical analysis of high SCE frequency cells in human lymphocytes". In: Tice R and Hollaender A (Eds): "Sister Chromatid Exchanges". Plenum, New York, 1984. Pp 469-480.

Moreschi C. "Beziehungen zwischen Ernährung und Tumorwachstum". Z. Immunitätsforsch 1909; 2:651-675.

Moses H, Tucker R, Leof E, Coffey R Jr, Halper J and Shipley G. "Type β-transforming growth factor is a stimulator and a growth inhibitor – In: J. Feramisco, B, Ozanne and C. Stiles (Eds.): Growth factors and transformation. Cancer Cells 3, 1985, pp 65-71. Cold Spring Harbor, NY: Cold Spring Harbor Press.

Moses H, Yang E and Pietenpol J. "TGF-β stimulation and inhibition of cell proliferation: new mechanistic insights". Cell 1990; 63: 245-247.

Motokura T and Arnold A. "Cyclins and oncogenesis". Biochim. Biophys Acta 1993; 1155:63-78.

Motokura T, Bloom T, Kim HG, Juppner H, Rudermant JV, Kroneberg HM and Arnold A. "A novel cyclin encoded by a *bcl*1-linked candidate oncogene". Nature (London) 1991; 350: 512-515.

Mukhopadhyay T, Tainsky M, Cavender AC and Roth JA. "Specific inhibition of k-*ras* expression and tumourigenicity of lung cancer cells by antisense RNA". Cancer Res. 1991; 51:1744-1748.

Muramatsu T. "Developmentally regulated expression of cell surface carbohydrates during mouse embryogenesis". Jl. Cell Biochem. 1988; 36:1-14.

Musset M. "LASA (Lipid Associated Sialic Acid): un nouveau traceur biologique de la néoplasie". Thesis Paris Sud-University, 1985. (In French).

Myrnes B, Giercksky KE and Krokan H. "Interindividual variation in the activity of O6- methylguanine-DNA methyl-transferase and uracil-DNA glycosylase in human organs". Carcinogenesis (London) 1983; 4: 1565-1568.

Nakachi K, Imai K, Hayashi S-i and Kawajiri K. "Polymorphisms of the CYP1A1 and Glutathione S-Transferase genes associated with susceptibility to lung cancer in relation to cigarrette dose in a Japanese population". Cancer Research 1993; 53:2994-2999.

Nathan CF. "Secretory products of macrophages". Jl. Clin. Invest, 1987; 79:319-326.

National Academy of Sciences (US). "Biologic Markers in Pulmonary Toxicology" – National Academy Press, Washington DC, 1989.

Nazar-Stewart V, Motulsky AG, Eaton DL, White E, Hornung SK, Leng Z-T, Stapleton P and Weiss NS. "The glutathione S-transferase μ polymorphism as a marker for susceptibility to lung carcinoma". Cancer Research 1993; 53:2313-2318.

Nebert DW, Petersen DD and Puga A. "Human AH locus polymorphism and cancer: inducibility of CYP1A1 and other genes by combustion products and dioxin". Pharmacogenetics 1991; 1:68-78.

Nishizuka Y. "Studies and perspectives of protein kinase C". Science 1986; 233:305-312.

Noda A, Ning Y, Venable SF, Perreira-Smith OM and Smith JR. "Cloning of senescent cell- derived inhibition of DNA synthesis using an expression screen". Exp. Cell Res. 1994; 211:90-98.

Nolori T, Miura K, Wu DJ, Lois A, Takabayashi K and Carson DA. "Deletions of the cyclin- dependent kinase-4 inhibitor gene in multiple human cancers". Nature 1994; 368:753- 756.

O'Brian C, Ward N, Wienstein IB, Bull A and Marnett L. "Activation of rat brain protein kinase C by lipid oxidation products". Biochem. Biophys. Res. Comm 1988; 155:1374-1380.

O'Brian CA and Ward NE "Biology of the protein kinase C family". Cancer and Metast. Rev. 1989; 8: 199-214.

O'Brian CA, Liskamp RM, Solomon DH and Weinstein IB. "Triphenylethylenes: a new class of protein kinase C inhibitors". Jl. Natl. Cancer Inst. 1986; 76: 1243-1246.

O'Brian CA, Vogel VG, Singletary SE and Ward NE. "Elevated protein kinase C expression in human breast tumour biopsies relative to normal breast tissue". Cancer Research 1989; 49:3215-3217.

Oesch F and Klein S. "Relevance of environmental alkylating agents to repair protein O^6-alkylguanine-DNA alkyltransferase: determination of individual and collective repair capacities of O^6-methylguanine". Cancer Res. 1992; 52:1801-1803.

Okey AB, Riddick DS and Harper PA. "The Ah receptor: mediator of the toxicity of 2,3,7,8-Tetrachlorodibenzo-p-dioxin (TCDD) and related compounds". Toxicology Letters, 1994; 70:1-22.

Paako P, Nuorva K, Kamel D, and Soini Y. "Evidence by *in situ* hybridization that c-*erb*B-2 proto-oncogene expression is a marker of malignancy and is expressed in lung adeno-carcinomas". Amer. J. Resp Cell. Mol. Biol. 1992; 7:325-334.

Papadopoulos N and 19 others, including de la Chapelle A and Vogelstein B. "Mutation of a *mut* L homolog in hereditary colon cancer". Science 1994; 263:1625-1629.

Pardee AB. "G1 events and regulation of cell proliferation" – Science (Washington DC), 1989; 246:603-608.

Payrastre B, van Bergen en Hennegouwen PMP, Breton P et al. "Phosphoinositide kinase, diacylglycerol kinase and phospholipase C activities associated to the cytoskeleton. Effect of epidermal growth factor". Jl. Cell Biol. 1991; 115:121-128.

Pelkonen O and Raunio H. "Individual expression of carcinogen metabolizing enzymes: Cytochrome P4502A". Jl Occup. Envir. Med. 1995; 37:19-24.

Peltomaki P, Aaltonen LA, Sistonen P, Pylkkänen L, Mecklin JP, Järvinen H, Green, JS, Jass JR, Weber JL, Leach FS, Petersen GM, Hamilton SR, de la Chapelle A and Vogelstein B. "Genetic mapping of a locus predisposing to human colorectal cancer". Science 1993; 260:810-812.

Penn I. "Secondary neoplasms as a consequence of transplantation and cancer therapy". Cancer Det. and Prev. 1988; 12:39-57.

Penno MB, August JT, Baylin SB, Mabry M, Linnoila RI, Lee VS, Croteau D, Yang XL and Rosada C. "Expression of CD44 in human lung cancers". Cancer Research 1994; 54:1381-1387.

Perdew GH. "Association of the Ah-receptor with the 90-KDa heat shock protein". J.Biol. Chem. 1988; 263:13802-805.

Perera F, Hemminki K, Grzybowska E, Motykiewicz G, Michalska J, Santella RM, Young TL, Dickey C, Brandt-Rauf P, De Vivo I, Blaner W, Tsai W-Y and Chorazy M. "Molecular and genetic damage in humans from environmental pollution in Poland". Nature 1992; 360:256-258.

Perera F, Mayer J, Jaretzki A, Hearne S, Brenner D, Young T, Fischman H, Grimes M, Grantham S, Tang M, Tsai W-Y and Santella R. "Comparison of DNA adducts and sister chromatid exchange in lung cancer cases and controls". Cancer Research 1989; 49:4446-4451.

Perera F. "Biological markers in risk assessment". In: CC Travis (Ed) "Carcinogen Risk Assessment", Plenum Press, New York, 1988; pp 123-138.

Perera F. "Biomarkers and molecular epidemiology of occupationally related cancer". Jl Toxicol. Envir. Health, 1993; 40:203-215.

Perera F. "The Potential Usefulness of Biological Markers in Risk Assessment". Envir. Health Perspect. 1987; 76:141-145.

Perera FP, Poirier MC, Yuspa SH, Nakayama J., Jaretzki A., Curnen MM, Knowles DM and Weinstein IB. "A pilot project in molecular cancer epidemiology. Determination of benzo[a] pyrene-DNA adducts in animal and human tissues by immunoassays". Carcinogenesis 1982; 3:1405-1410.

Pero RW, Roush GC, Markowitz MM and Miller DG. "Oxidative stress, DNA repair and Cancer susceptibility". Cancer Det. Prev. 1990; 14:555-561.

Pero RW; Johnson D; Markowitz M; Doyle G; Lund-Pero M; Halper M and Miller DG. "DNA repair synthesis in mono-nuclear leukocytes of individuals with and without a familial history of cancer". Carcinogenesis 1989; 10:693-697.

Perry P and Wolff W. "New Giemsa method for the differential staining of sister chromatids". Nature (London) 1974; 251:156-158.

Peto R, Doll R, Buckley JD and Sporn MB. "Can dietary β-carotene materially reduce human cancer rates". Nature 1981; 290:201-208.

Ploton D, Menager M, Jeanneson P, Himber G, Pigeon F and Adnet JJ. "Improvement in the staining and in the visualisation of the argyrophilic proteins of the nucleolar organising region at the optical level". Histochem. Jl. 1986: 18:5-14.

Pluygers E and Baldewyns P. "Tissue Polypeptide antigen (TPA) as a biomarler of the mesothelial cell and of mesothelioma". Eur. Respir. Rev. 1993; 3:47-49.

Pluygers E, Baldewyns P and Beauduin M. "Carcino-embryonic antigen as a marker of carcinogenesis". Jl. Cancer Res. Clinic. Oncol. 1990; 116 (Suppl):266 (abstract).

Pluygers E, Baldewyns P, Gourdin P, van de Weyer R, Minette P, Baleux C and Beauduin M. "Evaluation of the cancer risk associated with activities of the chemical industry in production, utilization and environmental pollution". In D. Breuer (Ed) "Occupational health in the chemical industry", published by Medichem and WHO, Regional Office for Europe, Copenhagen, 1992; pp 109-128.

Pluygers E, Baldewyns P, Minette P, Beauduin M, Gourdin S and Robinet P. "Biomarker assessments in asbestos-exposed workers as indicators for selective prevention of mesothelioma or bronchogenic carcinoma: rationale and practical implementations" Eur. Jl. Cancer Prevention, 1991-1992; 1:57-68 and 129-138.

Pluygers E, Beauduin M and Baldewyns P. "Tumour markers for cancer detection I and II". Cancer Det. and Prev., 1986; 9:495-504 and 505-509.

Pluygers E, Gourdin P, Dardenne G, Scoubeau B and Parfonry A. "Serum Biomarkers in the on-site evaluation of suspected cancer risk in humans residing near hazardous waste sites" - In: CC Travis (Ed) - "Use of Biomarkers in Assessing Health and Environmental Impacts of Chemical Pollutants" - NATO ASI series, volume 250 - Plenum Press, New York, 1993, pp 209-226.

Pluygers E. "Biomarkers". In: T.L. Guidotti (Ed) "A summary report of a workshop principles in epidemiological study designs". Medicina del Lavoro 1995;86:277-282.

Poulsen HE, Loft S and Wassermann K. "Cancer risk related to genetic polymorphisms in carcinogen metabolism and DNA repair". Pharmacol. Toxicol.1993; 72 (Suppl.); 93s-102s.

Prelich G, Tan CK, Kostura M, Mathews M, So AG, Downey K and Stillman B "Functional identity of proliferating cell nuclear antigen and DNA polymerase delta auxiliary protein". Nature (London) 1987; 326:517-520.

Prentice RL, Pepe M and Self SG. "Dietary fat and breast cancer: a quantitative assessment of the epidemiological literature and a discussion of methodological issues". Cancer Research 1989; 49:3147-3156.

Preston-Martin S, Pike MC, Ross RK, Jones PA and Henderson BE. "Increased cell division as a cause of human cancer": Cancer Research 1990; 50:7415-7421.

Quinn CM and Wright NA "The clinical assessment of proliferation and growth in human tumours: evaluation of methods and applications as prognostic variables". Jl. Pathol. 1990; 160:93-102.

Radman M and Wagner R. "Mismatch repair in *Escherichia coli*". Ann. Rev. Genet., 1986; 20:523-538.

Radman M, Taddei F and Halliday J. "Correction des erreurs dans l'ADN: de la génétique bactérienne aux mécanismes de prédisposition héréditaire aux cancers chez l'homme". Médecine/Sciences 1994; 10:1024-1030 (In French).

Ramael M, Jacobs W, Weyler J, Van Meerbeeck J, Bialasiewicz P, Vanden Bossche J, Buysse C, Vermeire P and Van Marck E. "Proliferation in malignant mesothelioma as determined by mitosis counts and immunoreactivity for proliferating cell nuclear antigen (PCNA). Jl. Pathol. 1994; 172:247-253.

Randerath K; Randerath E; Agarwal H; Gupta R; Schurdak and Reddy M. "Postlabelling methods for carcinogen DNA-adduct analysis" Envir. Health Perspct. 1985; 62: 57-65.

Ravitz MJ, Yan S, Herr KD and Wenner CE. "Transforming Growth Factor β-induced activation of Cyclin E-cdk 2 kinase and down regulation of p27kip1 in C3H loT 1/2 mouse fibroblasts". Cancer Research 1995; 55:1413-1416.

Reali Di, Marino F, Bahramandpour S, Carducci A, Barale R and Loprieno N. "Micronuclei in exfoliated urothelial cells and urine mutagenicity in smokers". Mutation Research 1987; 192:145-149.

Reed E, Ozols R, Tarone R, Yuspa SH and Poirier MC. "Platinum-DNA adducts in leukocyte DNA correlate with disease response in ovarian cancer patients receiving platinum-based chemotheraphy". Proc. Nat. Acad. Sci (US) 1987; 84:5024-5028.

Reed E, Ozols RF, Tarone R, Yuspa SH and Poirier MC. "The measurement of cisplatin - DNA adduct levels in testicular cancer patients". Carcinogenesis 1988; 9:1909-1911.

Reeve JC, Payne JA and Bleehen NM. "Production of immunoreactive insulin-like growth factor I (IGF-I) and IGF-I binding proteins by human lung tumours". Brit. J. Cancer 1990; 61:727-731.

Reisman D, Elkind NB, Roy B, Beamon J and Rotter V. "c-Myc trans-activates the p53 promoter through a required downstream CACGTG motif". Cell Growth Differ 1993; 4:57.

Reuterwall C, Hagmar L and the Nordic Study Group on the Health Risk of Chromosome Damage. "Increased cancer risk in humans predicted by increased levels of chromosomal aberrations in lymphocytes". Tenth International Symposium "Epidemiology in Occupational Health", Como, Italy, 1994. Abstract Book, p. 70.

Revel M. "Growth regulatory functions of IL6 and antitumour effects". Res. Immunol. 1992; 143:769-773.

Reyes H, Reisz-Porszasz S and Hankinson O. "Identification of the Ah-receptor nuclear translocator protein (Arnt) as a component of the DNA binding form of the Ah- receptor". Science 1992; 256:1193-1195.

Rhomberg L. "Use of biomarkers in quantitative risk assessment" – In: CC Travis (Ed) – "Use of Biomarkers in Assessing Health and Environmental Impacts of Chemical Pollutants" – NATO ASI series, volume 250 - Plenum Press, New York, 1993, pp 31-46.

Rinkus SJ and Legator MS. "Chemical characterization of 465 known or suspected carcinogens and their correlation with mutagenic activity in the Salmonella typhimurium system. Cancer Research 1979; 39:3289-3318.

Roberts TM "A signal chain of events". Nature 1992; 360:534-535.

Rodenhuis S and Slebos RJC. "The *ras* Oncogenes in Human Lung Cancer". Am. Rev. Respir. Dis 1990; 142:S27-S30.

Rodriguez C, Calle EE, Coates RJ, Miracle-Mc Mahill HL, Thun MJ and Heath CW, Jr. "Estrogen replacement Therapy and Fatal Ovarian Cancer". Am. Jl. Epidemiol. 1995; 141: 828-835.

Rodriguez JW, Kirlin WG, Ferguson RJ, Doll MA, Gray K, Rustan TD, Lee ME, Kemp K, Urso P and Hein DW. "Human acetylator genotype: relationship to colorectal cancer incidence and arylamine N-acetyltransferase expression in colon cytosol". Archiv. Toxicol. 1993; 67:445-452.

Roe, FJC, Lee PN, Conybeare G, Kelly D, Matter B, Prentice D and Tobin G. "The Biosure Study: influence of composition of diet and comsumption on longevity, degenerative diseases and neoplasia in Wistar rats studied for up to 30 months post weaning". Food Chem. Toxicol. 1995; 33 (Suppl. 1): 1s-100s.

Rogers MAM, Thomas DB, Davis S, Weiss NS, Vaughan TL and Nevissi AE. "A case-control study of oral cancer and pre-diagnostic concentrations of selenium and zinc in nail tissue". Int. Jl. Cancer, 1991; 48: 182-188.

Romain S, Chinot O, Klijn JGM, van Putten WLJ, Guirou O, Look M, Martin PM and Foekens JA. "Prognostic value of cytosolic tyrosine kinase activity in 249 node-positive breast cancer patients". Brit. Jl. Cancer 1994; 70: 304-308.

Rosin M, Dunn B and Stich H. "Use of intermediate endpoints in quantitating the response of precancerous lesions to chemopreventive agents". Canad. Jl. Physiol. Pharmacol.1987; 65:483-487.

Ross R, Yuan J-M, Yu M, Wogan GN, Qian G-S, Tu J-T, Groopman JD, Gao Y-T and Henderson BE. "Urinary aflatoxin biomarkers and risk of hepatocellular carcinoma". Lancet 1992; 339:943-946.

Ross R. "Platelet-derived growth factor". Lancet 1989, I:1179-1182.

Ross R. "The pathogenesis of atherosclerosis: a perspective for the 1990s". Nature (London) 1993; 362:801-809.

Rous P. "The influence of diet on transplanted and spontaneous mouse tumours". Jl. Exp. Med. 1914; 20:433-451.

Roussel P and Hernandez-Verdun D. "Identification of Ag-NOR proteins: markers of proliferation related to ribosomal gene activity". Exper. Cell Research 1994; 214: 465-472.

Routledge MN, Garner RC, Jenkins D and Cuzick J. "32P-Postlabelling analysis of DNA from human tissues". Mutation Research 1992; 260:139-145.

Rudiger HW, Schwarz U, Serrand E, Stief M, Krause T, Nowak D, Doerjer G and Lehnert G. "Reduced O^6-methylguanine repair in fibroblast cultures from patients with lung cancer". Cancer Research 1989; 49:5623-5626.

Rupa D, Rita P, Reddy P and Reddi O. "Screening of chromosomal aberrations and sister chromatid exchanges in peripheral lymphocytes of vegetable garden workers". Hum. Toxicology 1988; 7:333-336.

Rusch V, Klimstra D, Linkov I and Dmitrovsky E. "Aberrant expression of p53 or the epidermal growth factor receptor is frequent in early bronchial neoplasia and coexpression precedes squamous cell carcinoma development". Cancer Research 1995; 55:1365-1372.

Ryberg D, Kure E, Lystad S, Skang V, Stangeland L, Mercy I, Børresen A-L and Haugen A. "p53 mutations in Lung Tumours: Relationship to putative susceptibility markers for cancer". Cancer Research 1994; 54:1551-1555.

Sadowska A, Pluygers E, Narkiewicz M, Pawelczak A, Lata B. "Environmental genotoxicity and cancer risk in humans: a combined evaluation correlating the results of the Tradescantia micronucleus assay in the field and human biomarker assessments in serum. I. The TRAD-MCN assay". European Journal of Cancer Prevention; 1993, 3:69- 78.

Sakamoto J, Watanabe T, Tokumaru T, Takagi H, Nakazato H and Lloyd KO. "Expression of Lewis[a], Lewis[b], Lewis[x], Lewis[y], Sitalyl-Lewis[a] and Sialyl-Lewis[x] Blood group antigens in human gastric carcinoma and in nomal gastric tissue". Cancer Research 1989; 49:745-752.

Sakanoue Y, Hatada T, Kusunoki M, Yanagi H, Yamamura T and Utsunomiya J. "Protein Kinase C activity as a marker for colorectal cancer". Int J Cancer 1991; 48: 803-806.

Salonen JT, Alfthan G, Huttunen JK and Puska P. "Association between serum selenium and the risk of cancer". Amer Jl. Epidemiol. 1984; 120: 342-349.

Sanders BM, Jay M, Draper GJ and Roberts EM. "Non-ocular cancer in relatives of retinoblastoma patients". Brit J Cancer, 1989; 60:358-365

Santella RM. "DNA adducts in humans as biomarkers of exposure to environmental and occupational carcinogens" - Envir. Carcinog. Ecotox. Rev. 1991; cg: 57-81.

Sarasin A. "La réparation de l'ADN au centre de la biologie de la cellule". Médecine/Sciences 1994b; 10: 951-952. (In French).

Sarasin A. "Les génes humains de la réparation de l'ADN". Médecine/Sciences 1994a; 10: 43- 54. (In French).

Satoh MS and Lindahl T. "Enzymatic repair of oxidative DNA damage". Cancer Research (Suppl.) 1994; 54:1899s-1901s.

Satokata I, Tanaka K, Miura N, Miyamoto I, Satoh Y, Kondo S and OkadaY. "Characterization of a splicing mutation in group A xeroderma pigmentosum". Proc. Natl. Acad. Sci. USA 1990; 87: 9908-9912.

Savitsky K, Bar-Shira A, Gilad S, Rotman G, Ziv Y, Vanagaite L, Tagle DA, Smith S, Uziel T, Sfez S, Ashkenazi M, Pecker I, Frydmna M, Harnik R, Patanjali SR, Simmons A, Clines GA, Sratiel A, Gatti RA, Taylor R, Arlett CF, Miki T Weissman SM, Lovett M, Collins FS and Shiloh Y. "A single ataxia-telangiectasia gene with a product similar to PI-3 kinase". Science 1995; 268:1749-1753.

Schaeffer L, Roy R, Humbert S, Moncollin V, Vermeulen W, Hoeijmakers JHJ, Chambon P and Egly JM. "DNA repair helicase: a component of BTF2 (TFIIH) basic transcription factor". Science 1993; 260:58-63.

Schlichtholz B, Trédaniel J, Lubin R, Zalcman G, Hirsch A and Soussi T. "Analyses of p53 antibodies in sera of patients with lung carcinoma define immunodominant regions in the p53 protein". Brit. J Cancer 1994; 69:809-816.

Schlipkötter H-W, Baginski B and Krämer U. "The carcino-embryonic antigen (CEA) in urban populations. Epidemiological studies". Zbl. Bakt. Hyg. I Abt. Orig. B. 1978;166:136-143. (In German).

Schneider PM, Hung MC, Chiocca SM, Manning J, Zhao X, Fang K, and Roth JA. "Differential expression of the c-*erb*B-2 gene in human small cell and non-small cell lung cancer". Cancer Research 1989; 49:4968-4971.

Schoket B, Phillips DH, Hewer A and Vincze I. "32P-postlabelling detection of aromatic DNA adducts in peripheral blood lymphocytes from aluminium production plant workers". Mutation Research 1991; 260:89-98.

Schulte PA, Boeniger M, Walker J, Schober S, Pereira M, Gulati D, Wojciechowski J, Garza A, Froelich R, Strauss G, Halperin W, Herrick R and Griffith J. "Biologic markers in hospital workers exposed to low levels of ethylene oxide". Mutation Research 1992; 278: 237-251.

Schulte PA. "Contribution of biological markers to occupational health" – Keynote address at 23rd International Congress on Occupational Health, Montreal, September 1990 – In: volume of Keynote addresses, 23rd ICOH, Montreal, Canada, 1990 – Montreal, Communications 2000, pp 149-177.

Seidegård J, Pero RW, Markowitz MM, Roush G, Miller DG and Beattie EJ. "Isoenzyme(s) of glutathione transferase (class μ) as a marker for the susceptibility to lung cancer: a follow-up study". Carcinogenesis (London) 1990; 11:33-36.

Seidegård J, Vorachek WR, Pero RW and Pearson WR. "Hereditary differences in the expression of the human glutathione transferase active on *trans*-stilbene oxide are due to a gene deletion". Proc. Natl. Acadm. Sci., USA, 1988; 85:7293-7297.

Serrano M, Hannon GJ and Beach D. "A new regulatory motif in cell-cycle control causing specific inhibition of cyclin D/CDK4". Nature 1993; 366: 704-707.

Shamberger RJ, Rukenova E, Longfield AK, Tytko SA, Deodhar S and Willis CE. "Antioxidants and cancer: selenium in the blood of normals and cancer patients". Jl. Natl. Cancer Inst., 1973; 50:863-870.

Shamberger RJ. "Evaluation of water soluble and lipid soluble sialic acid levels as tumour markers". Anticancer Research 1986; 6:717-720.

Shamsuddin AK, Sinopoli NT, Hemminkikk, Boesch RR and Harris CC. "Detection of benzo[a]pyrene: DNA adducts in human white blood cells". Cancer Res. 1985; 45:66-68.

Shapiro GI, Edwards CD, Kobzik L, Godleski J, Richards W, Sugarbaker DJ and Rollins BJ. "Reciprocal Rb inactivation and p 16^{INK4} expression in primary lung cancers and cell lines". Cancer Research 1995; 55:505-509.

Shaw Rj, Benedict SH, Clark RA and King TE "Pathogenesis of pulmonary fibrosis in interstitial lung disease. Alveolar macrophage PDGF(B) gene activation and up-regulation by interferon γ" Am. Rev. Respir. Dis. 1991; 143:167-173.

Sherr CJ. "The ins and outs of Rb: coupling gene expression to the cell cycle clock". Trends Cell. Biol. 1994; 4:15-18.

Shi D, He G, Cao S, Pan W, Zhang HZ, Yu D and Hung MC. "Overexpression of the c-*erb*B-2/*neu*-encoded p185 protein in primary lung cancer". Mol. Carcinogen 1992; 5:213-218.

Shigenaga MK, Gimeno CJ and Ames BN. "Urinary 8-hydroxy-2'-deoxyguanosine as a biological marker of *in vivo* oxidative DNA damage". Proc Natl Acad Sci, USA, 1989; 86:9697-9701.

Shivji MKK, Kenny MK and Wood RD. "Proliferating cell nuclear antigen (PCNA) is required for DNA excision repair". Cell 1992; 69:657-676.

Shtivelman E and Bishop JM. "Expression of CD44 is repressed in neuroblastoma cells". Mol. Cell. Biol. 1991; 11:5446-5453.

Shuker D, Bailey E, Parry A, Lamb J and Farmer PB. "The determination of urinary 3- methyladenine in humans as a potential monitor of exposure to methylating agents" - Carcinogenesis 1987; 7:959-962.

Siess M-H, Le Bon AM and Suschetet M. "Dietary modification of drug-metabolizing enzyme activities: dose-response effects of flavonoids". Jl. Toxicol. Environ. Health 1992; 35:141-152.

Simic MG and Bergtold DS. "Dietary modulation of DNA damage in human". Muatation Research 1991; 250:17-24.

Singh N, McCoy M, Tice R and Schneider E. "A simple technique for quantitation of low levels of DNA damage in individual cells" - Exper Cell Research; 1988:184-191.

Singhal AK, Ørntoft TF, Nudelman E, Nance S, Schibig L, Stroud MR, Clausen H and Hakomori S. "Profiles of Lewis^{x}-containing glycoproteins and glycolipids in sera of patients with adenocarcinoma". Cancer Research 1990; 50:1375-1380.

Sinha A, Liscombe V, Gollapudi B, Jersy G and Flake R. "Cytogenetic variability of lymphocytes from phenotypically normal men: influence of age, smoking, season and sample storage". Jl. Toxicol. Envir. Health, 1986; 17:327-345.

Sinués B, Pérez J, Bernal ML, Sáenz MA, Lanuza J and Bartolomé M. "Urinary mutagenicity and N-acetylation phenotype in textile industry workers exposed to arylamines". Cancer Research 1992; 52:4885-4889.

Sivaraman L, Leatham MP, Yee J, Wilkens LR, Lau AF and Le Marchand L. "CYP1A1 genetic polymorphisms and *in situ* colorectal cancer". Cancer Research 1994; 54: 3692- 3695.

Skyberg K, Hansteen I-L, Jelmert Ø and Rønneberg A. A cytogenetic and haematological investigation of oil exposed workers in a Norwegian cable manufacturing company". Brit Jl Industr Med, 1989; 46:791-798.

Smith CA, Cooper PK and Hanawalt PC. "Measurement of repair replication by equilibrium sedimentation". In: EC Friedberg and PC Hanawalt (eds): "DNA repair. A Laboratory manual of research procedures". Vol. I, Part B, pp. 471-485. Marcel Dekker Inc., New York, 1981.

Smits A, Funa K, Vassbotn FS, Beausang-Linder M, Ekenstam F, Heldin CH, Westermark B and Nister M. "Expression of platelet-derived growth factor and its receptors in proliferative disorders of fibroblastic origin". Am. J. Pathol., 1992; 140:639-648.

Sorsa M, Anttila A and Järventaus H. "Styrene revisited-exposure assessment and risk estimation in reinforced plastics industry". In: New Horizons in Biological Dosimetry - Wiley-Liss, New York 1991, Pp 187-195.

Sorsa M, Pyy L, Salomaa S, Nyland L and Yager J. "Biological and environmental monitoring of occupational exposure to cyclophosphamide in industry and hospitals". Mutation Research 1988; 204: 465-479.

Sorsa M, Wilbourn J and Vainio H. "Human cytogenetic damage as a predictor of cancer risk". In: H Vainio, PN Maggee, DB Mc Gregor and AJ Mc Michael (Eds). "Mechanisms of Carcinogenesis in Risk Identification". International Agency for Research on Cancer, Lyon, 1992; pp. 543-554.

Soussi T, Caron de Fromentel C and May P. Structural aspects of the p53 protein in relation to gene evolution". Oncogene 1990; 5:945-952.

Soussi T, Legros Y, Lubin R, Ory K and Schlichtholz B. "Multifactorial analysis of p53 alteration in human cancer: a review". Int J Cancer 1994; 57:1-9.

Sozzi G, Miozzo M, Donghi R, Pilotti S, Cariani CT, Pastorino U, Della Porta G and Pierotti MA. "Deletions of 17p and p53 mutations in preneoplastic lesions of the lung". Cancer Research 1992; 52:6079-6082.

Sozzi G, Miozzo M, Taglialue E, Calderone C, Lombardi L, Pilotti S, Pastorino U, Pierotti MA and Della Porta G. "Cytogenetic abnormalities and overexpression of receptors for growth factors in normal bronchial epithelium and tumour samples of lung cancer patients". Cancer Research 1991; 51:400-404.

Sparnins VL, Barany G and Wattenberg LW. "Effects of organosulfur compounds from garlic and onions on benzo(a) pyrene induced neoplasia and glutathione S-transferase activity". Carcinogenesis (London) 1988; 9:131-134.

Stamatoyannopoulos G, Nute PE, Lindsley D, Farquhar M, Brice M, Nakamoto N and Papayannopoulou T. "Somatic cell mutation system based on human hemogloblin mutants". In: Ansari AA and de Serres FJ (Eds.) "Single Cell Monitoring Systems" (Topics in Chem. Mutag.) 1984; pp 1-35.

Stähelin HB, Gey KF, Eichholzer M and Lüdin E. "β-carotene and cancer prevention: the Basel study" Am Jl. Clin. Nutr. 1991; 53:265s-269s.

Stevens RG, Jones DY and Micozzi MS. "Body iron stores and the risk of cancer". New Engl. Jl. Med. 1988; 319:1047-1052.

Stich H and Rosin M. "Micronuclei in exfoliated human cells as a tool for studies in cancer risk and cancer intervention". Cancer Letters, 1984; 22:241-253.

Stich H, Curtis J and Parida B. "Application of the micronucleus test to exfoliated cells of high cancer risk groups: tobacco chewers". Int J. Cancer 1982; 30:553-559.

Stich H, Parida B and Brunnemann K. "Localized formation of micronuclei in the oral mucosa and tobacco-specific nitrosamines in the saliva of "reverse" smokers, khaini tobacco chewers and gudakhu users". Int J. Cancer 1992; 50:172-176.

Stiles AD and Moats-Staats BM. "Production and action of insulin-like growth factor/somatomedin C in primary cultures of fetal lung fibroblasts". Am. J. Respir. Cell Mol Biol 1989; 1:21-26.

Stolley P, Soper K, Galloway S, Nichols W, Norman S and Wolman S. "Sister-chromatid exchanges in association with occupational exposure to ethylene oxide". Mutation Research 1984; 129:89-102.

Sugimura T, Sato S, Nagao M, Xahagi T, Matsushima T, Seino Y, Takeuchi M and Kawachi T. "Overlapping of carcinogens and mutagens" – In: PN Magee, S Takayama, T Sugimura and T Matsushima (eds): "Fundamentals of Cancer Prevention", pp. 191-215. Univ. of Tokyo Press, Tokyo; Univ. Park Press, Baltimore, 1976.

Sundarensan V, Ganly P, Hasleton P, Rudd R, Sinha G, Bleehen NM and Rabbitts P. "p53 and chromosome 3 abnormalities, characteristic of malignant lung tumours, are detectable in preinvasive lesions of the bronchus". Oncogene 1992; 7:1989-1997.

Sutter TR and Greenlee WF. "Classification of members of the Ah gene battery". Chemosphere 1992; 25: 223-226.

Swift M, Reitnauer PJ, Morrell D and Chase CL. "Breast and other cancers in families with ataxia-telangiectasia". New Engl. Jl. Med. 1987; 316:1289-1294.

Taioli E, Crofts F, Trachman J, Demopoulos R, Toniolo P and Garte SJ. "A specific African- American CYP1A1 polymorphism is associated with adenocarcinoma of the lung". Cancer Research, 1995a; 55:472-473.

Taioli E, Trachman J, Chen X, Toniolo P and Garte SJ. "A CYP IAI. Restriction Fragment Length Polymorphism is associated with breast cancer in African-American women". Cancer Research 1995b; 55:3757-3758.

Tannenbaum A. "The genesis and growth of tumours. II: Effects of caloric restriction per se". Cancer Research 1942; 2:460-467.

Tannenbaum A. "The initiation and growth of tumours". Am. Jl. Cancer 1940; 38:335-350.

Tates AD, Bernini LF, Natarajan AT, Ploem JS, Verwoerd NP, Cole J, Green MHL, Arlett CF and Norris PN. "Detection of somatic mutants in man: HPRT mutations in lymphocytes and hemoglobin mutations in erythrocytes". Mutation Research, 1989; 213:73-82.

Teel RW. "Ellagic acid binding to DNA as possible mechanism for its antimutagenic and anticarcinogenic action". Cancer Letters 1986; 30:329-336.

Tennant RW, Margolin BH, Shelby MD, Zeiger E, Hasman JK, Spalding J, Caspary W, Resnick M, Stasiewicz S, Anderson B and Minor R. "Prediction of chemical carcinogenicity in rodents from *in vitro* genetic toxicity assays". Science 1987, 236:933-941.

Tennant RW. "Relationship between *in vitro* genetic toxicity and carcinogenicity studies in animals". In: C Maltoni and IJ Selikoff (eds) "Living in a chemical world - Occupational and environmental significance of industrial carcinogens" pp: 127-132. Annals of the New York Academy of Science, Vol 534. The New York Academy of Sciences, New York 1988.

Tenney D, Zabrecky J, Jarosz D and Carney WP. "Quantitation of the full length (p170) and truncated forms (p110) of the epidermal growth factor receptor EGFr using an ELISA format". Proc. Am. Ass. Cancer Res. 1993; 34:55.

Terheggen PM, Dykman R, Begg AC, Dubbelman R, Floot BG, Hart AA and den Engelse L. "Monitoring of interaction products of CIS-diammine dichloroplatinum (II) and CIS-diammine (1,1-cyclobutanedicarboxylato) platinum (II) with DNA in cells from platinum treated cancer patients" – Cancer Res., 1988; 48:5597-5603.

Thibodeau SN, Bren G and Schaid D. "Microsatellite instability in cancer of the proximal colon". Science 1993; 260:816-819.

Thiery JP and Boyer B. "Les molécules adhésives et la communication cellulaire". Pour la Science 1992; 179: 36-43. (In French).

Thiringer G, Granung G, Holmen A, Högstedt B, Järuholm B, Jönsson D, Wahlström J and Westin J. "Comparison of methods for the biomonitoring of nurses handling antitumour drugs". Scand. Jl. Work Environ. Health 1991; 17:133-138.

Thomale J, Seiler F, Müller MR, Seeber S and Rajewsky MF. "Repair of O^6-alkylguanines in the nuclear DNA of human lymphocytes and leukaemic cells: analysis at the single-cell level". Brit. Jl. Cancer 1994; 69: 698-705.

Thomas H, Nasim MM, Sarraf CE, Alison MR, Love S, Lambert HE and Price P. "Proliferating cell nuclear antigen (PCNA) immunostaining – a prognostic factor in ovarian cancer?". Brit. Jl. Cancer 1995; 71:357-362.

Thompson L. "Somatic cell genetics approach to dissecting mammalian DNA repair". Environ. Mol. Mutag. 1989; 14:264-281.

Thomson D, Krupey J, Freedman S and Gold P "The radio-immunoassay of circulating carcinoembryonic antigen of the human digestive system" Proc. Natl. Acad. Sci. USA 1969; 64:161-167.

Thorling EB. "Dietary non-nutritive cancer protective factors". Europ. Jl. Cancer Prev. 1993; 2:95-103.

Tkeshelashvili LK, McBride TJ, Spence K and Loeb LA. "Mutation spectrum of copper-induced DNA damage". Jl. Biol. Chem 1991; 266:6401-6406.

Törnqvist M. "Current research on Hemoglobin adducts and cancer risk: an overview" In: CC Travis (Ed.): "Use of Biomarkers in Assessing Health and Environmental Impacts of Chemical Pollutants". NATO ASI Series, volume 250. Plenum Press, New York, 1993: pp. 17-30.

Törnqvist M; Mowrer J; Jensen S and Ehrenberg L. "Monitoring of environmental cancer initiators through hemoglobin adducts by a modified Edman degradation method". Anal. Biochem 1986; 154:255-266.

Trauth BC, Klas C, Peters AMJ, Matzku S, Moller P, Falk W, Debatin KM and Krammer PH "Monoclonal antibody-mediated tumour regression by induction of apoptosis". Science 1989, 245:301-305.

Travis CC and Belefant H. "Promotion as a factor in carcinogenesis". Toxicology Letters 1992; 60:1-9.

Tretli S. "Height and weight in relation to breast cancer morbidity and mortality: a prospective study of 570.000 women in Norway". Int. Jl. Cancer 1989; 44:23-30.

Trosko JE and Chang CC "Stem cell theory of carcinogenesis". Toxicology Letters, 1989; 49:283-295.

Trosko JE and Yager JD. "A sensitive method to measure physical and chemical carcinogen- induced 'unscheduled DNA synthesis' in rapidly dividing eukaryotic cells". Exp. Cell Res. 1974; 88:47-55.

Trosko JE, Jone C and Chang CC. "The role of tumour promoters on phenotypic alterations affecting intercellular communication and tumourigenesis". Ann. NY Acad. Sci. 1983; 407:316-327.

Trosko JE. "A failed paradigm: carcinogenesis is more than mutagenesis". Mutagenesis 1988, 3:363-364.

Turley E and Auersperg N. "A hyaluronate binding protein transiently codistributes with p21k- *ras* in cultured cell lines". Exper. Cell. Research 1989; 182:340-348.

Uematsu F, Kikuchi H, Motomiya M, Abe T, Sagami I, Ohmachi T, Wakui A, Kanamaru R and Watanabe M. "Association between restriction fragment length polymorphism of the human Cytochrome P450 II E1 gene and susceptibility to lung cancer". Japn. Jl. Cancer Res., 1991; 82:254-256.

Vainio H. Sorsa M. and Hemminki K. "Biological monitoring in surveillance of exposure to genotoxicants". Amer J. Industr. Med. 1983; 4: 87-103.

Van Schooten FJ, van Leeuwen FE, Hillebrand MJX, de Rijke ME, Haret AAM, van Veen HG, Oosterink S and Kriek E. "Determination of benzo(a) pyrene diol epoxide-DNA adducts in white blood cell DNA from coke-oven workers: the impact of smoking". Jl. Nat. Cancer Inst. 1990; 82:927-933.

Van Sittert NJ. "Individual Exposure Monitoring from Plasma or Urinary Metabolite Determination". In "Biological Monitoring of Exposure and the Response at the Subcellular Level to Toxic Substances". Arch. Toxicology, 1989; Suppl. 13:91-100.

Vanparys P, Vermeiren F, Sysmans M and Temmerman R. "The micronucleus assay as a test for the detection of aneugenic activity". Mutation Research 1990; 244:95-103.

Vähäkangas K and Pelkonen O. "Host variantions in carcinogen metabolism and repair". In: Lynch HT and Hirayama T. (Eds) "Genetic Epidemiology of Cancer". CRC Press, 1990. Boca Raton, pp. 35-54.

Vähäkangas K, Haugen A and Harris CC. "An applied synchronous fluorescence spectrophotometric assay to study benzo[a]pyrene-diolepoxide DNA adducts". Carcinogenesis 1985; 6:1109-1116.

Vähäkangas KH, Samet JM, Metcalf RA, Welsh JA, Bennett WP, Lane DP and Harris CC. "Mutations of p53 and *ras* genes in radon-associated lung cancer from uranium miners". Lancet 1992; 339:576-580.

Västrik I, Mäkelä TP, Koskinen PJ, Klefstrom J and Alitalo K. "Myc protein: partners and antagonists". Crit Rev. Oncogenesis 1994; 5:59-68.

Vesalainen SLB, Lipponen PK, Talja MT, Alhava EM and Syrjänen KJ. "Proliferating cell nuclear antigen and p51 expression as prognostic factors in TI-2, Mo prostatic adenocarcinoma". Int. Jl. Cancer 1994; 58:303-308.

Vignaud J-M, Marie B, Klein N, Plénat F, Pech M, Borrelly J, Martinet N, Duprez A and Martinet Y. "The role of platelet-derived growth factor production by tumour-associated macrophages in tumour stroma formation in lung cancer". Cancer Research 1994; 54:5455-5463.

Vignaud JM, Allain M, Martinet N, Pech M, Plénat F and Martinet Y. "Presence of platelet-derived growth factor in normal and fibrotic lung is specifically associated with interstitial macrophages while both interstitial macrophages and alveolar epithelial cells express the c-*sis* proto-oncogene". Am. J. Respir. Cell. Mol. Biol. 1991, 5:531-538.

Vineis P, Caporaso N, Tannenbaum SR, Skipper PL, Glogowski J, Bartsch H, Coda M, Talaska G and Kadlubar F. "Acetylation phenotype, carcinogen-hemoglobin adducts and cigarrette smoking". Cancer Research 1990; 50:3002-3004.

Vineis P. "Uses of biochemical and biological markers in occupational epidemiology". Revue Epidem. et Santé Publique, 1992; 40:S63-S69.

Vleminckx C, Klemens W, Schriewer L, Joris I, Lÿsen N, Maes R, Ottogali M, Pays A, Planard C, Rigaux G, Ros Y, Vande Rivière M, Vandenvelde J, Verschaeve L, Deplaen P and Lakhanisky TL. "La Décharge de Mellery. Phase 2 de l'Enquête". Institut d'Hygiéne et d'Epidémiologie, Section Toxicologie, Brussels, 1994 (in French).

Vleminckx K, Vakaet L, Mareel M, Fiers W and van Roy F. "Genetic manipulation of E-cadherin expression by epithelial tumour cells reveals an invasion supressor role. Cell 1991; 66:107.

Vogelstein B, Fearon E, Hamilton S, Kern S, Preisinger A, Leppert M, Nakamura Y, Whyte R, Smits A and Bos J. "Genetic alterations during colorectal tumour development". N. Engl. J. Med. 1988; 319:525-532.

Volm M, Drings P, Mattern J and Wodrich W. "Prognostic value of oncoproteins for the survival of patients with non-small-cell lung carcinomas". J Oncol. 1993; 2:767-772.

Volm M, Efferth T and Mattern J. "Oncoprotein (c-*myc*, c-*erb*B-1, c-*erb*B-2, c-*fos*) and suppressor gene product (p53) expression in squamous cell carcinomas of the lung. Clinical and biological correlations". Anticancer Res. 1992; 12:11-20.

Waga S, Hannon GJ, Beach D and Stillman B. "The p21 inhibitor of cyclin-dependent kinases controls DNA replication by interaction with PCNA". Nature 1994; 369:574-578.

Wainfan E and Poirier L. "Methyl groups in carcinogenesis: effects on DNA methylation and gene expression". Cancer Research 1992; 52 (Suppl): 2071s-2077s.

Waldock A, Ellis IO, Armitage N, Turner DR, Hardcastle JD and Embleton J. "Differential expression of the Lewis Y antigen defined by monoclonal antibody C14/1/46/10 in colonic polyps". Cancer 1989; 64:414-421.

Walker C, Robertson LJ, Myskow MW, Pendleton N and Dixon GR. "p53 expression in normal and dysplastic bronchial epithelium and in lung carcinomas". Brit J Cancer 1994; 70:297-303.

Wang J, Coltrera MD and Gown AM. "Cell Proliferation in human soft tissue tumours correlates with platelet-derived growth factor B chain expression and immunohistochemical and in situ hybridization study". Cancer Res, 1994; 54:560-564.

Wang N, Yan K and Rasenick MM. "Tubulin binds specifically to the signal-transducing proteins Gs α and Giα1". Jl. Biol. Chem 1990; 265:1239-1242.

Wargovich MJ, Woods C, Eng VWS, Stephens LC and Gray K. "Chemoprevention of N-nitrosomethylbenzylamine-induced esophageal cancer in rats by the naturally occurring thioether, diallylsulfide". Cancer Research 1988; 48:6872-6875.

Warwick AP, Redman CWE, Jones PW, Fryer AA, Gilford J, Alldersea J and Strange RC. "Progression of cervical intra-epithelial neoplasia to cervical cancer: interactions of cytochrome P450 2D6 EM and glutathione S-transferase GSTM1-null genotypes and cigarette smoking". Brit Jl. Cancer 1994; 70: 704-708.

Washimi O, Nagatake M, Osada H. Veda R, Koshikawa T, Seki T, Takahashi To and Takahashi Ta. "*In vivo* occurrence of p16 (MTS1) and p15 (MTS2) alterations preferentially in non-small-cell lung cancers". Cancer Research, 1995; 55:514-517.

Waterfield MD, Serace GT, Whittle N, Stroobant P, Johnson A, Wasteson A, Westermark B, Heldin C-H, Huang JS and Deuel TF. "Platelet-derived growth factor is structurally related to the putative transforming protein p28 *sis* of simian sarcoma virus". Nature (London) 1983; 304:35-39.

Wattenberg LW, Sparnins VL and Barany G. "Inhibition of N-nitrosodiethylamine carcinogenesis by naturally organosulfur compounds and monoterpenes". Cancer Research 1989; 49: 2689-2692.

Wattenberg LW. "Chemoprevention of cancer". Cancer Research 1985; 45:1-8.

Wattenberg LW. "Inhibition of Carcinogenesis by Minor Dietary Constituents" – Cancer Research 1992; 52 (Suppl): 2085s-2091s.

Wattenberg LW. "Inhibition of neoplasia by minor dietary constituents". Cancer Research 1983; 43: 2448s-2453s.

Weber JL and May PE. "Abundant class of DNA polymorphisms which can be typed using the polymerase chain reaction". Ann. Hum. Genet., 1989: 44:338-396.

Webster NJG, Green S, Jin JR and Chambon P. "The hormone binding domains of the estrogen and glucocorticoid receptors contain an inducible transcription activation function". Cell. 1988; 54:199-207.

Wei Q, Matanoski GM, Farmer ER, Hedayati MA and Grossman L. "DNA repair and aging in basal cell carcinoma: a molecular epidemiology study". Proc. Natl. Acad. Sci, USA, 1993; 90: 1614-1618.

Wei Q; Matanoski GM; Farmer ER; Hedayati MA and Grossman L. "DNA Repair Related to Multiple Skin Cancers and Drug Use". Cancer Res. 1994; 54:437-440.

Weinberg RA. "The genetic origins of human cancer". Cancer 1988; 61: 1963-1968.

Weinberger C, Thompson CC, Ong ES et al. "The c-*erb*-A gene encodes a thyroid hormone receptor". Nature 1986; 284: 641-646.

Weiner DB, Nordberg J, Robinson R, Nowell PC, Gazdar A, Greene MI, Williams WV, Cohen JA and Kern JA. "Expression of the *neu* gene-encoded protein (p185 *neu*) in human non-small-cell carcinomas of the lung". Cancer Research 1990; 50:421-431.

Weinstein IB. "Growth Factors, Oncogenes and Multistage Carcinogenesis". Jl. Cell. Biochem. 1987; 33:213-224.

Weinstein IB. "The origins of human cancer: molecular mechanisms of carcinogenesis and their applications for cancer prevention and treatment" – Cancer Research 1988; 48:4135-4143.

Welsch CW. "Relationship between dietary fat and experimental mammary tumourigenesis: a review and critique". Cancer Research (Suppl.) 1992; 52:2040s-2048s.

Welshons WV, Leiberman ME and Gorski J. "Nuclear localization of unoccupied estrogen receptors". Nature, 1984; 307:747-749.

Westermark B and Heldin C-H. "Platelet-derived growth factor. Structure function and implications in normal and malignant cell growth". Acta Oncologica 1993; 32:101-105.

Wild CP; Jiang YZ; Sabbioni G; Chapot B and Montesano R. "Evaluation of methods for quantitation of aflatoxin-albumin adducts and their application to human exposure assessment". Cancer Research 1990; 50:245-251.

Wilson GD, McNally NJ, Dische S et al. "Measurement of cell kinetics in human tumours *in vivo* using bromodeoxyuridine incorporation and flow cytometry". Brit. Jl. Cancer 1988; 58:423-431.

Winter SF, Minna JD, Johnson BE, Takahashi T, Gazdar AF and Carbone DP. "Development of antibodies against p53 in lung cancer patients appears to be dependent on the type of p53 mutation". Cancer Research 1992; 52:4168-4174.

Wogan GN and Tannenbaum S. "Biological Monitoring of Environmental Toxic Chemicals" In: Lave LB and Upton AC (Eds): Toxic Chemicals, Health and the Environment. The Johns Hopkins University Press, Baltimore, 1987, pp 142-169.

Wogan GN. "Markers of Exposure to Carcinogens". Envir. Health Perspct. 1989; 9-17.

Wong WSF and Tattersall MHN "Immunohistochemical determination of tumour growth fraction in human ovarian carcinoma". Brit. Jl. Obstet. Gynaecol. 1989; 96:720-724.

Wyllie AH. "Apoptosis (The 1992 Frank Rose Memorial Lecture)". Brit. Jl. Cancer 1993; 67:205-208.

Xiong Y, Zhang H and Beach D. "Subunit rearrangement of the cyclin-dependent kinases is associated with cellular transformation". Genes Dev. 1993; 7:1572-1583

Xue K-X, Ma G-J, Wang S and Zhou P. "The *in vivo* micronucleus test in human capillary blood lymphocytes; methodological studies and effect of ageing". Mutation Research 1992a; 278:259-264.

Xue K-X, Wang S, Ma G-J, Zhou P, Wu P-Q, Zhang R-F, Xu Z, Chen W-S and Wang Y-Q. "Micronucleus formation in peripheral-blood lymphocytes from smokers and the influence of alcohol- and tea-drinking habits". Int. J. Cancer 1992 b; 50:702-705.

Xue K-X, Zhou P, Ma G-J and Wang S. "Improvement of method for counting micronucleated lymphocytes in human peripheral blood" Radiat. Protect, 1988; 8:224- 227.

Yager J, Rappaport S and Paradisin W. "Sister chromatid exchanges in peripheral lymphocytes of workers exposed to low concentrations of styrene". Environm. Mutagen, 1989; Suppl. 15:224.

Yamasaki H "Gap junctional intercellular communication and carcinogenesis". Carcinogenesis (London) 1990; 11:1051-1058.

Yokota AJ, Wad M, Shimosata Y, Tereda M and Sugimura T. "Loss of heterozygosity on chromosomes 3, 13 and 17 in-small-cell carcinoma and on chromosome 3 in adenocarcinoma of the lung". Proc. Natl Acad Sci USA. 1987; 84:9252-9256.

Yoshino I, Goedegebuure PS, Peoples GE, Parikh AS, Di Maio JM, Lyerly HK, Gazdar AF and Eberlein TJ. "HER2/*neu*-derived peptides are shared antigens among human non-small-cell lung cancer and ovarian cancer". Cancer Research 1994; 54:3387-3390.

Yotti LP, Chang CC and Trosko JE. "Elimination of metabolic cooperation in chinese hamster cells by a tumour promoter". Science 1979; 206: 1089-1091.

Yu S, Pritchard M, Kremer E, Lynch M, Nancarrow J, Baker E, Holman K, Mulley JC, Warren ST, Schlessinger D, Sutherland GR and Richards RI. "Fragile X genotype characterized by an unstable region of DNA". Science (Washington DC) 1991; 252:1179-1181.

Zakian VA. "ATM-related genes: what do they tell us about function of the human gene ?". cell 1995; 82:685-687.

Zeiger E. "Carcinogenicity of mutagens: predictive capability of the *Salmonella* mutagenesis assay for rodent carcinogenicity" Cancer Research 1987; 47:1287-1296.

Zhang L-X, Cooney RV and Bertram JS. "Carotenoids up-regulate Connexin-43 gene expression independent of their provitamin A or antioxidant properties". Cancer Research 1992; 52: 5707-5712.

Ziegler RG, Subar AF, Craft NE, Ursin G, Patterson BH and Granbard BI. "Does β-carotene explain why reduced cancer risk is associated with vegetable and fruit intake?". Cancer Research 1992 (suppl.) 52: 2060s-2066s.

Ziegler RG. "Vegetables, fruits and carotenoids and the risk of cancer". Am Jl. Clin. Nutr. 1991; 53:251s-259s.

Zielhuis RL. "Biological monitoring studies in occupational and environmental health". In: A. Castellani (editor). "Epidemiology and quantitation of environmental risk in humans from radiation and other agents". Plenum Press, New York-London, 1985; pp 291-306.

Chapter 5

THE MULTISTAGE MODEL OF CARCINOGENESIS: A CRITICAL REVIEW OF ITS USE

V.J. Cogliano[1], E.G. Luebeck[2], and G.A. Zapponi[3]

[1]U.S. Environmental Protection Agency, Washington DC, USA
[2]Fred Hutchinson Cancer Research Center, Seattle, USA
[3]National Institute of Health, Rome, Italy

5.1. INTRODUCTION

Dose-response models span a hierarchy that reflects an ability to incorporate different kinds of information. Models based on studies of a particular agent operating through an established mechanism of action provide the greatest specificity. An example is EPA's model (under development) of the receptor-mediated toxicity of dioxin (U.S. EPA, 1992).

Next are *general models of* mechanism *of action* that are used with parameter information from laboratory studies on a specific agent. Examples are the two-stage models of initiation, clonal expansion and progression first proposed by Moolgavkar, Venzon, and Knudson (Moolgavkar and Venzon, 1979; Moolgavkar and Knudson, 1981) and later extensions (Chen and Farland, 1991; Yang and Chen, 1991; Kopp-Schneider et al., 1991; Tan and Chen, 1991; Chen, 1993; Tan, 1991). The two-stage clonal expansion models are specifically examined in Chapter 6. The form of these model is built in dependence of the data. Therefore, such models generally require extensive data, also to determine how well they conform with the available observations.

Empirical models, which do not incorporate information about mechanism of action, form the rest of hierarchy. Empirical models are fitted to the available data in

[1]The views expressed in this chapter are those of the authors and do not necessarily reflect the views or policies of the U.S. Environmental Protection Agency.

order to describe the apparent dose-response relationship without reference to any specific mechanism of action. among these, *time-to-event models* (for example, time to death with or without tumor) incorporate longitudinal information of tumor development. Simple *quantal models* use only the final incidence at each dose level.

Several different models have been developed and used under the name "multistage model". An early formulation of the multistage model was proposed by Armitage and Doll, who described a process by which a normal cell becomes malignant through a sequence of transformations. Theirs is a model of a general mechanism of action. Later formulations of the multistage model, including the linearized multistage model used by regulatory agencies in the United States, are mostly empirical models that fit the available data without reference to a particular mechanism of action. Empirical multistage models may incorporate time-to-tumor information or may be quantal models based only on tumor incidence information.

The empirical models that have been used for cancer risk assessment are *stochastic* in nature; that is, they view the occurrence of cancer as a probabilistic event that cannot be predicted with certainty. All models are somehow "stochastic". However, certain "mechanisms" in biologically-based models are sometimes described deterministically, instead of stochastically (e.g., net cell growth).

Because the empirical multistage models do not have a basis in a mechanism of action, they cannot incorporate information about cell proliferation or the incidence of premalignant lesions. The more recent two-stage models of initiation, clonal expansion, and progression (which are described in chapter 6) can be considered to be mechanism-based extensions of the Armitage-Doll multistage model that incorporate information on cell population kinetics.

5.2. HISTORICAL ANTECEDENTS OF THE MULTISTAGE MODEL

Early attempts to model animal carcinogenicity studies used simple, empirical models. These models reflected the modest amount of data that was typically available. At that time, animal carcinogenicity studies often used only one dose level, which was kept constant throughout the duration of the experiment. Sometimes there was no control group. In most cases, there were no supplemental studies that could be used to identify a mechanism of action.

Some early empirical models were *tolerance distribution models,* which are based on the assumption that each individual in a population has a tolerance for the carcinogenic agent. Under this assumption, if the dose of a carcinogenic agent exceeds an individual's tolerance, a tumor will develop; if the dose is below the tolerance, there will be no tumor. Tolerances are assumed to vary from individual to individual, and tolerances across a population are assumed to follow a standard probability distribution, such as the lognormal distribution.

The *log-probit model* assumes that there are tolerances across a population that follow a lognormal distribution. This is equivalent to saying that the logarithms of the tolerances have a normal (bell-shaped) distribution, with mean μ and standard deviation σ. A tumor will develop if the dose exceeds the tolerance; the probability of this equals the portion of the distribution of log-tolerances lying below the logarithm of the dose (Finney, 1987):

$$P(d) = \int_{-\infty}^{(\log d-\mu)/\sigma} \exp -(z^2/2)/(2\pi)^{1/2} dz \,. \tag{5.1}$$

In practice, the tumor incidence data are plotted on log-probit paper (that is, the horizontal axis has a logarithmic scale and the vertical axis has a probit scale, whose axis is marked with divisions corresponding to standard deviations of a normal distribution). A straight line is then drawn through the tumor incidence data and used to extrapolate to lower doses. this model was used for rudimentary experiments without a control group, since the log-dose scale does not include 0.

The *Mantel-Bryan* model simplifies the log-probit model by assuming that the line has a slope of one probit unit per log unit. That is, for each 10-fold decrease in dose, the responding proportion decreases by one standard deviation of a normal distribution (Mantel and Brian, 1961). This assumption was intended to provide an upper bound on the risk; for a time it was used by regulatory agencies in the United States to set exposure standards protective of public health. The Mantel-Bryan model is particularly well suited to experiments conducted at only one dose level; in this case the log-probit slope could not be estimated from the data since at least two dose levels would be needed.

Other early empirical models were called "Mechanistic models", because they would postulate a hypothetical mechanism of action described in physical terms. These models, however, were used as empirical models, because tumor incidence data were fitted to a mathematically prescribed dose-response model and laboratory information was not used to validate the proposed mechanism and to determine the appropriate model and its parameter values.

The *One-hit model* is one such model; it postulates that cancer is the result of a single event in a single cell. The model has only one parameter and describes a dose-response relationship with a fixed shape that is virtually linear in the low and middle dose range.

$$P(d) = 1 - \exp(-qd), \quad q > 0 \tag{5.2}$$

The one-hit model was typically fitted to a single dose point, usually the lowest dose with an increased incidence of cancer. The one-hit model should not be used to fit a data set with more than one dose if the responses do not follow the model's fixed, linear shape (Whittemore and Keller, 1978).

The *multi-hit model* postulates that cancer is the result of a fixed number of identical events (or "hits") in a tissue (Rai and Van Ryzin, 1981). The shape of the model is governed by the number of hits assumed necessary for the induction of cancer. The more hits required, the lower the probability of cancer at low doses, but the faster that probability rises at higher doses. If k hits are required, the probability of a tumor developing is

$$P(d) = \int_0^{gd} z^{k-1} \exp(-z)/(k-1)!\, dz \,. \tag{5.3}$$

The *Weibull model* is another model with a shape parameter (Peto and Lee, 1973). It, too, is based on an analogy for how cancer develops: a tissue sustains "hits" at random, cancer occurs when a portion of the tissue sustains a fixed number of "hits"; cancer is observed when the first such portion has sustained the required number of "hits". The Weibull model can exhibit a dose-response relationship that is either sublinear (shape parameter $k > 1$), linear ($k = 1$) or supralinear ($k < 1$).

$$P(d) = 1 - \exp(-qd^k) \tag{5.4}$$

Around 1980 the limitations of many of these empirical models were apparent. Risk estimates spanning a wide range could be computed with these models, but there was no biological information to help in selecting one of these models over another. Several of these models were severely constrained in shape and were not adequate to empirically describe some data sets with multiple doses showing a nonlinear dose-response relationship. For example, the one-hit model was not adequate to describe state-of-the-art animal carcinogenicity studies with two or three dose groups plus a control group if the apparent dose-response relationship followed an "S"-shaped curve. Multistage models, which had been undergoing mathematical development, came into use as they were able to fit the newer animal carcinogenicity studies that tested several dose groups.

5.3. THE ARMITAGE-DOLL MULTISTAGE MODEL

The *Armitage-Doll Multistage model* was developed in the 1950s (Armitage and Doll, 1961) with the aim of mathematically describing the basic processes leading to the development of cancer, and it has been defined as one of the first significant steps towards biologically based modeling (Krewski et al., 1992). The purpose of proposing the multistage model was to appropriately take into account several factors – the rapid increase of cancer mortality and incidence rates with age, the principle that a specific number of changes (which may include the initiation-promotion sequence) is needed before the induction of a tumor, as well as some other findings resulting from cancer epidemiology and carcinogenic animal experiments and in vitro studies (Armitage, 1985). During the last few decades, a large number of studies have provided important contributions to the development of the mathematical theory of the model and of the computational methods; the model implications have also been investigated in detail (Armitage and Doll, 1961; Hartley and Sielken, 1977; Peto, 1977; Crump et al., 1977; Whittemore, 1977; 1978; Whittemore and Keller, 1978; Day and Brown, 1980; Armitage, 1982, 1985; Crump et al., 1984; Sielken 1991; Krewski et al. 1992;). The basic theory of multistage carcinogenesis has represented a key concept in the analysis of a large number of epidemiological data (e.g., Doll, 1971; Whittemore and Altshuler, 1976; Doll and Peto, 1978; Doll, 1978; Day and Brown, 1980; Armitage, 1985). However, the multistage model is well known mostly since it has been widely used for animal experiment based risk assessment by the US EPA and FDA, as well as by other national agencies, and by some expert groups of the World Health Organization (WHO) (US EPA 1980; WHO,1987; 1992; US EPA IRIS File).

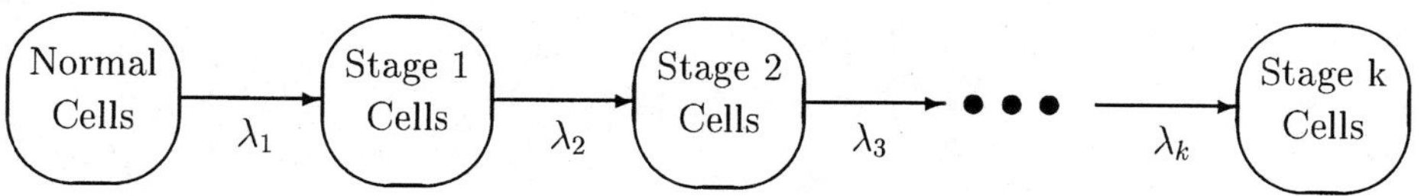

Figure 5.1: *Structure of the multistage model.*

The multistage model may be improved on in order to account for the pharmacokinetic processes which take place in specific cases, leading to a non-linear relationship between the applied dose, and the concentration of the active substance at the target tissue or organ (the latter may also be a metabolite of the applied dose). When measurements are available of concentrations of the active dose at the target, their values may be considered in the model. Moreover, mathematical functions may be included in the multistage model, which describe the specific metabolic process.

The multistage model is commonly employed for the assessment of risks deriving from exposure patterns which are constant, or nearly constant over time, even if its use may be extended to the case of variable exposure patterns (Kodell et al., 1987; Murdoch and Krewski, 1988). Recent developments of carcinogenic risk assessment indicate that the original form of this model cannot appropriately account for all the important components of chemical carcinogenesis. In particular, processes such as the growth and differentiation of normal and altered cells are not explicitly considered in the multistage model. This model, however, is still considered a default solution when other models may not be employed.

5.4. DERIVATION, RATIONALE AND MATHEMATICAL FORM OF THE MODEL

The multistage model is based on the assumption that a single normal cell may become fully malignant only after it has undergone a sequence of k irreversible heritable changes (k being higher or equal to the unity). It is assumed that the probability of each change is very low and that the tissue at risk is formed by normal cells, which have some comparable probability of progressing through the different stages. The sequence of stages or changes is generally assumed to take place according to a specific order.

The changes are assumed to occur spontaneously or to be induced by the environmental exposure to carcinogens. If the rate λ_i of occurrence of each i-th change ($1 \leq i \leq k$) is not dependent on the cell age (which may be assumed to be true in the hypothesis of a relatively constant lifetime exposure and of lifetime-constant spontaneous transition rates), and if the probability of any change in the involved cells is very small in the time period of interest (Armitage, 1985; Day and Brown, 1980; Brown and Chu, 1987), a suitable approximation of the event rate for the k-th change at the time

t may be given by:

$$f(t) \approx (\lambda_1\lambda_2 \ldots \lambda_k)t^{k-1}/(k-1)! \,. \tag{5.5}$$

The cumulative probability that the k-th change has occurred by the time t is obtained by integrating $f(t)$ over time, from 0 to t:

$$F(t) \approx (\lambda_1\lambda_2 \ldots \lambda_k)t^{k}/k! \,. \tag{5.6}$$

(The time lag between the k-th change and the growth of the tumor to a detectable size is assumed to be negligible; otherwise a time lag may be considered in the above formulas).

The mathematical justification of (5.5) and (5.6), which basically describe a form of a time-homogeneous birth process, has been given formally in various papers (Armitage, 1953; 1954; Moolgavkar, 1978); further details on this topic are presented in section 5.10.

Assuming that the specific tissue under examination contains N susceptible cells and defining the probability of a tumor to be detected in this tissue at time t as $P(t)$, the probability $1 - P(t)$ of not observing tumors at t will be:

$$1 - P(t) = (1 - F(t))^N \,, \tag{5.7}$$

which is practically equivalent to:

$$\begin{aligned} 1 - P(t) &\approx \exp(-NF(t)) & (5.8)\\ P(t) &\approx 1 - \exp(-NF(t)) & (5.9)\\ P(t) &= 1 - \exp(-N(\lambda_1\lambda_2 \ldots \lambda_k)/k!)t^k & (5.10)\\ P(t) &= 1 - \exp(At^k/k!) \,, & (5.11) \end{aligned}$$

where A is a constant equal to $N(\lambda_1\lambda_2 \ldots \lambda_k)$ (Armitage, 1985).

This implies a Weibull distribution for the time at which the first tumor is developed or detected.

The density function of $P(t)$ is:

$$P'(t) = NF'(t)\exp(-NF(t)) = Nf(t)\exp(-NF(t)) \tag{5.12}$$

and the hazard function (density of $P(t)$ divided by $1 - P(t)$) is:

$$h(t) = P'(t)/(1 - P(t)) = Nf(t) = At^{k-1}/(k-1)! \tag{5.13}$$

(Armitage, 1985).

According to the above discussed hypotheses and approximations, the hazard function $h(t)$ (5.13) may be assumed to describe the age-specific mortality rates or the age-specific incidence rates derived from epidemiological studies or cancer registries (Armitage, 1985).

From (5.5) and (5.13) it appears that the model assumes that the hazard function is proportional to the $(k-1)$st power of the age t, which, for k ranging from 2 to 6, is in agreement with many age-incidence curves derived from the epidemiological data available for many categories of tumors (Armitage, 1985; Murdoch and Krewski,

1988). On the log/log plane, the $h(t)$ function is represented by a straight line (i.e., $\log(h(t)) = constant + (k-1) \times \log(t)$), whose slope corresponds to $k-1$. This slope has often been used as an index of the number of the different stages possibly involved in the process (Armitage, 1985).

However, some observations may be made on this latter point (Armitage, 1985). First, there are many non-cancer diseases, which are not expected to follow a model like this, whose age-incidence curves might be described by a function like (5.13). Moreover, the event rates for the i-th change, indicated with λ_i in the model, might not be constant with time. As an example, the event rates could increase with age, or with the time from the last i-th change. In these cases, evidently, the slope of (5.13) on the log/log plane is not an indicator of the number of stages involved in the process.

However, as already mentioned, the multistage model generally appears to fit the time occurrence of many categories of human cancers remarkably well (Murdoch and Krewski, 1988). Moreover, support for the model is also given by its application to many animal experiment data, in which a constant exposure pattern has been adopted. In this case as well, the period of time up to the first tumor is generally well described by a Weibull distribution, that is, by a function such as (5.9).

Even if the multistage model has often been used to fit epidemiologically-derived dose-response data, its main application has been in the field of animal experiment dose-response analysis and in animal data-based cancer risk assessment. In this case, the generic event rate for change from the $(i-1)$-th to the i-th stage is assumed to be dose-dependent.

This dose-dependence is commonly assumed to be represented by a linear relationship (Armitage, 1985; Murdoch and Krewski, 1988; Krewski et al., 1991):

$$\lambda_i(d) = a_i + b_i d \; , \tag{5.14}$$

where the a_i and b_i coefficients respectively are positive and non-negative constants, and d represents the active dose of carcinogen.

It is worthwhile to notice that the assumption of a linear dose-dependence of the generic event rate, according to (5.14), has fundamental consequences on the definition of the low-dose behaviour of the model.

As a consequence of (5.14), the function $F(t)$ in (5.6) becomes the product of the $(t^k/k!)$ factor by k factors $(a_i + b_i d)$, corresponding to the k event rates:

$$F(t,d) = (a_1 + b_1 d)(a_2 + b_2 d) \ldots (a_k + b_k d)(t^k/k!) \; , \tag{5.15}$$

which may also be expressed as:

$$F(t,d) = (q_0 + q_1 d + q_2 d^2 + \ldots + q_k d^k)(t^k/k!) \; , \tag{5.16}$$

where the q_i are the coefficients of the k-th degree polynomial resulting from the product of the k factors $(a_i + b_i d)$.

If the data to which the model has to be fitted refer to lifetime exposure, the factor $(t^k/k!)$ reduces to a constant (t = lifetime), so that

$$P(d) = 1 - \exp[-(q_0 + q_1 d + q_2 d^2 + \ldots + q_k d^k)] \; , \tag{5.17}$$

where the constant $(t^k/k!)$ and the constant N in (5.9) may be considered to be absorbed in the values of the q_i parameters. It is worthwhile to notice that in usual long-term animal assays the condition of an exposure duration and of an observation period that are equal to the animal lifetime is only partially respected. Rather, the experiment duration is generally in the order of two years, which is lower than the rat average lifetime (up to three years) and relatively close to the mouse lifetime. Moreover, a briefer period is adopted for short-term assays. Therefore, as far as animal experiments are concerned, there is a distribution of the t parameter, rather than a single value. This has to be considered in risk assessment and modeling and in risk interspecies extrapolation.

The well known expression (5.17) represents the form of the multistage model which is commonly used for cancer experiment data fitting. The q_i parameters are commonly estimated through model fitting of experimental data by using the maximum likelihood method (Edwards, 1976; US EPA, 1980).

It is worthwhile to underline that in the Armitage-Doll formulation of the model the function $(q_0+q_1d+q_2d^2+\ldots+q_kd^k)$ is restricted to only those polynomials that can be factored into the product of linear terms a_i+b_id with $a_i>0$ and $b_i\geq 0$. Nonetheless, to simplify the mathematics, if the Armitage-Doll restrictions are substituted with the less stringent constraint that each $q_i\geq 0$, the resulting *generalized multistage model* is more flexible and can fit more data sets. That is, the Armitage-Doll formulation of the multistage model defines a rather limited set of models; relaxing the constraint that the polynomial be the product of linear factors admits a much larger class of models. This indicates that the generalized multistage model may theoretically provide suitable data fitting even in the case of dose-response curves which are generated by processes different from the one discussed above. In particular, this could happen if the logarithm of the specific experimental survival function $S(d)=1-P(d)$ is well fitted by a polynomial of the type discussed above. From this point of view, the generalized multistage model fitting of data may also be regarded as a "descriptive" or "empirical" interpolation; this, however, is not necessarily a negative feature of the model.

It is worthwhile to notice that if the q_1 parameter (linear coefficient of the dose) in (5.17) is positive, the function $P(d)$ will approach a linear function for d approaching zero (e.g., this emerges from the Taylor expansion of (5.17), when only the linear term is considered).

Generally, of interest is the *extra risk (excess risk)*, or the risk above background, defined as the increased risk in the population fraction which is not expected to develop tumors in the absence of exposure:

$$A(d)=\frac{P(d)-P(0)}{1-P(0)}=1-\exp[-(q_1d+q_2d^2\ldots+q_kd^k)]\ . \tag{5.18}$$

As the dose approaches 0, the marginal increase in the cancer risk for a small increment of exposure can be determined by the slope (or first derivative) of this latter curve evaluated at the dose $d=0$. Thus at low doses the incremental risk for a small dose sufficiently close to 0 is approximately:

$$A(d)\approx q_1d\ , \tag{5.19}$$

that is by the line which is tangent to the dose-response curve at the dose $d = 0$. For sufficiently low doses, this line is a close approximation of the dose-response curve.

5.5. THE "LINEARIZED MULTISTAGE MODEL"

As is evident from a statistical point of view, even if the maximum likelihood estimate of the "linear" coefficient q_1 of the multistage model is 0, a sufficiently small value of this parameter may still be compatible with the uncertainties of data and of the estimation procedure, so that a linear low-dose trend cannot be completely excluded (Armitage, 1985).

It is useful to examine in some detail the hypothesis of $q_1 = 0$, in the light of the Armitage-Doll formulation of multistage model, with reference to (5.15) and (5.17). The q_1 parameter is equal to the total of k terms, each represented by the product of the i-th parameter b_i by the $k-1$ parameters a_j whose j index is different from i (as an example, q_1 is equal to $a_1b_2 + a_2b_1$ for $k = 2$ and equal to $a_1a_2b_3 + a_2a_3b_1 + a_1a_3b_2$ for $k = 3$; in general, q_1 may be expressed as $q1 = [(b_1/a_1) + (b_2/a_2) + \ldots (b_k/a_k)](a_1a_2 \ldots a_k)$. Analogously, the q_0 constant will correspond to the product of all the a_i parameters. According to (5.14), the b_i parameters should be non-negative and the a_i parameters should be positive (i.e., $b_i \geq 0$ and $a_i > 0$ for all i) (Armitage, 1985; Murdoch and Krewski, 1988). Therefore, if a background incidence for the specific tumor exists (that is, according to the model, if the product of all the a_i parameters is positive) and if at least one transition rate is dose dependent, that is, at least one b_i is > 0, the q_1 parameter will be positive (more precisely, q_1 will be > 0 if at least one parameter b_i is > 0 and if all the a_j, with j different from i, are positive).

As is known, the statistical significance of dose-response trends may be evaluated by using appropriate statistical tests (e.g., for increasing/decreasing rate of occurrence of the end point with increasing dose level, for departure from a monotone relationship and/or from linearity, etc.) (Mantel, 1963; Mantel, 1980; IARC, 1986). In the case of a dose-response relationship monotonically increasing with the dose, at least one of b_i parameters of the multistage model is positive. Moreover, as largely attested by available human data, the large majority of carcinogen risk assessments regard cancer categories and mechanisms for which a positive, and often relatively high, background incidence exists in the human population (with the possible exception of some very rare categories of tumors). As is evident, according to (5.15) and (5.17), this implies a positive value of the q_0 coefficient, and consequently, a positive value of all the a_i parameters. Therefore, under rather general conditions, the low-dose behavior of the multistage model should be linear, at least if Armitage-Doll multistage theory discussed above holds. A different behavior should be the exception, rather than the rule. As a consequence, in conditions such as the ones discussed above, an estimated null value of the q_1 parameter could very likely be the consequence of the uncertainty of the data, of the whole computation method and of approximations made.

The maximum likelihood estimates of q_1 have been seen to be relatively unstable, with a considerable variability even in the case of small perturbations to the data to which the model is fitted (Krewski et al., 1991). The possibility of lacking identification of a non-null q_1 parameter in the multistage model may be easily explored through model fitting of computer simulated dose-response curves, which are generated from a pre-fixed theoretical model which is linear for low doses. Exploration of this kind may easily show that a lack of identification of the linear component of the multistage model cannot be excluded and is more likely when the q_1 theoretical value is very low, when the number of "stages" is high, the number of the experimental points is low, the number of subjects per experimental group is limited, and/or, in general, when the quality of the experiment is low (Reichard et al., 1990). Moreover, also in the case of objective experimental dose-response curves, comparison of the results obtained through model fitting to the whole set and to different subsets of the available points frequently shows significant variations of the q_i coefficient estimates; this variability may include cases in which a coefficient estimate ranges from a positive to a null value, and viceversa. As an example, in the case of the 2-acetylaminofluorene dose-response curve presented by Staffa and Mehlman (1979), multistage model fitting of all the eight experimental points essentially indicates a linear and quadratic component (q_1 and $q_2 > 0$), while only a quadratic component is identified ($q_2 > 0$ and $q1 = 0$) when model fitting is limited to the first four experimental points (Reichard et al., 1990).

It is important to note that the "qualitative" type and not only the quantitative type of the low-dose trend of the model will change if the value of the q_1 parameter changes from a positive to a null value and viceversa (e.g., transition from a linear to a quadratic or higher order low-dose trend, or viceversa). It is quite evident that the low-dose extrapolations based on a model that is linear for low doses may lead to low-dose risk estimates different up to several orders of magnitude from the ones based on dose-risk models whose low-dose behaviour is markedly non-linear (e.g., in the case of a model whose low-dose trend is $P(d) \approx kd^3$ in the dose region of interest, a reduction of the dose by a factor 100 will lead to a reduction of the risk estimated value in the order of 100^3, while, in the same conditions, the reduction of the risk estimated with a linear model will obviously be only 100).

In general, as already discussed in section 5.2, depending on their mathematical form, models are usually classified as "linear" (i.e.,for $d \to 0, P(d) \approx kd$), "sublinear" (i.e., for $d \to 0, P(d) \approx kd^q$ with $q > 1$), "supralinear" (i.e., for $d \to 0, P(d) \approx kd^q$ with $q < 1$) in the low-dose range. These "qualitative" differences among low-dose behaviours of mathematical models are generally the cause of the largest differences observed among low-dose extrapolations obtained with different models fitted to same experimental data. These differences, that are easily explained by differences among the theories adopted for data modeling, sometimes have been underlined as an indication of a lack of reliability of the whole cancer risk assessment methodology here discussed. However, the analysis of cancer risk models in the light of basic biological concepts and experimental findings, and the inclusion of more biology in mathematical modeling of cancer processes may provide solid ground to overcome these difficulties: the scope of this report is exactly to provide some contribution in this direction; these aspects will be examined in detail in chapter 6.

If the above hypothesis of an intrinsic low-dose linearity of the multistage model is assumed, the behavior of this model is defined 'a priori' for low doses, at least qualitatively. Independently from the model adopted, sound theoretical and biological reasons have been proposed in favor of low-dose linearity of carcinogenic dose-response relationships, especially for "genotoxic" carcinogens.

As is known, most of data relative to the dose-response trend of DNA-adduct formation indicate a linear low-dose trend, providing further support to the low-dose linearity hypothesis (Perera, 1988; Buss et al., 1990). This argument provides strong support of the hypothesis of a linear dose-response relationship for low doses of genotoxic carcinogens. Moreover, many saturable metabolic processes involved in the carcinogenic process, which may result in being remarkably non-linear for high doses, are substantially linear for doses far below the saturation region. This may hold for saturable Michaelis-Menten processes which include the formation of active metabolites as well as for detoxification and excretion processes (Garrett in Tardiff and Rodricks, 1987). In such conditions, such processes may not induce non-linearities for low doses.

Based on analyses of carcinogenic experiments, Cohen and Ellwein (1990) have proposed a classification scheme for carcinogens, according which the existence of thresholds is considered unlikely for genotoxic carcinogens, questionable for cell receptor-mediated non-genotoxic mechanisms, and likely for non-genotoxic mechanisms which do not involve reactions with cell receptors. Moreover, it has also been underlined that if a carcinogen accelerates an endogenous process leading to spontaneous tumor formation, a linear proportion between the dose and the tumor induction may be hypothesized, independently of the mechanism of action (Lutz, 1990). This argument may be extended to background exposure-related carcinogenic processes. According to some opinions, this may be assumed for both genotoxic and non-genotoxic carcinogens (estrogenic compounds and 2,3,7,8-tetrachlorodibenzo-p-dioxin have been indicated as possible examples of the second category; Lutz, 1990). (It may be interesting to note that the hypothesis of an intrinsic low-dose linearity of the multistage model holds when the a_i parameters are all positive: as above discussed, this implies that the dose-dependent events have an endogenous or background counterpart). Arguments giving support to the low-dose linearity hypothesis have been extensively discussed in the last few years (e.g., Guess et al., 1977; Crump et al., 1976).

It has also been pointed out that the heterogeneity of the human populations may have a "linearizing" effect on the population dose-response relationship even if non-linear trends are hypothesized to exist for the mechanisms involved in the carcinogenic processes under study. According to this hypothesis, if the sensitivity of individuals to a chemical carcinogens is governed by a relatively high number of genes, of life-style factors and of past exposure patterns, and if all these factors are significantly different in the population under study, a smoothing effect may result on the dose-response trend, which tends to lead to a substantially linear trend even if in the case of a completely homogeneous population this relation would be non-linear (Lutz, 1990).

These considerations may provide the rationale for a conservative assessment procedure based on the adoption of the "linearized multistage" model, commonly used by US EPA as well as by other national and international agencies.

The form of the linearized multistage model is simply based on the use of the "upper bound" (upper confidence limit) of the parameter q_1, instead of its maximum likelihood estimate. The upper bound of the linear coefficient q_1, denoted as q_1^*, is computed as follows. Let L be the maximum value of the log-likelihood function. Define L^* by the equation $2(L - L^*) = \chi_1^2(0.90)$, the cumulative percentile of the chi-square distribution with one degree of freedom, which corresponds to a 95%, one-sided, upper confidence limit. Increase q_1 until the log-likelihood function, holding q_1 fixed at its increased value, has a maximum value of L^*. This increased value of q_1 is the upper bound (95% upper confidence limit) of q_1.

It has been shown that relatively small differences are found among low dose estimates based on models which are linear for low-doses (Krewski et al., 1991). This may mean that in the case of a carcinogenic response which is linear for low doses, a linear form of the multistage model could still provide a reliable conservative low-dose estimate of risk even if it does not explicitly consider all the aspects of the carcinogenic process.

Lastly, it may be useful to underline that the use of the "linearized multistage" model generally leads to risk extrapolations (based on the upper confidence limit of the "linear component") which appear fairly reproducible. In fact, low-dose risk extrapolations obtained through "linearized multistage" model fitting to different experimental data relative to the same chemical and the same animal species are often consistent, while this does not occur when the full multistage model is used (Reichard et al., 1990). This is true, for example, in the case of different experiments concerning sodium saccharine (IRDC, 1983; Tayler and Friedman, 1974) and vinyl chloride (Lee et al., 1978; Keplinger et al., 1975; Maltoni, 1977). The relative insensitivity of the linearized multistage model estimates in relation to changes in the data on which they were based has been criticized (Krewski et al., 1991). However, from the point of view discussed here, this may be considered a positive aspect. Reproducibility of estimates is always desirable and if this also implies a higher degree of conservatism, it may be preferable to more complicated modeling.

5.6. TIME-DEPENDENT NON-CONSTANT EXPOSURE PATTERNS: THEIR INFLUENCE ON MULTISTAGE-DERIVED RISK ESTIMATES

In the above discussion, the "event rates" for the i-th change in the multistage model are assumed to be independent of time. In particular, when the model is used for describing a carcinogenic process which depends on the dose d of the specific agent, the generic dose-dependent rate for the i-th change, that is $(a_i + b_i d)$, is usually considered to be constant over time. This implies a value of the dose d which is substantially constant over time. This assumption is generally true in the case of carcinogenic experiments, in which experimental animals are exposed to a constant dose for approximately a lifetime, and may also be true for some patterns of human exposure to environmental carcinogens. However, this might not be considered as a general rule: effective human exposure to carcinogenic factors certainly exist which might not be classified, at least in a strict sense, as constant over a lifetime.

The use of the multistage model has been extended to the case of non-constant exposure patterns (Crump and Howe, 1984). The consequences of a time dependent exposure pattern, in the hypothesis of a multistage carcinogenic process such as the one discussed here, have been investigated in detail by several authors (Crump and Howe, 1984; Kodell et al., 1987; Day and Brown, 1980; Murdoch and Krewski, 1988).

Multistage model versions and computational methods exist, which allow the use of this model in the case of time-dependent exposure or dosing patterns (e.g, by specifying the dose rate at time t through a function $d(t)$ and/or representing $d(t)$ as a sequence of piecewise continuous functions approximated by step functions) (Crump and Howe, 1984).

When only a single stage is dose-dependent and the dose or exposure varies over time, reference in the multistage model to the time-weighted average exposure may lead to an underestimation of low-dose risk, whose upper bound has been demonstrated not to exceed a factor equal to the whole number k of stages assumed by the model (Kodell et al., 1987). Murdoch and Krewski (1988) have demonstrated that this also holds in the low-dose region when more stages are dose dependent. Also in this case, in the low-dose range the factor k represents the upper bound of the possible underestimation of the low-dose risk, when the time-weighted average of a time-dependent exposure is used in the multistage model.

Moreover, this kind of analysis confirms what could be intuitively expected: early exposures exert a more intense effect when affecting a dose-dependent early stage, and late exposures when affecting a dose-dependent late stage.

In any case, the above mentioned upper bounds may be of great help in multistage model-based risk evaluations, when the exposure pattern is non-constant and time-dependent. The use of a time-weighted average of the exposure together with the reference to the appropriate upper bound factor may consent the derivation of conservative estimates, without necessitating complex calculations. Moreover, this simple approach may be the only one available when the time pattern of the exposure under study may not be appropriately defined and, consequently, the time rate of dosing cannot be considered in the model.

5.7. CONSIDERATION OF PHARMAKOKINETICS IN MULTISTAGE MODELING

Today, the inclusion of pharmacokinetic data and models in carcinogenic risk assessment is considered an essential step. First, the pharmacokinetic processes which govern the absorption, distribution, accumulation, detoxification, excretion, as well as the chemical transformation of the exposure dose may largely influence the shape of carcinogenic dose-response relationships. This aspect is very important when the available dose-response data are interpreted in terms of specific mathematical models of carcinogenesis. In this case, the dose-response shape is not only determined by the characteristics of the carcinogenic processes taking place at the target, which are expected to be described by the model, but also by other processes, generally not accounted for by models of carcinogenesis. In the case of the multistage model, this implies that the dose-response characteristics are not necessarily determined only by the number and types of the different carcinogenic stages hypothesized, but also by other parameters.

Pharmacokinetic processes and parameters need to be appropriately defined in order to correctly use the mathematical models of carcinogenesis (at least the models which do not explicitly include pharmacokinetics) when pharmacokinetics is to be included.

As is well known, reference to pharmacokinetic theory and data has made it possible to give a suitable and satisfactory explanation and interpretation of the shape of some specific classes of dose-response curves, as well as to appropriately extend the application of multistage and other mathematical models to the analysis of these curves (Gehring et al., 1979; Anderson et al., 1980).

Pharmacokinetics may be accounted for in cancer risk modeling by considering it within the model (therefore, by modifying the model) (Anderson et al., 1980). In practice, the exposure dose parameter d (chronically administered dose) of the multistage model (or of other models) is substituted by a function $g(d)$ describing, in function of the exposure dose d, the concentration of the substance that is estimated to be active at the target. The form of this function depends upon the pharmacokinetics of the involved chemical.

Alternatively, pharmacokinetics is simply accounted for by making reference to the doses effectively active at the target, that are estimated through pharmacokinetic data and models. These two approaches will be briefly discussed.

As an example, inclusion of pharmacokinetics in multistage and "One Hit" models has allowed satisfactory fitting of these models to experimental dose-response relationships, whose "downward" curvature (convexity) and "supralinear" trend could be explained by the hypothesis that a main carcinogenic agent was an active metabolite of the applied dose, which was produced by a saturable metabolic process (Anderson et al., 1980; Gehring et al., 1979). In order to appropriately take into account metabolic processes which are described by the Michaelis-Menten law, whose final product is an active carcinogenic metabolite, the multistage model may be simply modified by substituting, (Anderson et al. 1980; Gehring et al., 1979) the exposure dose parameter with a function assumed to represent the concentration of the substance active in the involved target:

$$g(d) = d/(1 + Kd) \ , \qquad (5.20)$$

(K being a constant) which may describe a Michaelis-Menten process, that, under steady state conditions, is assumed to lead to a concentration of the active metabolite in the target tissue represented by $C = k_1 d/(1 + k_2 d)$ (k_1 and k_2 being constants) (Garrett in Tardiff and Rodricks, 1987). This function indicates that the ratio of the concentration at the target to the exposure dose is decreasing with increasing exposure dose. Only one constant is considered in (5.20) because the constant in the numerator of this function is assumed to be absorbed by the multistage model constants.

It is interesting to note that this modification of the model does not influence low-dose linearity. In the low-dose region, when $d \ll 1/K$ the function (5.20) is substantially linear, and, therefore, does not change the low-dose mathematical form of the original multistage model or of other models used. Moreover, it should be kept in mind that using the above expression (5.20) in the multistage model, instead of the dose parameter d, generally leads to more conservative estimates (higher values for the q_1 coefficient and its upper bound) (Reichard et al., 1990).

Saturable kinetics may also govern the elimination processes of the active dose. If this saturation process is a Michaelis-Menten one, the steady state concentration at the target organ may be described by $C = k_1 d/(k_2 - d)$, for $d < k_2$ (k_1 and k_2 being constants) (Garrett in Tardiff and Rodricks, 1987). The ratio of the plasma or target concentration to the exposure dose will increase with increasing exposure dose (very rapidly for d approaching the saturation level). In the low dose range (for $d \ll k_2$) the concentration C is practically equivalent to $k_1 d/k_2$, so that it is linearly proportional to the applied dose, and this kind of process may not be expected to change the low-dose dose mathematical qualitative form of the multistage model.

These simple considerations are certainly limited to a small part of the pharmacokinetics and pharmacokinetic modeling in carcinogenic risk assessment. However, it is important to point out that saturation processes taking place only at high doses (present in some animal experiments) may not be expected to cause significant nonlinearities at very low doses, provided that they are ruled by laws as the ones discussed above. Rather, in such hypothesis, in the low dose region, according to the hypotheses discussed above, the concentration active at the target may be expected to be substantially a linear function of the exposure dose (Garrett in Tardiff and Rodricks, 1987).

Lastly, it may also be observed that modification of the multistage model according to (5.17) does not create particular problems in the calculation procedure. Available pharmacokinetic data, parameters and models may be easily incorporated in the model (Anderson et al., 1980).

As already mentioned, an alternative approach for taking the relevant pharmacokinetic processes into account is to directly insert into the model the values of the doses which are determined or estimated as effectively active at the target organ or tissue. This procedure is relatively simple if data are available which allow the determination of the dose parameters to be used in the model (see the example of tetrachloroethylene (PCE) risk assessment discussed in section 8.7). It also has the advantage of stimulating a specific and risk oriented study of metabolic processes: recent experience has shown the importance of producing, evaluating and using metabolic data in risk assessment. Lastly, reference to specific evaluations of the dose-at-the-target may be particularly useful for inter-species extrapolation purposes.

The well-known Physiologically-Based-PharmacoKinetic models (PBPK models) (Travis, 1988) may provide extremely useful information in this field.

Pharmacokinetic models and the inclusion of pharmacokinetics in cancer risk assessment are discussed in chapter 6. The discussion here is limited to more general considerations.

5.8. THE PROBLEM OF MULTIPLE EXPOSURE: MULTISTAGE CARCINOGENESIS THEORY AND ADDITIVE AND MULTIPLICATIVE MODELS

The joint effect of more carcinogens has been considered with reference to the multistage theory and model. In the absence of biochemical interactions, it is generally hypothesized that if two carcinogens affect the same stage of carcinogenesis, an additive model may be expected, while if the two carcinogens act on different stages, a multiplicative model may be expected. This latter assumption is considered to be true only in the case of a substantially constant exposure to the two carcinogens, lasting for the time of life (Brown and Chu, 1987; Gibb and Chen, 1986).

The importance of the time-pattern of the exposure has been underlined; in the hypothesis of a time-limited exposure to two carcinogens which affect different stages, the relative risk predicted by the multistage model in the absence of biochemical interaction is between additive and multiplicative (Brown and Chu, 1987). It is concluded that while the observation of a multiplicative relative risk relationship in an epidemiological study concerning the joint exposure to two carcinogens will support the hypothesis of an action on different stages, the observation of an additive risk relationships may not be immediately interpreted in terms of an action on the same stage. In this case, the time pattern of exposure need to be considered for more reliable conclusions (Brown and Chu, 1987).

Moreover, the general observation has to be considered, that in the range of very low doses a multiplicative risk model may be expected to practically lead to results comparable to the ones which may be derived from an additive risk model (Krewski and Thomas, 1992).

The examination of the effects of biochemical interactions and other types of interaction is out of the scope of this brief discussion.

In any case, it may be observed that the multistage model has been and may be used for the analysis of the response to more carcinogen factors, providing reasonable hypotheses in the examination of the epidemiological and animal experiment data.

5.9. CRITICAL REVIEW OF THE MODEL

Despite the fact the Armitage-Doll model does not explicitly consider the cell kinetics, it is still widely used for data analysis and in cancer risk assessment. The model has intuitive appeal and is mathematically straightforward. Here we would like to review this model in order to introduce the key quantities that are used in time-to-tumor data analysis and to point out potential pitfalls that can be encountered in the use of this particular model.

It has been observed that for many human carcinomas the age-specific incidence rate increases roughly like a power of the age, i.e., $I(t) \cong ct^k$, and the Armitage-Doll model, as already mentioned, was originally proposed to explain this observation. The age-specific incidence rate is a measure of the rate of appearance of tumors in a previously tumor-free tissue. The appropriate statistical concept is that of the hazard function.

First, for the tissue of interest, let T be a random variable representing the time of appearance of a malignant tumor. We define $P(t)$ as the probability that a malignant tumor has occurred by the time t, i.e., $P(t) = \text{Prob}[T \leq t]$. The hazard function, $h(t)$, is then defined by

$$h(t) = \lim_{\Delta t \to 0} \frac{1}{\Delta t} \text{Prob}[t < T \leq t + \Delta t | T > t] = P'(t)/(1 - P(t)) \qquad (5.21)$$

and represents the rate of change in $P(t)$ conditional on there being no tumor present prior to time t. Obviously, $S(t) = 1 - P(t)$ is the probability of no tumor at time t, also termed the survival function.

Suppose that there are N cells susceptible to malignant transformation in the tissue of interest and let us assume that these cells are independents. Let $p(t)$ be the probability that a specific susceptible cell is malignant by time t. It can be shown that the overall hazard is the sum of all the individual hazards, i.e.

$$h(t) = Np'(t)/(1 - p(t)) \qquad (5.22)$$

as seen in Fig. 5.1. A malignant tumor arises when a single susceptible cell sustains a number of critical insults (say n) that take it from a normal tissue cell to a malignant cell, which grows after a short lag time into a malignant tumor. The waiting time distribution for the cell to go from stage i to stage $i + 1$ is assumed to be exponential with parameter λ_i. Let $p_i(t)$ be the probability that a cell is in the stage i. The expression (5.22) can be rewritten as $h(t) = Np_n'(t)/(1 - p_n(t))$. If we now assume that malignancy (at the level of the cell) is a rare event, i.e. $p_n(t) \cong 0$, we may approximate the hazard function by

$$h(t) \approx Np_n'(t).$$

In this case, Taylor series expansion (Moolgavkar 1978, 1991) leads to the approximation

$$h(t) \approx Np_n'(t) = \frac{N\lambda_0 \ldots \lambda_{n-1}}{(n-1)!} t^{n-1} [1 - \bar{\lambda} + f(\lambda, t)] \,, \qquad (5.23)$$

where $\bar{\lambda} = \sum_{i=0}^{n-1} \lambda_i / n$ is the mean of the transition rates, and $f(\lambda, t)$ involves second and higher order moments of the transition rates.

Retention of only the first non-zero term in this series expansion leads to the Armitage-Doll approximation, namely

$$h(t) \approx \frac{N\lambda_0 \ldots \lambda_{n-1}}{(n-1)!} t^{n-1} \,. \qquad (5.24)$$

Thus, with the two approximations made (1) $p_n(t) \approx 0$ and (2) $|\bar{\lambda} t + f(\lambda, t)| \ll 1$, this model predicts an age specific incidence curve that increases with a power of age that is one less that the number of distinct stages involved in malignant transformation.

Since the Armitage-Doll model does not allow for cell death, it is immediately clear that any susceptible cell eventually becomes malignant with probability 1. Further, since the waiting time distribution to malignant transformation is the sum of n exponential waiting time distributions, it follows that $h(t)$ is a monotone increasing function. Moreover, it can be shown that $h(t)$ has a finite asymptote: $\lim_{t\to\infty} h(t) = N\lambda_{\min}$, where $\lambda_{\min}$ is the minimum of the transition rates. Thus, the Armitage-Doll approximation, which grows without bound, becomes progressively worse with increasing age.

It is instructive to rephrase the Armitage-Doll approximation in mathematical terms that involve the expectation of the occupancy in each stage. For this purpose, let $X_i(t)$ be a sequence of random variables associated with each cell such that $X_i(t) = 1$ if the cell is in stage i at time t and 0 otherwise. Since the probability $p_n(t)$ of a cell to become finally malignant obeys the Kolmogorov equation

$$p_n'(t) = \lambda_{n-1} p_{n-1}(t),$$

the hazard can also be written as

$$h(t) = Np_n'(t)/(1 - p_n(t)) \equiv N\lambda_{n-1}\mathrm{E}[X_{n-1}(t)|X_n(t) = 0]\ , \tag{5.25}$$

where E denotes the expectation. In words, the hazard or incidence is proportional to the expected (or mean) number of cells in the penultimate stage, conditional on there being no cells that are malignant. When $p_n(t)$ is close to zero or, equivalently, when the transition rates are small enough, the conditional expectation may be approximated by the unconditional expectation, and

$$h(t) \approx Np_n'(t) = N\lambda_{n-1}\mathrm{E}[X_{n-1}(t)]. \tag{5.26}$$

Thus the Armitage-Doll approximation consists of replacing the conditional expectation of $X_{n-1}(t)$ by the unconditional expectation and then retaining only the first non-zero term in the Taylor series expansion of the unconditional expectation. Expressions similar to (5.22) and (5.23) can also be written for the hazard function of the two-mutation clonal expansion model.

Obviously, for the Armitage-Doll model to hold, $\bar{\lambda}$, and thus each λ_i, must be small enough. An example of how poorly this approximation may do is discussed in Moolgavkar (1978, 1991). In addition, in animal experiments, the probability of tumor may be too large for $p_n(t) \cong 0$ to hold in which case the approximation should be avoided altogether.

In order to model the action of environmental carcinogens, one or more of the transition rates can be made functions of the dose of the agent in question. Usually, the transition rates are modeled as linear functions of the dose, so that $\lambda_i = a_i + b_i d$. The assumption of first order kinetics may be justified, at least for carcinogens that interact directly with DNA to produce mutations. Then, using the Armitage-Doll approximation Eq.(5.24), the hazard function at age t and dose d can be written as $h(t,d) = g(d)t^{n-1}$, where $g(d)$ is a polynomial in dose, and the probability of tumor is approximately given by $P(t,d) = 1 - \exp[g(d)t^n]$. Note that $g(d)$ is a product of linear terms. As already mentioned, it is in this form, called the linearized multistage model, that the Armitage-Doll model is commonly applied to the problem of low-dose extrapolation. Generally, the proportion of animals developing tumors at a specified age at each of three different dose levels is known. The linearized multistage model is fitted to the data and the estimated parameters used to extrapolate risk to lower doses. There are formally at least two problems with this procedure. First, as noted above, the Armitage-Doll approximation holds only when the probability of tumor is low and this condition is not satisfied in the usual animal experiments used for risk assessment. Second, as far as the above discussed "generalized multistage model" is concerned, in the statistical analysis $g(d)$ is treated as a general polynomial rather than a product of linear terms.

The discussion above applies only when the exposure to a carcinogen starts at birth or very early in life, and continues at the same constant level throughout the period of observation. With time-dependent exposures the hazard function can no longer be couched in the form of Eq.(5.23). A starting point for the mathematical development is the set of Kolmogorov differential equations. However, the papers in the literature use approximation Eq.(5.24) as the starting point (see, e.g., Whittemore, 1977; Day and Brown, 1980; Crump and Howe, 1984; Brown and Chou, 1987; Freedman and Davidi, 1989). As noted above, this approximation is inappropriate unless one has reason to believe that each of the transition rates is small enough. The approximation is almost inappropriate when applied to experimental data.

5.10. DISCUSSION

The multistage model of carcinogenesis has a long history, and has been largely used in low-dose practical risk assessment and carcinogen regulation, as well as for the analysis of the results of a large number of epidemiological studies. The multistage theory and the multistage model have been studied, discussed, criticized and applied for more than 20 years, and theoretical and practical developments of the various details and correlated aspects have been going on since 1970, so that a large "corpus" of knowledge has been accumulated on the subject.

It is clear today that the multistage model cannot account for all the relevant processes in carcinogenesis. For instance it is unable to incorporate data on cell proliferation. Also, time dependent exposures (e.g., fractionation of the dose) are not easily incorporated. Except for the Armitage-Doll model, it is impossible to include information from mutation assays in the other forms of the multistage model because the biological significance of the parameters is lost. However, the multistage model as an empirical model has its place in risk assessment. The inclusion of cell proliferation into the Armitage-Doll model produces a new class of models which are discussed in Chapter 6.

5.11. REFERENCES

Anderson M.W., Hoel D.G. and Kaplan N.L. (1980): A general scheme for the incorporation of pharmacokinetics in low-dose risk estimation for chemical carcinogens: Example - Vinyl Chloride, Toxicol. and Appl. Pharmacol., 55, 154-161

Armitage P. and Doll R. (1961): Stochastic models for carcinogenesis, Proceedings of the 4th Berkeley Symposium on Mathematical Statistics and Probability, Vol. IV, (J. Neyman ed.) University of California Press, Berkeley and Los Angeles, pp 19-38.

Armitage P. (1982): The assessment of low-dose carcinogenicity, Biometrics, 38 (Suppl.), 119-129.

Armitage P. (1985): Multistage Models of Carcinogenesis, Environmental Health Perspectives, 63, 195-201.

Brown C. and Chu K. (1987): Use of multistage models to infer stages affected by carcinogenic exposure: Example of lung cancer and cigarette smoking, J. Chronic Disease 40 (Suppl. 2), 171S-179S.

Brown C.C. and Chu K.C. (1989): Additive and multiplicative models and multistage carcinogenesis theory, Risk Analysis, 9, 99-105.

Buss P., Caviezel M. and Lutz W.K. (1990): Linear dose-response relationship for DNA adducts in rat liver from chronic exposure to aflatoxin B1, Carcinogenesis, 11, 12, 2133-2135.

Cohen M.S. and Ellwein L.B. (1990): Cell proliferation ion carcinogenesis, Science, 249, 1007-1011.

Crump K.S., Hoel D.G., Langley C.H. and Peto R. (1976): Fundamental carcinogenic processes and their implications for low-dose risk assessment, Cancer Research, 36, 2973-2979.

Crump K.S., Guess H.A., and Deal K.L. (1977): Confidence intervals and tests of hypotheses concerning dose response relations inferred from animal carcinogenicity data, Biometrics, 33, 437-451.

Crump K.S. and Howe R.B. (1984): The multistage model with a time dependent dose pattern: application to carcinogenic risk assessment, Risk Analysis, 4, 163-176.

Day N.E. and Brown C.C. (1980): Multistage models and primary prevention of cancer, JNCI, 64, 977-989.

Doll R. (1971): The age distribution of cancer: implications for models of carcinogenesis, J.Roy. Statist. Soc., A134, 133-166.

Doll R. and Peto R. (1978). Cigarette smoking and bronchial carcinoma: dose and time relationships among regular smokers and life-long non-smokers, J. Epidemiol. Commun. Health, 32, 303-313.

Doll R. (1978): An epidemiological perspective on the biology of cancer, Cancer Res., 38, 3573-3583.

Edwards A.W. (1976): Likelihood, Cambridge University Press, London and N.Y..

Finney D.J. (1987): Statistical Method in Biological Assay, Oxford University Press, Oxford.

Freedman D.A. and Davidi W. (1989): Multistage models for carcinogenesis, Environ. Health Persp., 81, 169-188.

Garrett E.R. (1987): Toxicokinetics, in Tardiff R.G. and Rodricks J.V., eds.: Toxic substances and human risk, Plenum Press, N.Y. and London, pp. 153-236.

Gehring P.J., Watanabe P.G. and Park C.N. (1979): Risk of angiosarcoma in workers exposed to vinyl chloride as predicted from studies in rats, Toxicol.Appl. Pharmacol., 49,15.

Gibb H.J. and Chen C.W. (1986): Multistage interpretation of additive and multiplicative carcinogenic effects, Risk Analysis, 6, 167-170.

Guess H., Crump K. and Peto R. (1977): Uncertainty estimates for low-dose-rate extrapolations of animal carcinogenicity data, Cancer Research, 37, 3475-3483.

Hartley H.O. and Sielken R.L. Jr. (1977): Estimation of 'safe doses' in carcinogenic experiments, Biometrics, 33, 1-30.

IARC - International Agency for Research on Cancer (1986): The design and analysis of long-term animal experiments, IARC Scientific Publications No. 79, IARC, Lyon.

IRDC - International Research and Development Corporation (1983): evaluation of the dose-response and in utero exposure of saccharin in rats, IRDC, Mattawan, Michigan.

Keplinger M., Goode J.W, Gordon D.E., and Calandra J.C. (1975): Interim results of exposure of rats, hamsters and mice to vinyl chloride, Ann. N.Y. Acad. Sci., 246, 219-224.

Kodell R.L., Gaylor D.W., and Chen J.J. (1987): Consequences of using average lifetime dose rate to predict risks from intermittent exposures to carcinogens, Risk Analysis, 7, 339-345.

Krewski D., Gaylor D. and Szyszkowicz M. (1991): A model-free approach to low-dose extrapolation, Environmental Health Perspectives, 90, 279-285.

Krewski D., Goddard M.J. and Zielinski J.M. (1992): Dose-response relationships in carcinogenesis, in H. Vanio, P.N. Magee, D.B. McGregor and A.J. McMichael eds.: Mechanisms of carcinogenesis in risk identification, pp. 579-599, IARC, Lyon.

Krewski D. and Thomas D. (1992): Carcinogenic mixtures, Risk Analysis, 12, 105-113.

Lee C.C., Bhaudar C., Winston J.M., House W.B., Dixon R.L. and Woods J.S. (1978): Carcinogenicity of vinyl chloride and vinyliden, J. Toxicol. Environ. Health, 4, 11-30.

Lutz W.K. (1990): Commentary: Dose-response relationship and low dose extrapolation in chemical carcinogenesis, Carcinogenesis, 8, 1243-1247. Maltoni C. (1977): Vinyl chloride carcinogenicity: An experimental model for carcinogenicity studies, in Hiatt H.H. et al., eds,: Origins of human cancer.A, Cold Spring Lab., Cold Spring Harbor, N.Y. pp. 119-146.

Mantel N. and Brian W. (1961): Safety testing of carcinogenic agents, J. Natl.Cancer Inst., 27, 455-470.

Mantel N. (1963): Chi-square tests with one degree of freedom: extensions of the Mantel-Haenszel procedure, J. Amer. Statistical Association, 58, 690-700.

Mantel N. (1980): Assessing laboratory evdence for neoplastic activity, Biometrics, 36, 381-399.

Moolgavkar S.H. (1978): The multistage theory of carcinogenesis and the age distribution of cancer in man, J. Natl. Cancer Inst., 61, 49-52.

Moolgavkar S.H. and Venzon D.J. (1979): Two-event models for carcinogenesis: Incidence curves of childhood and adult tumors, Math. Biosci., 47, 55-77.

Moolgavkar S.H. and Knudson A. (1981): Mutation and cancer: A model for human carcinogenesis, Journal of the National Cancer Institute, 66, 1037-1052.

Moolgavkar S.H. (1991): Stochastic models of carcinogenicity, Rao C.R. and Chakraborty R., eds.: Handbook of Statistics, Vol. 8, Elsevier Science Publishers B.V., 373-393.

Murdoch D.J. and Krewski D. (1988). carcinogenic risk assessment with time-dependent exposure patterns, Risk Analysis, 4, 1988.

Perera F.P. (1988): Biological markers in risk assessment, in C.C. Travis ed.: Carcinogen risk assessment, Plenum Press, N.Y..

Peto R. and Lee P.N. (1973): Weibull distributions for continuous-carcinogenesis experiments, Biometrics, 29,457-470.

Peto R. (1977): Epidemiology, multistage models and short-term multigenicity tests, in H.H. Hiatt, J.D. Watson and J. A. Watson eds: Origins of Human cancer, book C: Human Risk Assessment, Cold Spring Harbor Laboratory, Cold Spring Harbor.

Rai K. and Van Ryzin J. (1981): A generalized multi-hit dose-response model for low-dose extrapolation, Biometrics, 37, 341.

Reichard E., Cranor C., Raucher R. and Zapponi G. (1990): Groundwater contamination risk assessment, International Association of Hydrological Sciences-IAHS, Wallingford, Oxfordshire, UK.

Staffa J.A. and Mehlman M.A. (1979). Innovation in cancer risk assessment. Park Forest South, IL, Pathotocs Publishers Inc.

Tayler J.M. and Friedman l. (1974): Combined chronic feeding and three-generation reproduction study of sodium saccharin in the rat, toxicol. appl. Pharmacol., 29, 154 (abstract 200).

Travis C.C. (1988): Pharmacokinetics in Travis C.C., edr.: Carcinogenic Risk Assessment, Plenum Press, N.Y..

US EPA (1980): Water Quality Criteria Documents, Federal Register, 45, 231, 79319-79378.

Whittemore a. and Altshuler B (1976): Lung cancer incidence in cigarette smokers: further analysis of Doll and Hill's data for British physicians, Biometrics, 32, 805-816.

Whittemore A. (1977): The age distribution of human cancers for carcinogenic exposures of varying intensity, Am. J. Epidemiol., 106, 418-432.

Whittemore A. (1978): Quantitative theories of carcinogenesis Adv. Cancer Res., 27, 55-58.

Whittemore A. and Keller J. (1978): Quantitative theories of carcinogenesis, SIAM Rev., 20, 1-30.

WHO (1987): Air Quality Guidelines for Europe, WHO, Geneva.

WHO (1992): Revision of Drinking Water Guidelines (Summary Report), WHO, Geneva.

Chapter 6

BIOLOGICALLY BASED MODELS OF CARCINOGENESIS

E. G. Luebeck[1], K. Watanabe[2], and C. Travis[2]

[1]Fred Hutchinson Cancer Research Center, Seattle, USA
[2]Tulane University Medical Center, New Orleans, USA

6.1. INTRODUCTION

Recent advances in molecular biology in understanding the causes of cancer make it clear that cancer is the outcome of complex genetic (and possibly epigenetic) changes. Some of these changes are hereditary in nature or are related to predisposing traits. However, the majority of events are believed to happen by chance (in soma) under the influence of environmental factors.

This chapter is primarily about mechanistic models of carcinogenesis, describing toxicokinetic as well as toxicodynamic aspects of the carcinogenic process. It should be pointed out that the models described here are, by in large, hypothetical in character and are not meant to represent 'true' descriptions of the underlying biological processes which may not yet be fully understood. However, the goal of using biologically based models is to incorporate as many relevant and plausible mechanisms in order to arrive at better predictions for cancer risk and to generate new hypotheses that can be tested by future experiments.

Why are mechanistic or biologically motivated models better than statistical ones? One answer is that the parameters that define mechanistic models are endowed with biological significance. They represent quantities that, at least in principle, can be measured by experiment.

Since the endpoint of interest, namely cancer, is related to (epi)genetic changes in the cell, model parameters are used to describe the responses to toxic agents on the tissue level, on the cellular level, and on the level of the genome (DNA).

Physiologically based toxicokinetic models are used to understand how external

Perspectives on Biologically Based Cancer Risk Assessment, edited by Cogliano *et al.*
Kluwer Academic/Plenum Publishers, New York, 1999.

exposure translates into tissue dose and how the agent is metabolized by the cell. Toxicodynamic models are then used to describe how cells respond to the action of the toxicant. Primarily, one is concerned with the effect of the agent on cell kinetics (cell proliferation, apoptosis or necrosis) and the kind of DNA-damage inflicted, if the agent is mutagenic. Ultimately, biologically based models can be chosen that identify probable sequences of mutational events on the pathway to cancer. Some of these events may be affected by the agent in question. Some models have also been developed that explicitly consider DNA repair.

Better understanding of carcinogenic processes is an iterative process. Mechanistic modeling of cellular effects by putative carcinogens, and data analysis based upon these models, leads to new hypotheses. The hypotheses generated are for exposures and in situations were no experimental data are yet available. Data analysis (estimation of response functions) may point to new features or mechanisms previously not recognized. Consequently, better experiments are designed that result in improved models. This 'cyclic' process may be recognized as the 'principle' that drives scientific progression.

In the following, we provide a brief history of biologically based models of carcinogenesis. This will lead us to a qualitative and quantitative discussion of the two-mutation clonal expansion model, the 'outgrowth' of Knudson's recessive oncogenesis model. The later part of the chapter is devoted to the issue of practical cancer risk assessment, the use of toxicokinetic models and interspecies extrapolation. A perspective on low-dose extrapolation is offered in the last section.

6.2. A BRIEF HISTORY OF BIOLOGICALLY-BASED CANCER MODELS

Several mathematical models have been developed over the past 40 years that are biologically motivated, beginning with the models by Nordling (1953), and Armitage and Doll (1954). A common trait of these models is the basic assumption that malignant tumors arise from a single cell that has sustained a number of irreversible critical insults to its genome. Thus, the fundamental unit of description is the susceptible target cell as a carrier of the genome, together with its probability of malignant transformation. The idea of a multistage nature of the carcinogenic process is well supported by modern laboratory observations (Land et al., 1983, Bishop, 1991; IARC, 1992).

The model that first explored the consequences of the multistage nature of carcinogenesis mathematically is the Armitage-Doll multistage model (see Chapter 5 of this report). The model is popular with risk assessors because it is intuitive, mathematically tractable and yields age specific tumor incidence curves that resemble the incidence patterns of many adult human carcinomas. However, there are serious drawbacks in the use of this model, as discussed in Chapter 5. In some situations, especially when the probability of tumor is high, commonly made approximations fail.

A central aspect of carcinogenesis was recognized with the discovery of tumor suppressor genes, such as the *Rb* (retinoblastoma) gene and the *p*53 gene (Knudson, 1971; Hollstein et al., 1991; Levine et al., 1991). Both genes have been shown to play important roles in the control of the cell cycle.

Knudson (1971) showed that a two-mutation recessive oncogenesis model could explain both the sporadic and inherited form of the retinoblastoma childhood cancer. According to this model the sporadic form of this cancer is due to the somatic loss (or loss in function) of both copies of the *Rb* gene while the hereditary form of the cancer is caused by a germ line transmission of a missing or defective copy of the *Rb* gene and the loss of the remaining copy in soma.

For most adult cancers the situation is less clear and they seem not to follow the recessive oncogenesis model described above. For instance, laboratory work suggests that a small number (3-4) of mutations are involved in colorectal carcinoma implicating three tumor suppressor genes (APC, p53 and DCC) and one proto-oncogene (K-ras) (Fearon and Vogelstein, 1990; Moolgavkar and Luebeck, 1992). Another example is the Li-Fraumeni syndrome, which increases the risk of divers tumor types, but does not convey the same high risk as the *Rb* defect, that affects people at very young age. The syndrome is caused by a *p*53 germline mutation. Clearly, differences in the developmental function of the genes are quite important and strongly influence the onset of tumorigenesis.

Since tumor progression is often accompanied by genetic instability it is difficult to pin down the exact number of rate-limiting steps that lead to the occurrence of a malignant tumor. Some mutational events may occur late in the development of a tumor and should not be considered rate-limiting or necessary for malignant conversion. In this context the recent finding of a 'mutator gene' on the long arm of chromosome 2 is of interest. The dysfunction of this gene seems to be responsible for a good fraction of familial colorectal cancers and causes a strong increase in genomic instability in tumor cells (Aaltonen et al, 1993).

The Armitage-Doll model adequately describes the incidence of many human carcinomas (Cook, Fellingham and Doll, 1969; Renan, 1993). However, this model cannot be applied to experimental situations were the endpoints are intermediate in nature, such as the appearance of preneoplastic lesions in the rat liver or the appearance of papillomas on mouse skin. A comprehensive description of these phenomena will necessarily have to include a description of the underlying growth processes that result in the *observable* lesions or tumors of interest. The analysis of data obtained from initiation and promotion protocols requires the incorporation of cell kinetics into the model. This leads to the notions of *clonal expansion* (or net cell proliferation) and *clonal extinction*. Both aspects will be discussed in detail below. A logical extension of the Armitage-Doll model that includes a stochastic description of proliferating intermediate cell populations is provided by the two-mutation clonal expansion model as promulgated by Moolgavkar and colleagues (Moolgavkar and Knudson, 1981; Moolgavkar et al., 1988). It provides a useful framework in which both aspects, the multistage nature of carcinogenesis and the property of intermediate (initiated) cell populations to proliferate, are modeled explicitly. Intermediate cells are assigned specific probabilities to either divide, to die or to differentiate, or to divide asymmetrically into one cell of the same lineage and one cell that has suffered another critical event on the pathway to cancer. A comprehensive review of stochastic models of carcinogenesis can be found in the book by Tan (Tan, 1991).

6.3. TWO-MUTATION CLONAL EXPANSION MODEL

Let us begin with a list of important points that have emerged over the last 10 years that are pertinent to carcinogenesis. In order to account for the experimental observations in multistage carcinogenesis, biologically based cancer models will need to address these points. This list is likely to increase as more details of the underlying biological processes are uncovered.

- Cancer is a *multistep* process that involves the *clonal expansion* of intermediate and malignant cell populations.
- Model parameters should be biologically significant or represent biological observables that can, at least in principle, be measured or tested by experiment. Parameters of interest are those that describe processes affected by environmental agents. Dose-response relationships of cellular responses should be described by physiologically based toxicodynamic models.
- The model should provide a unified framework for the analysis of epidemiological and experimental data, so that the maximal benefit can be drawn from animal experiments for human carcinogenesis research. Mechanisms that manifest themselves on the cellular level may be similar between species and may help species extrapolation of the carcinogenic response. In certain situations, similarities may be absent and the use of a certain species, for human cancer risk assessment, may not be justified. It is important, however, to understand the origins of the differences.
- The model should account for the observed phenomena in initiation-promotion (IP) experiments, such has the induction and promotion of enzyme altered foci in the rat liver or the occurrence of papillomas on mouse skin after painting with a promoter substance. Here the focus is on the number of lesions caused by a certain dose of a specific initiating compound and on the growth kinetics of intermediate lesions under the influence of the promoter.
- Last, but not least, the incorporation of time and dose dependent exposure patterns of carcinogens should not pose great mathematical difficulty.

The two-mutation clonal expansion model shown in Fig. 6.1 and formalized by Moolgavkar and colleagues (Moolgavkar et al., 1988; Dewanji et al., 1989; Moolgavkar and Luebeck, 1990), starts to address these points by providing an interface for their incorporation. Slightly different versions of the model have been considered in the past by Neyman and Scott (1967), Kendall (1960) and more recently by Portier and Kopp-Schneider (1991).

The model can be viewed as a mathematical generalization of the recessive oncogenesis model of Knudson (Knudson, 1971; Moolgavkar and Knudson, 1981), according to which the inactivation of both alleles of a specific tumor suppressor gene leads to cancer. The main feature of the model is the transition of target stem cells into cancer cells via an intermediate, premalignant, stage in two rare rate-limiting mutational steps. The mutations are considered irreversible, although the possibility of cell death through apoptosis may effectively remove the mutation on the tissue level.

In addition, the model also accounts explicitly for the growth kinetics of normal and intermediate cells. Growth of normal target cells is assumed to be deterministic. This is a reasonable assumption because the number of normal cells is large and probably still under tight homeostatic control, whereas intermediate or initiated cells are assumed to undergo a stochastic process because their numbers are small compared to the number of normal cells in the tissue. Furthermore, the process of initiation likely results in the loosening of homeostatic control leading to the positive net growth of intermediate lesions with rates that are typically increased over background rates. As a result, statistical fluctuations become more important in the intermediate compartment and need to be considered.

Here we summarize the basic assumptions required for the mathematical development of the model. Let $X(t)$ be the number of normal target cells at time t. Then, initiated cells arise from normal cells according to an inhomogeneous Poisson process with intensity $\nu(t)X(t)$, where $\nu(t)$ is the first mutation rate. Intermediate cells then either divide with rate $\alpha(t)$, die (or differentiate) with rate $\beta(t)$ or divide into one intermediate and one malignant cell with rate $\mu(t)$. Due to the presence of cell death, however, intermediate cells or their clones may become extinct before giving rise to malignant progeny. Further mathematical details can be found in Dewanji et al. (1989, 1991) and Moolgavkar and Luebeck (1990). Fig. 6.1 is a graphical representation of the model.

Note, in its present form the model assumes that the occurrence of the first malignant cell will inevitably lead to a tumor, possibly after a certain lag time. This, of course, is an oversimplification that most likely leads to underestimation of the mutation rates. Several problems that can arise from this assumption were considered by Luebeck and Moolgavkar (1994). For instance, it was found from computer simulations that the data analysis of tumor incidence data, within the framework of the two-stage model, was not sensitive to the length of the time lag, defined as the lag between the occurrence of the first malignant cell and the crossing of the generated clone of a certain viability threshold. In the simulations viability was assumed when the probability of extinction of the tumor became less than 10^{-3}. In the following, unless stated otherwise, we will assume that the tumor is synonymous with the first malignant cell in the tissue.

In general, promoters are defined as either exogenous or endogenous agents that stimulate cell proliferation. For the purpose of modeling their effect on cell kinetics, both, cell division rates α and cell death rates β, can be made functions of dose and time. Obviously, if an agent increases the net cell proliferation rate, $\alpha - \beta$, the pool of intermediate cells that are susceptible to malignant transformation will increase and hence the cancer risk. However, there are distinct modes of action of so called promoter carcinogens. An increase in $\alpha - \beta$ may come about through an increase in the cell division rate only. In this case a corresponding increase in the second mutation rate is expected. On the other hand, when the increase in $\alpha - \beta$ originates from the decrease of cell loss (death or differentiation) no accompanying increase is expected in the transformation rate μ.

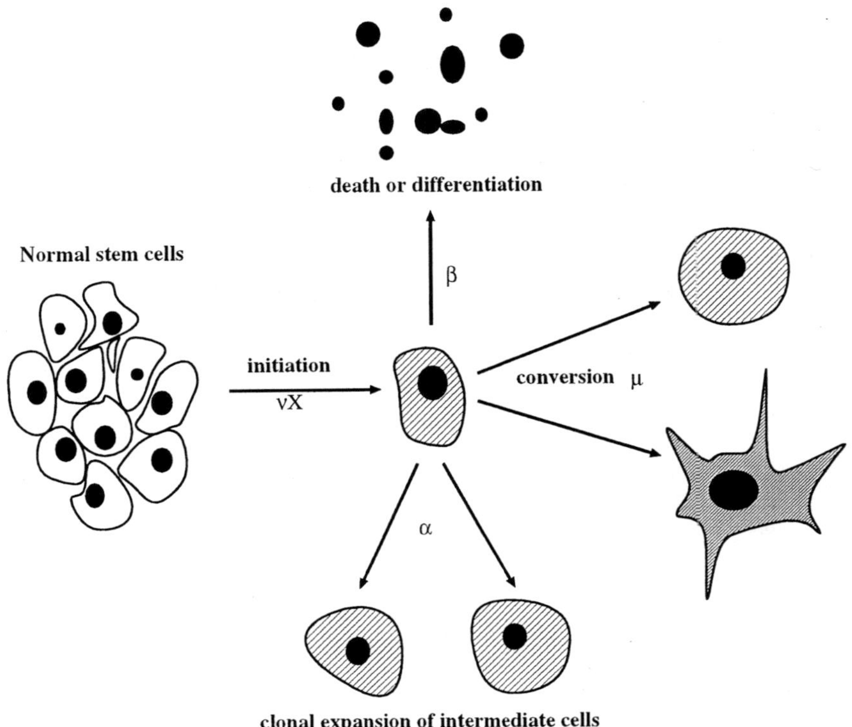

Figure 6.1: *Pictorial representation of the two-mutation clonal expansion model.*

In the framework of the model, a promoter can be categorized entirely in terms of its effects on the parameters α and β. The effects on cell death or differentiation, however, can also be couched in terms of the ratio β/α. When both α and β are constant in time and when $\alpha > \beta$, this ratio equals the asymptotic probability of extinction, namely the probability that a clone together with all its progeny ultimately becomes extinct. When $\alpha \leq \beta$ this probability is 1, i.e. given enough time, a clone will become extinct with certainty.

In this context it is interesting to note that quantitative analyses of enzyme altered foci in rat liver (Moolgavkar et al., 1990a; Luebeck et al., 1991) and of papillomas on mouse skin (Kopp-Schneider and Portier, 1992) all result in $\beta/\alpha \simeq 1$. This indicates that homeostatic control among intermediate cell populations remains strong. In the mouse papillomas there is actually indication that homeostatic control is protective, i.e. $\alpha < \beta$. However, under the influence of the promoter this protective effect seems to be abrogated, i.e. β/α(with promoter) $< \beta/\alpha$(without promoter). The finding that $\beta/\alpha \simeq 1$ in these analyses underlines the importance of the stochastic nature of the underlying clonal expansion processes. When $\beta/\alpha \simeq 1$, the net growth is slow or close to zero on average, but depending on the absolute values of α or β, large fluctuations around the mean may occur.

A simulation-based approach for the analysis of intermediate and tumor data, within the context of the model presented here, was formulated by Cohen and Ellwein (see Ellwein and Cohen, 1992, and references therein). This approach is motivated by the fact that cellular responses, and hence respective model parameters, may vary greatly with time over the course of an experiment. Variability of this kind is difficult to treat explicitly in the mathematical formulation of the model presented above. However, if the time behavior of these parameters is known, the effect on the outcome of interest can be studied straightforwardly by simulation. Cohen and Ellwein have developed a discrete time model for two-stage carcinogenesis that comprises cell proliferation kinetics in the normal, intermediate and malignant compartment. In their model, however, the stochastic birth and death process described in the foregoing is replaced by a deterministic recursion formula that computes expected clone and population sizes only. The view taken is that information about cell kinetics in each stage and related dose-response mechanisms can be obtained (ultimately) from experiment and be used directly for risk assessment. Obviously, this method has intuitive appeal and is able to deal with rather complicated experimental situations. At present, however, few ancillary data come with typical carcinogenesis data that help in specifying the unknown model parameters. Thus, parameter estimation is necessary, but no formal statistical procedures are available to determine the uncertainty of the estimates in the Cohen and Ellwein model. Another shortcoming of the Cohen and Ellwein approach is that only (unconditional) expectations are used in fitting the data. The stochastic nature of the data is ignored altogether. This, it can be shown, leads to an erroneous expression of the tumor incidence function. Yet, simulation based approaches are useful for exploratory data analysis and for model validation procedures with simulated data.

6.4. MODES OF ACTION OF CARCINOGENS

The distinction between the *concepts* of initiation, promotion and the *action* of specific environmental agents should be kept in focus. For example, while promotion is defined within the framework of the model as clonal expansion of initiated cells, an agent deemed to be a promoter may have other effects as well. It could cause hyperplasia of the normal tissue and, as pointed out above, indirectly increase the mutation rates. Other promoting agents may induce enzyme systems that produce reactive oxygen species that are mutagenic (Cerutti, 1985). See also the discussion by Moolgavkar on the action of environmental agents (Moolgavkar, 1983).

Within the context of the biologically-based model discussed here the terms initiation and promotion can be given precise meaning depending on the effect of a particular agent on the mutation rates ν and μ, and the effects on the cell kinetic rates α and β. Note, the definitions given here deviate form those given earlier in Chapter 3 where they were based mainly on the evaluation of short term bioassay data. Based on the model described here, the following classification scheme for the mode of action of a carcinogenic/anti-carcinogenic agent can be given:

promoter: An agent that increases the net cell proliferation rate $\alpha - \beta$. Thus a mitogen that increases α, but not β, is a promoter. Other substances, that do not change α, the cell division rate, but lower the death or differentiation rate β, are also promoters. PCBs and phenobarbital (in long term assays) seem to fall into this category.

(**anti-promoter:** An agent that lowers the net cell proliferation rate $\alpha - \beta$.)

initiator: An agent that increases the first mutation rate ν, leading to an increase in the number of intermediate clones. If the two critical events refer to the same locus on homologous chromosomes, then both rates, ν and μ, are deemed to be affected equally by the agent. However, they could also be affected differently by secondary processes following the first event.

completer: An agent that increases the rates of the remaining steps towards malignancy, without necessarily increasing the probability of the first (initiation) step. In the framework of the two-stage model, this implies an increase in the rate μ. Thus, there could be agents, that are not promoters, as defined above, but still increase the probability of the second event, without affecting the first event. An agent that favors mitotic recombination, for instance, may belong to this class.

inhibitor: An agent that lowers the background rates of ν and/or μ. Spontaneous rates of initiation or progression can be caused by endogenous factors, DNA replication errors or by the presence of very low doses of natural carcinogens in the environment. An inhibitor, by definition, would have a protective effect and lower these background rates.

It must be kept in mind that a single agent alone can be initiating, promoting, and completing the carcinogenic process, as discussed above. Even non-genotoxic compounds, that do not directly interact with DNA, may act as mutagens by increasing cell replication rates, overriding cell cycle check points that are important for DNA repair. Still, the above classification scheme is found useful in describing the primary modes of action of putative carcinogens. Physiologically based toxicodynamic models, as discussed further below, may then be used to understand each of these roles in detail.

6.5. QUANTITATIVE FORMULATION OF THE MODEL

For the analysis of epidemiological and experimental data in which the endpoint of interest is the appearance of malignant tumors we need expressions for the hazard function and the probability of tumor. However, initiation-promotion experiments often also yield data on the number and size of intermediate lesions such as the papillomas on the epidermis of the mouse or the enzyme altered foci in the rat liver. These data provide important information on the cell kinetics of intermediate lesions. We first introduce the essential mathematical expressions for the analysis of tumor incidence data and then discuss the analysis of intermediate lesions.

The following discussions focus on model fitting procedures using the maximum likelihood principle. The likelihood function reflects the probability of the total observed outcomes of an experiment or a human study given a probabilistic model for the endpoints of interest with degrees of freedom that describe all relevant covariates. In many epidemiological cohort studies covariate information is available on an individual basis, and the endpoint of interest is the appearance of tumors in members of the cohort. In this case the probability density of tumor (if the tumor is rapidly fatal or immediately diagnosed) or the probability of tumor (if the tumor is incidental) and the survival function are required to construct the likelihood. When aggregate data on groups of individuals are available the hazard (incidence) function is required.

Several analyses have employed an approximate solution to the two-stage model (analogous to the Armitage-Doll approximation discussed in Chapter 5), i.e. replacing the conditional expectation value for the number of intermediate cells by the unconditional one. Here we will not belabor the problems associated with this approximation. However, it is worth pointing out that the use of the approximate hazard function, in the opinion of the authors, does not offer any real conceptual or computational advantages over the use of the exact hazard function. It can be shown that the approximate solution depends on two parameter combinations, the first being the net cell proliferation $\alpha - \beta$, the second being the product $\nu X \times \mu$. From this nothing can be learned about the roles of α or β alone. In the light of the discussion above, this constitutes a serious shortcoming. We shall see further below that the computation of the exact hazard can be couched as a recursive procedure in the case of piecewise constant model parameters. The situation of piecewise constant exposure patterns is indeed the most frequently encountered among epidemiological and experimental data. For instance, see the discussion of the Colorado Plateau uranium miners' cohort in Chapter 8.

Some experimental data also provide information on the number and size of intermediate lesions, such as the enzyme altered foci in the rat liver or the papillomas on the skin of the mouse. In this case expressions for the number and size distribution of *non-extinct* lesions need to be derived. Because these data usually come from 2-dimensional sectional observations on histological slides the construction of the likelihood requires that the resulting stereological problem to be addressed first.

6.5.1. The Probability of Tumor

Likelihood based analyses of tumor (incidence) data require a definition of the probability of tumor. From it the probability density function and the hazard function can be derived. Here, only an outline of the mathematical steps that lead to these key concepts is given. More details can be found in a review by Moolgavkar and Luebeck (1990). Let $Y(t), Z(t)$, represent the number of intermediate and malignant cells, respectively, at time t and let

$$\Psi(y, z; t) = \sum_{j,k} P_{j,k}(t) y^j z^k$$

be the probability generating function with

$$P_{j,k}(t) = Prob\ [Y(t) = j, Z(t) = k \mid Y(0) = 0, Z(0) = 0].$$

Then the process $(Y(t), Z(t))$ is Markovian, and Ψ satisfies the Kolmogorov forward differential equation

$$\Psi'(y, z; t) = \frac{\partial \Psi(y, z; t)}{\partial t} = (y - 1)\nu(t)X(t)\Psi(y, z; t)$$

$$+\{\mu(t)yz + \alpha(t)y^2 + \beta(t) - [\alpha(t) + \beta(t) + \mu(t)]y\}\frac{\partial \Psi}{\partial y}, \tag{6.1}$$

with initial condition $\Psi(y, z; 0) = 1$. $S(t) = \Psi(1, 0; t)$ is the survival function and $P(t) = 1 - S(t)$ the probability of tumor for this model. As for the Armitage-Doll model (see Chapter 5), the hazard (incidence) function is then given by

$$h(t) = P'(t)/(1 - P(t)) = -\Psi'(1, 0; t)/\Psi(1, 0; t). \tag{6.2}$$

It follows immediately from the Kolmogorov equation that

$$\Psi'(1, 0; t) = -\mu(t)\frac{\partial \Psi}{\partial y}(1, 0; t),$$

and thus

$$h(t) = \mu(t)E[Y(t) \mid Z(t) = 0], \tag{6.3}$$

where E denotes the expectation and where we have used the relationship

$$E[Y(t) \mid Z(t) = 0] = \frac{\partial \Psi}{\partial y}(1, 0; t)/\Psi(1, 0; t).$$

Two approaches can be used to obtain the exact solution to the two-mutation model. The first approach involves solving the characteristic equations associated with the Kolmogorov equation. The second approach is somewhat more general, and is not described here, but can be found in Moolgavkar and Luebeck (1990). Specifically, the characteristic equations associated with Eq.(6.1) are

$$\frac{dy}{du} = -R(y, u) = -\{\mu(u)yz + \alpha(u)y^2 + \beta(u) - [\alpha(u) + \beta(u) + \mu(u)]y\} \tag{6.4}$$

$$\frac{dz}{du} = 0 \quad (z \text{ is constant along characteristics})$$

$$\frac{dt}{du} = 1, \quad \text{and} \quad \frac{d\Psi}{du} = (y - 1)\nu(u)X(u)\Psi.$$

The ordinary differential equation for Ψ may be solved along characteristics to yield

$$\Psi(y(t), z, t) = \Psi_0 \exp \int_0^t [y(u, t) - 1]\nu(u)X(u)du, \tag{6.5}$$

where $\Psi_0 = \Psi(y(0), z, 0) = 1$ is the initial value of Ψ. We are interested in computing $\Psi(1, 0; t)$ for any t, and thus we need to find the values of Ψ along the characteristic through $(y(0), 0, 0)$ where $y(0)$ is the initial value of y and $y(t) = 1$. Now, along the characteristic, Y satisfies the differential equation $dy/du = -R(y, u)$ and this is just a Ricatti equation which can be readily integrated in closed form if the parameters of the model are piecewise constant. To be precise, the Ricatti equation for y can be solved to yield a value for $y(u)$ for any u, with initial condition $y(t) = 1$. Note that y depends on u and t.

Thus, the survival function

$$S(t) = \Psi(1, 0; t) = \exp \int_0^t [y(u, t) - 1]\nu(u)X(u)du, \tag{6.6}$$

where the explicit dependence of y on u and t is acknowledged. The hazard function then is given by

$$h(t) = -\Psi'(1, 0; t)/\Psi(1, 0; t) = -\int_0^t \nu(u)X(u)y_t(u, t)du, \tag{6.7}$$

where y_t denotes the derivative of y with respect to t.

6.5.1.1. Solution for Piecewise Constant Parameters Assume there are n intervals $[t_{i-1}, t_i]$ with $i = 1, 2, ..., n$, covering the time period $[t_o = 0, t_n = t]$. Then the solution of Eq.(6.4), $y(u, t)$, can be computed recursively starting from $u = t = t_n$ using the boundary condition $y(t, t) = 1$. For $u \in [t_{i-1}, t_i]$ we have (see Moolgavkar and Luebeck, 1990)

$$y(u, t) = \frac{B_i - A_i \frac{y(t_i,t)-B_i}{y(t_i,t)-A_i} \exp[\alpha_i(A_i - B_i)(u - t_i)]}{1 - \frac{y(t_i,t)-B_i}{y(t_i,t)-A_i} \exp[\alpha_i(A_i - B_i)(u - t_i)]}, \tag{6.8}$$

where A_i (B_i) are the lower (upper) root of the quadratic form: $\alpha_i x^2 - [\alpha_i + \beta_i + \mu_i]x + \beta_i$. The constant parameters α_i, β_i and μ_i refer respectively to the cell division, cell death and second mutation rate in the time interval $[t_{i-1}, t_i]$. When $\nu(u)X(u)$ is also piecewise constant over time, the time integral in Eq.(6.6) can be computed in explicit form. For $u \in [t_{i-1}, t_i]$ we can rewrite the integrand $[y - 1]$ as

$$y(u, t) - 1 = \frac{C_i}{1 - r_i \exp[\delta_i(u - t_i)]} + (A_i - 1),$$

where $C_i = B_i - A_i$, $r_i = (y(t_i, t) - B_i)/(y(t_i, t) - A_i)$ and $\delta_i = \alpha_i(A_i - B_i)$. The survival function Eq.(6.6) can then be computed as

$$S(t) = \exp[-\sum_{i=1}^{n} H_i] \quad \text{with} \tag{6.9}$$

$$H_i = -\nu X_i \int_{t_{i-1}}^{t_i} [y(u, t) - 1]du \tag{6.10}$$

$$= -\nu X_i \Big[(B_i - 1)(t_i - t_{i-1}) + \ln\Big(\frac{1 - r_i}{1 - r_i \exp[-\delta_i(t_i - t_{i-1})]}\Big)/\alpha_i\Big]. \tag{6.11}$$

Thus, the survival function can be computed in explicit form in the case of piecewise constant model parameters. The probability density function for a tumor at time t is the time derivative of the tumor probability $P(t) = 1 - S(t)$, i.e. $P'(t) = -S'(t)$.

6.5.1.2. Identifiability of Model Parameters It is interesting to note that for constant cell division rates α the probability of tumor is only dependent on three combinations of the four parameters α, β, νX and μ. Thus, for instance, in the situation of constant exposures, tumor data alone are not sufficient to estimate all the biological parameters of the model. To see this, consider the cumulative hazard H and the solution $y(u, t)$ of the Ricatti equation (6.4) defined above. Obviously, $y(u, t)$ solves an equation of the form $y' = -\alpha(A - y)(B - y)$, where A and B are the two (time dependent) roots of the Ricatti equation (6.4). It is easy to see that the transform $w = \alpha(y - 1)$ solves a similar equation when α is constant, that is $w' = -[\alpha(A - 1) - w][\alpha(B - 1) - w]$. Therefore the solution w depends only on the two modified roots $\alpha(A-1)$ and $\alpha(B-1)$ and the hazard only on $\nu X/\alpha$ and these two roots. Of course, other parametrizations can be given that are merely combinations of the three functions arrived here. However, to lowest order in the parameter μ, we recover familiar quantities

$$-\alpha(A - 1) = \alpha - \beta + \mathcal{O}(\mu) \tag{6.12}$$

and

$$\alpha(B - 1) = \frac{\mu}{1 - \beta/\alpha} + \mathcal{O}(\mu^2). \tag{6.13}$$

It is worthwhile pointing out that the non-identifiability inherent in the two-stage model may also be used to strengthen the risk estimates in chronic exposure tumor bioassays. The non-identifiability in the two-stage model was first pointed out by W. Heidenreich (1996).

6.6. LIKELIHOOD CONSTRUCTION AND ESTIMATION

The likelihood contribution of an individual in a study that monitors the incidence or appearance of a specific kind of malignant tumor can be constructed as follows: Let t_i be the time of observation at which the subject i develops the tumor, dies (with or without tumor), or is lost to follow-up. Then subject i contributes the term $\mathcal{L}_i(t_i)$ to the entire likelihood which is given by $\mathcal{L} = \prod \mathcal{L}_i(t_i)$ with

$$\mathcal{L}_i(t_i) = \begin{cases} P(t_i) & \text{if malig. tumor was incidental} \\ P'(t_i) & \text{if malig. tumor was fatal} \\ S(t_i) = 1 - P(t_i) & \text{if free of tumor.} \end{cases}$$

If individual level information is not available then the hazard function is needed. Since the derivative $y_t(u, t)$ in Eq.(6.7) is cumbersome to compute using the chain rule repeatedly, it is probably faster to compute $P'(t)$ numerically with a midpoint formula. The hazard is then computed according to $h(t) = P'(t)/(1 - P(t))$. For examples see Moolgavkar et al. (1990b) and Moolgavkar and Luebeck (1992).

For many studies one has to consider several different time intervals defined by a specific exposure pattern. On each of these intervals the parameters of the model can be assumed constant. The roots A_i and B_i of the quadratic polynomial (see 6.8) on interval i are functions of the parameters of the model and thus also of the exposure rate variables. There is no limitation on the number of intervals in the recursive scheme for the computation of the probability of tumor outlined above.

Maximizing $\mathcal{L}$ over the parameter space yields the maximum likelihood estimates (mle's) of the model parameters. An efficient method is the Davidon-Fletcher-Powell (DFP) algorithm (Press et al., 1986). Stability of the maximum likelihood estimates can be determined by running a modified Newton-Raphson method after convergence with the DFP algorithm and by checking for 'positive definiteness' of the Hessian. 95% confidence intervals can either be based on the information matrix, or, better, should be computed using the profile-likelihood method (Venzon and Moolgavkar, 1988).

6.7. QUANTITATIVE ANALYSIS OF INTERMEDIATE LESIONS

Many initiation-promotion (IP) experiments have been designed to provide information on intermediate endpoints such as the papillomas in mouse skin painting experiments or the enzyme altered foci (EAF) in rodent hepatocarcinogenesis experiments. Next to the number of lesions their size and particular phenotype is often determined as well. It is generally believed that at least some of these lesions represent clones of initiated cells that are precursors to malignant tumors. In the following we will focus our attention onto rodent hepatocarcinogenesis. Most of the mathematical results necessary to analyze such data have been derived in Dewanji et al. (1989) and in Moolgavkar et al. (1990a). An application of the methods to mouse skin papillomas can be found in Kopp-Schneider and Portier (1992). The following sections are meant to serve as an introduction to the statistical analysis of foci data. See Chapter 3 for a description of such data and a discussion of the role of cell kinetics in the growth of EAF.

6.7.1. Modeling Initiation and Promotion of EAF

There are numerous discussions in the literature of biochemical and physiological aspects and of the role of EAF in hepatotumorigenesis (Emmelot and Scherer, 1980; Farber, 1980; Goldfarb and Pugh, 1981; Kunz et al., 1982; Goldsworthy et al., 1986; Buchmann et al., 1987; Pitot et al., 1987).

Assume that at time s one ml liver contains a number $X(s)$ of normal hepatocytes which transform into altered cells with rate $\nu(s)$. The change in enzyme expression in transformed hepatocytes is considered a hereditary and irreversible trait of the altered cell. The number of initiated cells that arise from normal hepatocytes is then modeled as a Poisson distribution with mean $\int_0^t \nu(s)X(s)ds$.

Promotion is the clonal expansion of such altered cells and is mathematically described by a non-homogeneous (time dependent) birth-death process (Cox and Miller, 1972) with birth rate $\alpha(s)$ and death (or differentiation) rate $\beta(s)$. As before, this means that altered cells either divide into two altered cells with rate $\alpha(s)$ or die (or differentiate) with rate $\beta(s)$. The third possibility, namely that altered cells divide asymmetrically into one altered and one further progressed (toward malignancy) cell, is not explicitly considered here. However, when simultaneous information on the occurrence of malignant tumors is available, the model can be extended to incorporate this information.

The parameter $\nu(s)$ is to be interpreted as the rate at which normal cells are altered to express a particular enzyme phenotype. It is, of course, conceivable that the initiated cell corresponds only to a subset of the particular phenotype in question or that other phenotypes, not under study, can be transformed into malignancies as well. Thus, at this point, we simply view the enzyme alteration as a surrogate marker for initiation.

As formulated the model does not yet distinguish killed cells from differentiated cells, or from cells that are quiescent; all are assumed absent from the proliferating (actively cycling) intermediate cell pool.

Dewanji et al. (1989) derive mathematical expressions for the number of altered foci and their size distribution. Luebeck and Moolgavkar (1991) give a slightly more general derivation of these results that allows for an extension to Gompertzian growth of intermediate lesions (see below). Here only general formulas and their relationship to cell kinetic parameters are presented. Let us define the two functions

$$g(t, s) = \exp\left[-\int_s^t (\alpha(u) - \beta(u))\, du\right] \tag{6.14}$$

and

$$G(t, s) = \int_s^t \alpha(u)\, g(u, s)\, du. \tag{6.15}$$

Then the expected number of non-extinct foci at time t can be written as

$$\Lambda(t) = \int_0^t \nu(s)X(s)\frac{1}{G(t, s) + g(t, s)}\, ds \tag{6.16}$$

and the probability, $p_m(t)$, of finding a non-extinct clone consisting of exactly m cells at time t, as

$$p_m(t) = \frac{1}{\Lambda(t)}\int_0^t \nu(s)X(s)\frac{g}{G^2}\left(\frac{G}{G+g}\right)^{m+1} ds. \tag{6.17}$$

The inverse function $g^{-1}(t, s)$ represents the expected size of a clone at time t starting off with one cell at time s. The above integrals can also be computed in closed form when constant or piecewise constant parameters are assumed, see Kopp-Schneider (1992) and Luebeck et al. (1994). The more general case of Gompertzian growth of intermediate lesions is discussed below. It assumes that cell replication and death behave exponentially with time.

In many IP experiments initiation is induced by an acute exposure to a mutagenic carcinogen followed by an application of a promoter substance. Unless the promoter is a pure promoter, in the sense that it doesn't cause any increases in the transformation rates leading to cancer, one needs to control for promoter induced initiation in the analysis of the data. Thus, proper control groups (animals which were not exposed to the

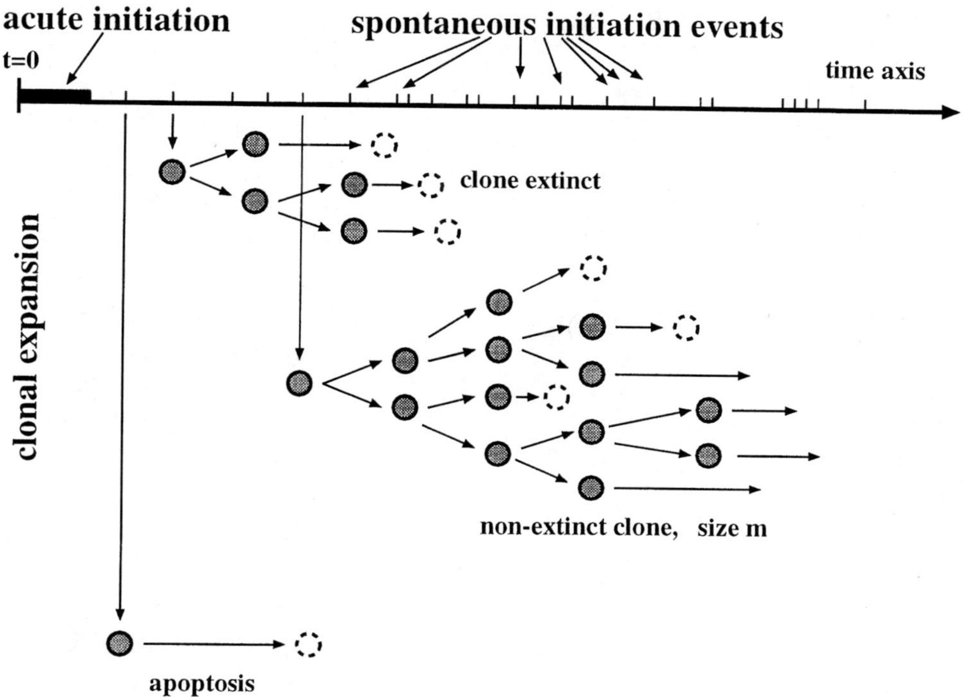

Figure 6.2: *Pictorial representation of initiation and promotion. Normal cells are initiated either spontaneously or by application of a chemical agent. These cells may either divide or undergo apoptosis. If all the cells in a clone undergo apoptosis, the focus becomes extinct. The probability of this occurring is high when the focus is small.*

primary initiator) should be included in the analysis whenever available. To capture this situation mathematically, the initiation rate $\nu(s)$ is composed of an acute rate, say ν_o, conveniently expressed by a Dirac delta-function, and a spontaneous background rate, say ν_1. Once initiated, a cell will follow the stochastic birth and death process described above. The stochastic nature of the clonal expansions is portrayed schematically in Fig. 6.2. The model is then fit to the observed number and size distribution of non-extinct foci seen at the various time points.

6.7.2. Gompertz Growth

The assumption of exponential mean growth may well be an oversimplification. Cellular responses to promoting agents are often more pronounced at the beginning of the treatment, accompanied by a spurt in focal cell replication which, as the treatment continues, may be slowed by adaptive responses (Schulte-Hermann et al., 1990). For instance, a significant slowing of exponential growth of EAF was observed in female Wistar rats initiated acutely with DEN and treated continuously with PB (Luebeck et al., 1991). Hence, we would like to relax the assumption of constant or piecewise constant parameters α and β. A straightforward generalization arises when α and β

are assumed to depend on time exponentially so that, beginning at some time s

$$\alpha(u) = \alpha_o \exp[-a(u-s)], \qquad \beta(u) = \beta_o \exp[-a(u-s)] \tag{6.18}$$

Here α_o, β_o and a are constants. These definitions imply that the ratio of cell death and cell birth rates, β/α, is also a constant. It follows (Tan, 1986; Luebeck and Moolgavkar, 1991) that the resulting mean growth is Gompertz-like, following the curve

$$g^{-1}(u) = \exp[(\alpha_o - \beta_o)(1 - \exp(-a(u-s)))/a]. \tag{6.19}$$

When $a = 0$ then $\alpha - \beta =$ constant and the mean growth is exponential. Thus, the Gompertz model introduces one extra parameter, a, which measures departures from exponentiality of the mean growth. When $a = 0$, mean growth is exponential; when $a > 0$, mean growth is Gompertzian (subexponential); when $a < 0$, mean growth is superexponential. The hypothesis $a = 0$ can be tested using standard likelihood based procedures such as the likelihood ratio test.

6.7.3. Statistical Analysis

Unfortunately, Equations (6.16) and (6.17) are not yet sufficient to compute the overall likelihood of the experimental outcome, because the number of non-extinct foci and their sizes are not directly observable (see Chapter 3). Instead, what is known is the number and the size (in terms of area or radius) of 2-dimensional transections on histological slides stained for some enzyme marker activity. Hence, Eqs.(6.16) and (6.17) need to be translated into expressions describing the mean number of focal transections per unit area, say $n_2(t)$, and a probability density, $f_2^{\epsilon}(y)$, for finding an observable transection of size $y > \epsilon$. Here ϵ is a lower bound below which transections cannot be reliably detected.

For spherical objects, the stereological problem was solved by Wicksell (1925). Wicksell's formula relates the distribution of radii of 3-dimensional spheres to the distribution of radii of transectional disks observed in 2-dimensional sections. Thus, Wicksell's formula requires the 3-dimensional probability density function, $f_3(r)$, for finding a 3-dimensional sphere of radius r, as input. Hence, we need to relate 3-dimensional radii to the number of (actively cycling) cells in the foci denoted by m.

If all cells in a spherically shaped focus are actively cycling the number of cells can simply be inferred from the ratio of clone volume to cell volume: $m(r) = r^3/r_c^3$. However, there is some indication from pulse labeling data that cell replication is inhomogeneous across individual foci, showing higher mitotic activity in the outer parts of the foci (Buchmann, personal communication). In general, the shape of $m(r)$ should be determined from labeling index measurements that also provide information on the positions of the cell divisions within individual foci.

After taking into account the Jacobian of the transformation ($m \to r$), which is given by the derivative $dm(r)/dr$, Wicksell's formula can be written as

$$f_2^{\epsilon}(y) = \frac{y}{\mu_\epsilon} \int_y^{\infty} \frac{f_3(r)}{\sqrt{r^2 - y^2}} dr, \tag{6.20}$$

where

$$f_3(r) = \frac{dm(r)}{dr} p_{m(r)}(t), \tag{6.21}$$

with $p_{m(r)}$ given by Eq.(6.17) and with the (adjusted) mean radius, μ_ϵ, given by

$$\mu_\epsilon = \int_\epsilon^\infty \sqrt{r^2 - \epsilon^2} f_3(r)\, dr. \tag{6.22}$$

Furthermore, the number of non-extinct transections (per unit area) is also assumed to be Poisson distributed with mean $n_2(t)$ and related to $\Lambda(t)$, its 3-dimensional equivalent (see Eq.(6.16)), by means of

$$n_2(t) = 2\mu_\epsilon \Lambda(t), \tag{6.23}$$

where $\Lambda(t)$ is given by (6.16). For more details, see Moolgavkar et al. (1990a).

If one also chooses to condition the analysis to foci that are smaller than a prescribed size, say radius R, then the above formulae need to be modified accordingly. It can be shown that in this case μ_ϵ in the equations above is replaced by $\mu_\epsilon - \mu_R$, with μ_R defined like μ_ϵ, correctly taking into account the new condition: $\epsilon \leq r \leq R$. The values of ϵ, the smallest transection radius reliably detected, and of R, the largest size admitted, are in general determined by the experimenter.

The likelihood for the experimental data is constructed as a product of the contributions each animal makes. For each animal we have the Poisson probability of its section (area A) showing a total of $N_2 = n_2(t)A$ transections with radii between ϵ and R (Eq.(6.23)) and the probability density $f_2^\epsilon(y)$ that a particular transection is actually of size y (Eq.(6.20)). The total likelihood is the product of the likelihood contributions made by each animal.

In Chapter 8 we provide the reader with two examples of analyses of EAF data. The first example is a chronic exposure experiment with N-nitrosomorpholine (NNM). The second example presents the analysis of data from a typical initiation-promotion experiment with a number of PCB congeners as promoters. More examples can be found in the literature.

6.7.4. Joint Analysis of Premalignant and Malignant Lesions

Many rodent experiments provide information on both malignant and benign tumors. If the benign tumors lie on the pathway to malignancy then they should also be considered in any analysis of the data. Frequently, however, no use is made of premalignant lesions or benign tumors, or they are thrown in with the malignant lesions. Obviously, valuable information is lost if these data are ignored. On the other hand, if premalignant and malignant lesions are not distinguished, the cancer model might crossly overestimate the risk.

Recently, attempts have been made to quantify the appearance of 'foci within foci', i.e., the appearance of small islands, presumably clonal, of cells within altered hepatic foci, characterized by a second phenotypic change. Foci within foci may represent the earliest stage of malignancy. A similar situation arises when simultaneous information is available on foci and whether or not a malignant tumor is present in the tissue of interest. The mathematical tools required for analyses of data in which information on both premalignant and malignant lesions is available are currently being developed (Dewanji et. al., 1991; de Gunst and Luebeck, 1994).

6.8. TOXICOKINETICS IN BIOLOGICALLY BASED RISK ASSESSMENT

In the absence of epidemiological data, cancer risk assessments need to rely on the use of animal data to predict the risk of chemical exposures to the human population. Interspecies extrapolation is a necessary element in this process and has been performed by scaling the doses used in a dose-response relationship according to body weight or surface area. That is, a dose represented in the appropriate units, mg/kg/day (body weight scaling) or mg/m^2 (surface area scaling), is assumed to result in the same cancer incidence across species. As an improvement to the risk assessment process, physiologically based pharmacokinetic models have been used to estimate target tissue doses and facilitate interspecies extrapolation. In the remainder of this text we refer to these models as physiologically based toxicokinetic (PBTK) models since we are concerned with toxicants rather than therapeutic drugs.

Physiologically based toxicokinetic models provide a means of describing the disposition of a xenobiotic in the body. These models have been used to predict the dose of a xenobiotic to a target tissue or a dose surrogate more closely related to the incidence of cancer than the external dose. PBTK models have been developed for styrene (Ramsey and Andersen, 1984), methylene chloride (Andersen et al., 1987), carbon tetrachloride (Paustenbach et al., 1988), tetrachloroethylene (Bois et al., 1990; Ward et al., 1988), chloroform (Corley et al., 1990), benzene (Bois et al., 1991; Medinsky et al., 1989; Spear et al., 1991; Travis et al., 1990a; Woodruff et al., 1992), and ethyl acrylate (Frederick et al., 1992). This list is not comprehensive but demonstrates the abundance of research devoted to PBTK models.

In the following, we review the use of PBTK models in risk assessment. We then describe the framework of a biologically based risk assessment and the mathematical formulation of a PBTK model.

6.8.1. Physiologically-based Toxicokinetic Models in Risk Assessment

There have been several studies utilizing PBTK models in risk assessment (Bailer and Hoel, 1989; Beliles and Totman, 1989; Bois et al., 1990; Cox and Ricci, 1992; Fisher and Allen, 1993; Leung and Paustenbach, 1990; Reitz et al., 1990a; 1990b; Travis et al., 1989). The role of a PBTK model has been: 1) to predict a measure of animal tissue dose used in the dose-response curve; and 2) to determine the human administered dose corresponding to a tissue dose at a given level of risk. Inherent in 2) is the assumption that the PBTK model is valid at the low dose identified by the cancer model. The underlying question is whether or not the model, parameterized under higher dose conditions, provides a reasonable representation of the kinetics at low doses. To answer this question, kinetic data obtained at low administered doses are required and would improve the risk assessment process by eliminating the uncertainty introduced by the high to low dose extrapolation of the PBTK model. Furthermore, PBTK models would yield better estimates of target tissue doses.

The following steps outline the use of a PBTK model in cancer risk assessment:

1. The PBTK model is used to calculate the effective dose (dose surrogate) in the animal;
2. A cancer model is fitted to the cancer incidence (bioassay data) versus dose surrogate (from PBTK model) in animals;
3. The value of the animal dose surrogate at a specified risk level is determined from the cancer model. It is assumed that the dose surrogate has the same effect across species or scales allometrically to determine the human dose surrogate value;
4. The PBTK model for humans is used to determine the administered dose corresponding to the dose surrogate value at the specified risk level.

Variations of this basic methodology have been employed in the following examples.

6.8.2. Multistage Modeling

Travis et al. (1989) compared risks calculated from "classical" risk assessment methodology (U.S. Environmental Protection Agency, 1986) and an approach separating toxicokinetics and toxicodynamics for tetrachloroethylene. A physiologically based toxicokinetic model (Ward et al., 1988) was used to predict the effective dose of carcinogen (dose surrogate) via a nonlinear metabolic pathway. These doses were then scaled to human doses using both body weight and surface area scaling since the relationship between metabolized dose per gram of mouse tissue and its toxicodynamic effect (cancer) is uncertain. The linearized multistage model was used for the high to low dose extrapolation of the dose-response curve. Travis et al. reported that the incorporation of toxicokinetics reduces the risk estimate at low exposures regardless of the method of interspecies dose extrapolation (see Section 8.7 for calculations).

Beliles and Totman (1989) incorporated toxicokinetics through their calculation of metabolized dose in a risk assessment of occupational benzene exposure. Michaelis-Menten kinetics were used to describe the relationship between the applied dose and metabolized dose in rats and mice. Human equivalent doses were then scaled allometrically from the rodent metabolized doses corresponding to cancer bioassay exposures. Beliles and Totman used the multistage model to estimate the lifetime cancer risk in humans. Agreement in the estimated risks regardless of the route of exposure, endpoint, or animal species was attributed to the incorporation of experimental data rather than default allometric procedures.

Along the same lines, Bailer and Hoel (1989) used Michaelis-Menten kinetics to represent the relationship between applied dose and metabolized dose in rats and mice. The multistage model was used to estimate the 95% lower bound on dose having an added risk of 10^{-6} (VSD). They compared VSDs based on applied dose and internal metabolized dose. The internal dose determined by the multistage model was converted back to an applied VSD with the Michaelis-Menten relationship. Bailer and Hoel found that the internal dose based risk assessment yielded higher estimates of risk than the applied dose method. They also calculated human lifetime cancer risks for an occupational benzene exposure. First, the exposure was converted into species equivalent dose units (mg/kg/day) and the internal dose calculated from the animal kinetic relationship. Then, the internal dose based multistage model was used to predict the risk.

More recently, Cox and Ricci (1992) re-examined the cancer risks calculated by Bailer and Hoel and used a PBTK model as an alternative to calculating internal dose. Using the PBTK model to calculate internal doses resulted in lower risk estimates than the administered dose approach and Bailer and Hoel's internal dose approach.

The use of physiologically based toxicokinetics and the multistage model in risk assessment have been reported for chloroform (Reitz et al., 1990b), dioxane (Leung and Paustenbach, 1990; Reitz et al., 1990a), and trichloroethylene (Fisher and Allen, 1993) . In general, the procedure outlined by Travis et al. was used with compound and investigator dependent dose surrogates and the assumption that the amount of carcinogen per mass of tissue results in the same cancer response across species. For chloroform and dioxane the risk specific dose determined by incorporating toxicokinetics is greater than that determined by the classical risk assessment methodology. Fisher and Allen also found the risk specific dose to be higher than EPA's estimate using the lifetime average daily total amount of trichloroethylene metabolized as the dose surrogate. However, a second dose surrogate (lifetime average area under the concentration versus time curve for trichloroacetic acid in plasma) resulted in a lower risk specific dose than the classical approach.

A distributional method was used by Bois et al. (1990) to investigate the precision of incorporating a PBTK model in the risk assessment of tetrachloroethylene. Distributions were obtained for the PBTK model parameters, carcinogenic potency, and the estimated risks for humans. Monte Carlo sampling was used to convolve distributions of cancer potency and metabolized dose (predicted from the PBTK model), to obtain the distribution of human risk. They reported percentiles for the cancer risk estimate of an individual exposed continuously to 1 ng/L of tetrachloroethylene in air.

We believe that incorporation of PBTK models in risk assessment provides a more realistic basis for determining human risks from data obtained in animals. Based on the literature reviewed, PBTK models do not consistently lower or raise the human risk estimate relative to the classical approach. Instead, the results are largely dependent on the choice of a dose surrogate. See Section 6.9 for a discussion on selecting a dose surrogate.

6.8.3. Biologically-based Risk Assessment

Physiologically based toxicokinetic models can be used to obtain a target tissue dose as described previously, then linked to a biologically-based cancer model. An early example of this was reported by Liu (1990). A PBTK model of tetrachloroethylene (Ward et al., 1988) was used to correlate tissue metabolized doses with DNA synthesis data (Schumann et al., 1980). The increase in DNA synthesis above background was assumed to be proportional to the mitotic rate increase in the cancer model.

Similarly, Bogen (1990) calculated human virtually safe doses for three chlorinated methanes, carbon tetrachloride, chloroform, and methylene chloride. PBTK models were used to establish relationships between administered dose and target tissue dose. Then, an approximate two-stage cell-kinetic-multistage (CKM) model (Bogen, 1989) based on the 'fully stochastic' multistage model of Moolgavkar (1983) was used to simulate tumor incidence data in mice. The cell proliferation effects of the compounds were incorporated through the growth parameters in the CKM model. That is, increased growth parameter values were assumed to be proportional to increased compound-induced cellular proliferation. Finally, assuming that the cell proliferation effects are the same in mice and humans, human virtually safe doses associated with an increased cancer risk of 10^{-6} were calculated for each of the three compounds.

Conolly and Andersen (1991; 1993) outlined an approach to mechanism-based cancer risk assessment. They proposed the use of three submodels: 1) a PBTK model to predict tissue dosimetry; 2) an early tissue response model to establish a relationship between the target tissue dose and its effects (e.g., DNA damage, cytolethality, mitogenic stimulation); and 3) a cancer model to simulate tumor responses based on the early tissue effects of the active xenobiotic. At times it may be difficult to clearly define the beginning of the early tissue response submodel and the end of the PBTK submodel (e.g., Reitz et al. (1990b) modeled cytotoxicity in their PBTK model for chloroform).

More recently, Mills and Andersen (1993) described a biologically based dose-response model for dioxin induced liver tumors in rats. A PBTK model, a toxicodynamic model, and a stochastic model for cell growth were linked in an effort to simulate the data from exposure to tumorigenic response. The PBTK and toxicodynamic models included protein binding in the liver compartment and simulation of altered gene expression. Additionlly, Mills and Andersen outlined the need for more complete representations of gene regulation in toxicokinetic and toxicodynamic models and the need for elucidation of the mechanisms by which alterations in growth regulating factors cause growth regulatory responses in tissues.

As noted by Conolly and Andersen (1993), the need remains for a better understanding of the 'early tissue response' or cellular response. That is, we must identify how the target tissue dose damages DNA to increase the probability of genetic mutation, stimulates or depresses cell division or cell death. Toward this end, we must first collect data on these cellular responses at different dose levels. Once the mechanism(s) of action is understood at the cellular level, predictive mechanistic models can be developed to improve the biologically based risk assessment.

6.8.4. Model Development and Parameterization

The physiologically based toxicokinetic model is constructed to represent the salient features of toxicant disposition in the body. Compartments represent a 'well-stirred'

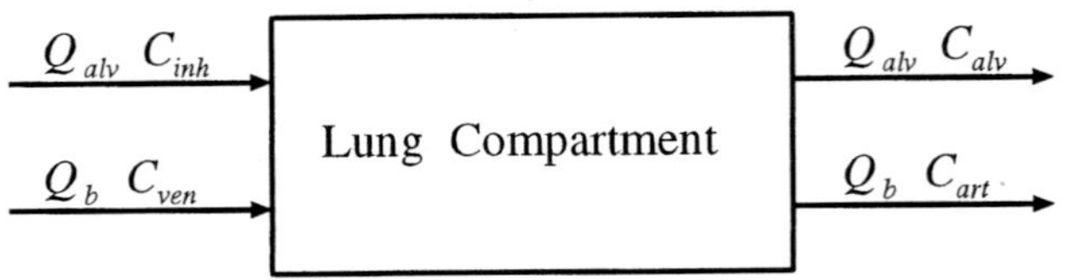

Figure 6.3: *Diagram of the flows into and out of the lung compartment in a physiologically based toxicokinetic model.*

mixture of blood and tissue(s) that impacts the distribution of the compound of interest through storage, metabolism, or elimination from the body.

Ramsey and Andersen (1984) developed a PBTK model for styrene which has become the prototype for perfusion-limited models of suspected carcinogens. Their model consists of 5 compartments: lung; fat; muscle; richly perfused tissue; and liver. Mass balances across each compartment define the governing differential equations for the system. The following describes the mathematical formulation of a PBTK model.

For the inhalation route, the compound is inspired at concentration C_{inh} with a flow rate equal to the alveolar ventilation rate, Q_{alv}. The model assumes that there is no gas storage in the lungs and that ventilation of the alveoli is continuous, rather than cyclic (Figure 6.3). The lung compartment is described individually here because the venous blood enters and the arterial blood leaves this compartment.

Conservation of mass requires that the flow of chemical entering the lungs be equal to the flow leaving the lungs:

$$Q_{alv}(C_{inh} - C_{alv}) = Q_b(C_{art} - C_{ven}), \tag{6.24}$$

where Q_b is the total blood flow rate, the C_{alv}, C_{ven} and C_{art} are the alveolar, mixed venous blood, and arterial blood concentrations, respectively. The compound in the alveolar air is assumed to equilibrate instantaneously with pulmonary capillary blood so that the compound concentration in lung blood and in alveolar air leaving the lungs maintains a constant ratio specified by the blood/gas partition coefficient, λ_b:

$$\lambda_b = C_{art}/C_{alv}. \tag{6.25}$$

In the body tissues, conservation of mass requires that the amount of chemical entering via the arterial blood in an interval of time, dt, be equal to the quantity gained by each tissue group, dA_i, plus the amount leaving (e.g., in the venous blood, through metabolism or through elimination). Some compartments neither metabolize nor eliminate chemicals, thus, the mass balances across these compartments are simplified. Figure 6.4 pictures a hypothetical tissue compartment and equation (6.26) is its corresponding mass balance.

$$\frac{dA_i}{dt} = Q_i(C_{art} - C_{vi}) - \frac{dA_{mi}}{dt} - K_r C_{vi} V_i, \tag{6.26}$$

where A_i is the amount of compound in the tissue, Q_i is the blood flow rate through tissue group i, dA_{mi}/dt is the rate of metabolism in tissue i, K_r is the elimination rate constant in tissue i, and V_i is the tissue volume. Equation (6.26) assumes first order

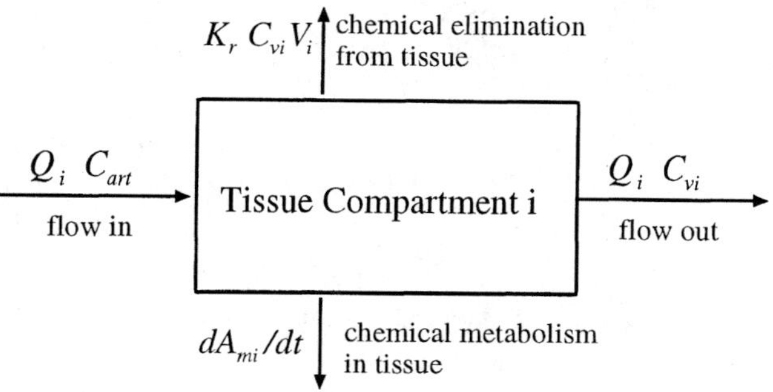

Figure 6.4: *Representation of a tissue compartment with theoretical flows in and out of the compartment labeled by the arrows.*

chemical elimination, but other representations may be appropriate. The concentration of chemical in venous blood leaving tissue group i is assumed to satisfy the equilibrium equation:

$$C_{vi} = \frac{C_i}{\lambda_i} = \frac{A_i}{V_i \lambda_i}, \tag{6.27}$$

where λ_i is the tissue/blood partition coefficient.

Assuming a combination of Michaelis-Menten and first-order reaction kinetics, the metabolic rate is expressed in terms of the concentration of the chemical in venous blood leaving the tissue (C_{vi}) as:

$$\frac{dA_{mi}}{dt} = \frac{V_{max} C_{vi}}{K_m + C_{vi}} + K_f C_{vi}, \tag{6.28}$$

where V_{max} is the maximum metabolic rate constant, K_m is the concentration at one-half V_{max}, and K_f is the linear metabolic rate constant.

The concentration of the chemical in the mixed venous blood returning to the lungs is formulated as the sum of the venous contribution from each of the tissue groups:

$$C_{ven} = \sum \{(Q_i C_{vi})/Q_b\}. \tag{6.29}$$

By combining equations (6.24) and (6.25), the equation for arterial blood concentration is:

$$C_{art} = \frac{Q_{alv} C_{inh} + Q_b C_{ven}}{Q_b + Q_{alv}/\lambda_b}. \tag{6.30}$$

Thus, the toxicokinetics of the parent compound are described by the system of equations, (6.24-6.30). These equations are numerically integrated to provide concentrations of the toxicant in each compartment over time. Physicochemical characteristics unique to individual toxicants may require a different set of model assumptions and modified equations. The toxicokinetics of metabolites can be included in the model by following the mass balance principles described above.

A gavage exposure involves absorption of the compound from the gut into the liver. This can be modeled as a first order kinetic process. Equation (6.26) is modified as follows:

$$\frac{dA_l}{dt} = Q_l(C_{art} - C_{vl}) - \frac{dA_{ml}}{dt} + kD_0 e^{-kt}, \tag{6.31}$$

where k is the first order absorption rate constant and D_0 is the total quantity of compound administered. In equation (6.31), elimination of the chemical has been omitted.

Parameterization

Traditionally, PBTK model parameters are derived from population averages. As discussed in Chapter 3, publications exist (Arms and Travis, 1988; Davies and Morris, 1993; Fiserova-Bergerova, 1983; Fiserova-Bergerova and Diaz, 1986; Fiserova-Bergerova et al., 1984; Perbellini et al., 1985) which compile measurements of PBTK model parameters in an effort to identify the average value. If data are unavailable for a certain parameter, the parameter is estimated by fitting the model to the toxicokinetic data. Both visual fits (Leung and Paustenbach, 1990; Medinsky et al., 1989; Paustenbach et al., 1988; Ramsey and Andersen, 1984; Travis et al., 1990a; Ward et al., 1988) and formal methods of parameter estimation (Andersen et al., 1987; Bois et al., 1991; 1990; Corley et al., 1990; Fisher et al., 1991; Reitz et al., 1990a) have been performed.

Monte Carlo simulations have been used to find multiple parameterizations that are consistent with the data while allowing for population variability and measurement uncertainty (Bois et al., 1991; Spear et al., 1991; Watanabe, 1993; Woodruff et al., 1992). Parameter ranges are randomly sampled according to a statistical distribution in an effort to determine a set of model parameterizations. A uniform distribution is used if only the parameter maximum and minimum are known (Tiwari and Hobbie, 1976). A criterion function defining an upper and lower bound around each data point is used to assess the goodness-of-fit. Each parameter vector allowing the model to satisfy the criterion function can be interpreted as representing a feasible member of the population given the uncertainty and variability in the data.

6.9. INTERSPECIES EXTRAPOLATION

6.9.1. Scaling Physiologic and Metabolic PBTK Model Parameters

Many of the physiologic and metabolic parameters used in toxicokinetic modeling are directly correlated to the body weight of the particular organism. These physiologic parameters generally vary with body weight (BW) according to a power function expressed as:

$$y = aBW^b \tag{6.32}$$

where y is a physiological parameter of interest, and a and b are constants (Davidson et al., 1986; Lindstedt, 1987). If b equals one, the physiologic parameter y correlates directly with body weight. If b equals two-thirds, the parameter y correlates with surface area. The following is a review of the empirical scaling laws for physiologic and metabolic parameters found in equations (6.24-6.31).

Organ Volumes

Organ volumes tend to scale across species with the first power of body weight. Fiserova-Bergerova and Hughes (1983) and Mordenti (1986) tabulate the constants, a and b, for a number of organs. Examples are total blood volume which scales across species with the 1.02 power of body weight (Stahl, 1967) and the mass of the mammalian heart which scales with powers of body weight ranging from 0.87 to 1.04 (Fiserova-Bergerova and Hughes, 1983; Mordenti, 1986; Prothero, 1979). The liver scales with powers of body weight ranging from 0.83 to 0.99 (Fiserova-Bergerova and Hughes, 1983; Mordenti, 1986; Stahl, 1965). Following the National Academy of Sciences (National Research Council, 1986), the scaling law for volume of a tissue group is:

$$V_i = V_{i\theta} BW^{1.0}, \tag{6.33}$$

where $V_{i\theta}$ is a species-independent allometric constant.

Cardiac Output

Cardiac output is defined as the volume of blood pumped by each ventricle of the heart per minute. Stahl (1967) and Günther (1975) reported cardiac output scaling with the 0.81 and 0.79 powers of body weight, respectively. There is considerable evidence, though, that cardiac output is related to metabolic rate (Guyton, 1986) and that metabolic rates across species are related to the 0.75 power of body weight (Fiserova-Bergerova and Hughes, 1983; Schmidt-Nielsen, 1970). Hence, the most commonly assumed scaling law for cardiac output has the form:

$$Q_b = Q_{b\theta} BW^{0.75}, \tag{6.34}$$

where $Q_{b\theta}$ is a species-independent allometric constant.

The fraction of cardiac output distributed to different organs is approximately constant across species (Arms and Travis, 1988). Thus, arterial blood flow to tissue group i, Q_i, has the form:

$$Q_i = Q_{i\theta} BW^{0.75}, \tag{6.35}$$

where $Q_{i\theta}$ is a species-independent allometric constant.

Alveolar Ventilation

Ventilation is a cyclic process of circulation and the exchange of gases in the lungs that is basic to respiration. Total ventilation or minute volume is defined as the volume of air exhaled per minute. The fraction of minute volume available for gas exchange in the alveolar compartments is termed the alveolar ventilation rate. Minute volume and, hence, alveolar ventilation has been shown to scale across species with powers of body weight ranging from 0.74 to 0.80 (Fiserova-Bergerova and Hughes, 1983). The most commonly assumed scaling law for alveolar ventilation rate has the form:

$$Q_{alv} = Q_{alv\theta} BW^{0.75}, \tag{6.36}$$

where $Q_{alv\theta}$ is a species-independent allometric constant.

Renal Clearance

Renal clearance relates the kidneys' rate of elimination of a given compound to the concentration of the compound in the blood. Adolph (1949) first showed that renal clearance of inulin in four species scaled with body weight to the 0.77 power. Based on glomerular filtration rate, Weiss et al. (1977) suggest that renal clearance scales with body weight to the 0.82 power. However, studies by Brody (1945), Edwards (1975), Lindstedt and Calder (1981), Boxenbaum (1982), Schmidt-Nielsen (1984), and Mordenti (1986) support a general scaling law for renal clearance:

$$K_r = K_{r\theta} BW^{0.75}, \tag{6.37}$$

where $K_{r\theta}$ is a species-independent allometric constant.

Metabolic Parameters

Oxygen consumption rates have been shown to scale across species approximately with the 0.75 power of body weight (Benedict, 1938; Brody, 1945; Kleiber, 1932; Lindstedt, 1987; Lindstedt and Calder, 1981; McMahon, 1973; Schmidt-Nielsen, 1984). Limited data exist on interspecies scaling of metabolic enzymatic activity. Weiss et al. (1977) support 0.73 as the power of body weight for scaling hepatic metabolic clearance based on the allometric equation for enzyme activity. Cytochrome oxidase has been found to scale with the 0.75 power of body weight (Jansky, 1961; 1963; Kunkel et al., 1956). The number of mitochondria in mammalian liver scales with the 0.72 power of body weight (Smith, 1956), and mitochondria densities in 13 species of mammals have been shown to closely parallel maximal rates of oxygen consumption (Mathieu et al., 1981). However, information on interspecies scaling of metabolic parameters is inadequate and further studies are needed. Nevertheless, it has been assumed that the appropriate scaling law for metabolic parameters (see definitions given after equation (6.28)) is:

$$V_{max} = V_{max\theta} BW^{0.75}, \tag{6.38}$$

and

$$K_f = K_{f\theta} BW^{0.75}. \tag{6.39}$$

The Michaelis-Menten constant, K_m, is generally assumed to be approximately constant across species (National Research Council, 1986).

Partition Coefficients

Partition coefficients are an expression of a chemical's solubility in tissues. The partition coefficient of a given chemical between two media is defined as the ratio of the equilibrium chemical concentration in the first medium to the chemical concentration in the second medium. The most common measurements are blood/air and tissue/air partition coefficients with tissue/blood derived as the ratio of tissue/air to blood/air. Tissue/air partition coefficients tend to be constant across species (National Research Council, 1986); while blood/air partition coefficients show some species-dependent variability. As a general rule, however, partition coefficients are approximately constant across species (National Research Council, 1986).

6.9.2. Discussion of Allometric Scaling

Travis et al. (1990b) assume that certain physiological and metabolic processes scale across species with the 0.75 power of body weight. While there is a substantial body of empirical data to suggest that this assumption is at least approximately correct, it is far from universally accepted. Recently, Hayssen and Lacy (1985) have criticized Kleiber's (1932) original work establishing 0.75 as the allometric exponent for basal metabolic rates. They argue that Kleiber's data were insufficient in number, unrepresentative of the class Mammalia and incorrectly analyzed statistically. They analyzed data on 293 mammalian species and found an exponent of 0.7, but note that 22% of the species fell more than 50% above or below the line. Yates and Kugler (1986) argue that allometric scaling based on a single variable (e.g., body weight) oversimplifies chemically reactive hydrodynamic systems. Instead, they propose establishing a physical basis for allometry.

Physiological Time

The presence between species of a biologically variable time scale has been asserted by several authors (Adolph, 1949; Boxenbaum, 1982; Brody, 1945; Carrell, 1931; Dedrick, 1973; Hill, 1950; Mordenti, 1986; Yates and Kugler, 1986). Hill (1950) first suggested that body size served as the regulating mechanism for an internal biological clock, making the rate of all biological events constant across species when compared per unit physiological time. His conclusions are supported by Adolph (1949), Stahl (1967), Günther and Leon de la Barra (1966), Calder (1968), Dedrick (1973), Lindstedt and Calder (1981), Boxenbaum (1982; 1986), Mordenti (1986) and Lindstedt (1987), who have shown that breath duration, heartbeat duration, longevity, pulse time, breathing rates, and blood flow rates are approximately constant across species when expressed in internal time units. These time units have been termed physiological time (t') and can be defined in terms of chronological time (t) and body weight (BW) as:

$$t' = \frac{t}{BW^{0.25}}. \tag{6.40}$$

Thus, while chronological time is the same for all species, physiological time is different for each species. The value of this concept is that all species have approximately the same physiological and metabolic rates when measured in the physiological time frame (Boxenbaum, 1986; Dedrick, 1973; Lindstedt, 1987; Mordenti, 1986; Yates and Kugler, 1986).

6.9.3. Choice of a Dose Surrogate

There can be little disagreement that the most precise measure of dose to target tissue is the time profile of the concentration of the toxic moiety in the target tissue. That is, two individuals within the same species will receive the same dose to target tissue, if and only if, the time course of the tissue concentration curve is the same in both individuals. However, this is rarely the case and it is inconvenient to compare tissue concentration curves at all points Therefore, the area under the tissue concentration curve (AUC) of the toxic moiety is often used as a convenient surrogate. Historical experience indicates that this measure is appropriate when standardizing dosing schedules for the purpose of intraspecies extrapolation of chronic effects. However, its use is questionable for interspecies extrapolation.

Travis et al. (1990b) propose that individuals from different species will receive the same dose to target tissue, if and only if, the time profiles in physiological time of the concentration of toxic moiety in target tissue are the same. Support for this definition is based upon observations that the rate of biological events across species is approximately constant when compared per unit of physiological time (Boxenbaum, 1986; Dedrick, 1973; Lindstedt, 1987; Mordenti, 1986; Yates and Kugler, 1986). Thus, toxicodynamic processes should be approximately constant in physiological time across species if doses to target tissue for different species are constant in physiological time.

A convenient surrogate metric would be area under the tissue concentration curve in physiological time of the toxic moiety ($AUC\ t'$). To clarify this concept, consider the definition of AUC.

$$AUC = \int_0^\infty C_1(t)dt$$

Using a change of variable from chronological time to physiological time,

$$AUC = \int_0^\infty C_1(t')dt' BW^{0.25}. \tag{6.41}$$

Thus, $AUC\ t' = AUC/BW^{0.25}$. Within a species, no difficulty arises from assuming that toxic effect is proportional to AUC rather than $AUC\ t'$ since the two measures of dose differ by a constant. For interspecies extrapolation, however, the two different dose measures produce different results. Travis et al. (1990b) assume that the proper surrogate measure of dose to target tissue is $AUC\ t'$.

Under the assumption that the time profile of the tissue concentration curve in physiological time is the most appropriate metric for dose to target tissue, Travis et al. (1990b) investigated the question of whether or not it is possible to choose a measure of administered dose so that tissue concentration curves are species-independent when measured in physiological time. They demonstrate that if toxic response is a function of the target tissue concentration in physiological time and the toxic moiety is metabolically deactivated, then, regardless of the mechanism of action (direct-acting, reactive metabolite, or stable metabolite), the appropriate dose metric is mg kg^{-1} t'^{-1}. At low doses, this measure is equivalent to mg $\text{kg}^{-0.75}$ day^{-1}. In addition, the interspecies scaling metric at low doses for reactive metabolites that are spontaneously deactivated is mg kg^{-1} day^{-1}.

Reitz et al. (1990a) discuss six feasible types of dose surrogates for dioxane eliminating four of them for various reasons. The two dose surrogates investigated were the area under the dioxane concentration curve in liver (AUC-Liver) and the average area under the metabolite concentration time curve for the whole body (AUC-Met). Comparison of the two dose surrogates and tumor incidence for male and female mice, and the no-effect levels in drinking water studies for rats resulted in AUC-Liver more closely representing the observed tumor frequencies than AUC-Met. The Virtually Safe Doses (VSDs) calculated based on AUC-Liver were consistently higher than those based on AUC-Met.

Reitz et al. (1990b) used two dose surrogates in their hazard evaluation of chloroform: 1) average daily molecular binding (AVEMMB); and 2) cytotoxicity resulting from binding of reactive metabolites to macromolecules in liver cells (PTDEAD). The two dose surrogates were found to yield vastly different VSDs for liver tumors following lifetime continuous exposure in air or water. Thus, correlations between the dose surrogates and the incidence of liver tumors were investigated in greater detail. Reitz et al. concluded that PTDEAD provided the most reliable estimates of liver cancer risk due to chloroform exposures.

More recently, Fisher and Allen (1993) investigated the use of three dose measures in their risk assessment of trichloroethylene: 1) lifetime average daily total amount of TCE metabolized (AMET); 2) lifetime average daily amount of trichloroacetic acid formed (FCTCA); and lifetime average daily area-under-the-concentration curve for trichloroacetic acid in plasma (AUCTCA). A PBTK model was used to output values of these dose surrogates at the doses tested in the cancer bioassay. AMET was selected as a plausible dose surrogate by visual comparison of the liver cancer incidence and the dose surrogates. AUCTCA was selected as the alternate because of its strong correlation to extra risk of liver tumor in female mice by both gavage and inhalation exposures ($r^2 = 0.95$). FCTCA showed little correspondence with liver cancer rates.

The effect of toxicokinetics on the dose-response curve is largely dependent on the choice of a dose surrogate. Fisher and Allen (1993) selected the lifetime average daily total amount of trichloroethylene metabolized because it was consistent with liver cancer rates despite a nonlinear relationship. Their alternate dose surrogate was linearly correlated to extra cancer risk in female mice only.

6.9.4. Interspecies Extrapolation of Toxicokinetics

Interspecies extrapolation of toxic effect attempts to find a measure of administered dose (i.e., mg kg^{-1} day^{-1} or mg m^{-2} day^{-1}) which produces the same measure of effect in all species. It is understood that any such extrapolation procedure is only approximately correct and should be used only when species-specific data are unavailable. Historically, it has been assumed that a single extrapolation procedure would work for all chemicals regardless of their mechanism of action. More recently, Andersen et al. (1987) and the National Academy of Sciences (National Research Council, 1986; 1987) suggested that interspecies extrapolation rules should depend on the mechanism of action. They distinguished three classes, depending on whether the parent compound, stable metabolite, or reactive metabolite produces the toxic response. Since then, Travis et al. (1990b) demonstrated that it is not necessary to make such distinctions if the toxic moiety is metabolically deactivated. Regardless of mechanism of action, the appropriate metric was found to be dose (mg/kg) per unit of physiological time which, at low doses, is equivalent to mg $kg^{-0.75}$ day^{-1}.

6.10. IMPLICATIONS FOR LOW-DOSE EXTRAPOLATION

We have seen that the parameters in the models presented here have biological significance describing biological processes and responses at the level of the tissue and the cells involved. Model parameters can be assumed to be functions of dose and time to allow for the varying influence of specific carcinogens on cell transformation and/or cell kinetics. Whenever possible, detailed dose-response modeling on the cellular level should be based on mechanistic considerations that are consistent with experimental data. Because the problem of low-dose extrapolation is now shifting from the macroscopic level of the (observable) cancer to a microscopic level of cellular responses on the pathway to cancer, the problem of low-dose extrapolation may now stand a better chance.

The task is to identify first the metabolic pathway(s) and to determine the dose of the active metabolites responsible for the carcinogenic response in the tissue of interest. Thus, the carcinogenesis models used should be combined with pharmaco- or toxicokinetic 'front-ends', that derive the tissue levels of the participating metabolites from the level of the agent in the environment. The importance of toxicokinetic modeling in quantitative risk assessment is now widely appreciated.

What do we hope to gain from such refinement for assessing risk? The cellular mechanisms considered in this chapter are assumed to be intermediate in character, i.e. are on the pathway to cancer, and are obviously more sensitive to low dose stimuli. The occurrence of premalignant lesions likely precedes the formation of malignancies and, hence, leads to an 'amplification' of the dose effect, provided these lesions can be identified and their correlation with malignant tumors can be established (at least in a statistical way). In the rodent liver, for instance, many thousand enzyme altered foci (EAF) can be seen before animals die of liver cancer. The correlation between hepatocellular carcinomas and appearance of EAF is well established empirically.

What would the amplification be? Assuming, very conservatively, that the first malignant transformation leads inevitably to an observable tumor, the number of non-extinct intermediate clones that are present at time t would roughly equal $\nu X(1-\beta/\alpha)t$. Here, the product νX is the number of initiated premalignant progenitor cells and the factor $(1 - \beta/\alpha)$ is the asymptotic probability of survival of a generated clone. Of course, some intermediate clones may give rise to malignant tumors before they become extinct. To be specific, let us give an example: In their analysis of the number and size distribution of EAF (in rat liver) of rats that were treated with various levels of N-nitrosomorpholine (NNM), Moolgavkar et al. (1990a) estimated that $\nu X \sim 200$ per day per liver at the 1 ppm dose level. The parameter β/α, measuring clonal extinction, was estimated to be near 0.99. Thus, after 1 year of treatment with a dose of 1 ppm NNM, we have an 'amplification' factor of 200x(1-.99)x365=730. This is likely a lower bound since none of the animals that were not sacrificed for the EAF ascertainment developed hepatocellular carcinomas in this dose group. Furthermore, it is unlikely that the first malignant cell generated in the tissue leads to a tumor, so that many more intermediate clones may be needed, on average, to yield a malignant tumor during the animal's life span. Admittedly, this example is very crude but exemplifies the idea.

6.11. REFERENCES

Aaltonen, L.A., Peltomaki, P., Leach, F.S., Sistonen, P., Pylkkdnen, L., Mecklin, J.-P., Jdrvinen, H., Powell, S.M., Jen, J., Hamilton, S.R., Peterson, G.M., Kinzler, K.W., Vogelstein, B., and de la Chapelle, A. (1993): Clues to the pathogenesis of familial colorectal cancer. Science 260, 812-816.

Adolph, E. F. (1949): Quantitative relations in the physiological constitutions of mammals. Science 109, 579-585.

Andersen, M. E., Clewell III, H. J., Gargas, M. L., Smith, F. A., and Reitz, R. H. (1987): Physiologically based pharmacokinetics and the risk assessment process for methylene chloride. Toxicol. Appl. Pharmacol. 87, 185-205.

Armitage, P. and Doll, R. (1954): The age distribution of cancer and a multistage theory of carcinogenesis. Br. J. Cancer 8, 1-12.

Arms, A. D., and Travis, C. C. (1988): Reference Physiological Parameters in Pharmacokinetic Modeling. (Report #EPA/600/6-88/004). United States Environmental Protection Agency.

Bailer, A. J., and Hoel, D. G. (1989): Metabolite-based internal doses used in a risk assessment of benzene. Environ. Health Perspect. 82, 177-184.

Beliles, R. P., and Totman, L. C. (1989): Pharmacokinetically based risk assessment of workplace exposure to benzene. Regul. Toxicol. Pharmacol. 9, 186-195.

Benedict, F. G. (1938). Vital Energetics: A Study in Comparative Basal Metabolism. Carnegie Institute of Washington, Washington, D.C..

Bishop, J.M. (1991): Molecular themes in oncogenesis. Cell 64, 235-248.

Bogen, K. T. (1989): Cell proliferation kinetics and multistage cancer risk models. J. Nat. Cancer Inst. 81, 267-277.

Bogen, K. T. (1990): Risk extrapolation for chlorinated methanes as promoters vs initiators of multistage carcinogenesis. Fund. Appl. Toxicol. 15, 536-557.

Bois, F. Y., Woodruff, T. J., and Spear, R. C. (1991): Comparison of three physiologically based pharmacokinetic models of benzene disposition. Toxicol. Appl. Pharmacol. 110, 79-88.

Bois, F. Y., Zeise, L., and Tozer, T. N. (1990): Precision and sensitivity of pharmacokinetic models for cancer risk assessment: Tetrachloroethylene in mice, rats, and humans. Toxicol. Appl. Pharmacol. 102, 300-315.

Boxenbaum, H. (1982): Interspecies scaling, allometry, physiological time, and the ground plan of pharmacokinetics. J. Pharmacok. Biopharm. 10, 201-227.

Boxenbaum, H. (1986): Time concepts in physics, biology and pharmacokinetics. J. Pharm. Sci. 75, 1053-1062.

Brody, S. (1945): Bioenergetics and Growth: With Special Reference to the Efficiency Complex in Domestic Animals. Reinhold, New York.

Brown, C. and Chu, K. (1987): Use of multistage models to infer stages affected by carcinogenic exposure: Example of lung cancer and cigarette smoking. J. Chronic Disease 40 (Suppl.2), 171S-179S.

Buchmann, A., Schwarz, M., Schmitt, R., Wolf, C.R., Oesch, F. and Kunz, W. (1987): Development of cytochrome P-450 altered preneoplastic and neoplastic lesions during nitrosoamine-induced hepatocarcinogenesis in the rat. Cancer Research 47, 2911-2918.

Buchmann, A., Ziegler, S., Wolf, A., Robertson, L.W., Durham, S.K. and Schwarz, M. (1991): Effects of polychlorinated biphenyls in rat liver: Correlation between primary subcellular effects and promoting activity. Toxicol. Appl. Pharmacol. 111, 454-468.

Bursch, W., Lauer, B., Timmermann-Trosiener, I., Barthel, G., Schuppler, J. and Schulte-Hermann, R. (1984): Controlled death (apoptosis) of normal and putative preneoplastic cells in rat liver following withdrawal of tumor promoters. Carcinogenesis 5, 453-458.

Bursch, W., Taper, N.S., Lauer, B. and Schulte-Hermann, R. (1985): Quantitative histological and histochemical studies on the occurrence and stages of controlled cell death (apoptosis) during regression of rat liver hyperplasia. Virchows Archiv (Cell Pathol.) 50, 153-166.

Bursch, W., Putz, B., Barthel, G. and Schulte-Hermann, R. (1990): Determination of the length of the histological stages of apoptosis in normal liver and in altered hepatic foci of rats. Carcinogenesis 11, 5, 847-853.

Calder, W. A. (1968): Respiration and heart rates of birds at rest. Condor 70, 358-365.

Carrell, A. (1931): Physiological time. Science 74, 618-621.

Cerutti, P.A. (1985): Prooxidant states and tumor promotion. Science 227, 375-381.

Conolly, R. B., and Andersen, M. E. (1991): Biologically based pharmacodynamic models: Tools for toxicological research and risk assessment. Annu. Rev. Pharmacol. Toxicol. 31, 503-523.

Conolly, R. B., and Andersen, M. E. (1993): An approach to mechanism-based cancer risk assessment: formaldehyde. Environ. Health Perspect. 101, 169-176.

Cook, P., Doll, R. and Fellingham, S.A. (1969): A mathematical model for the age distribution of cancer in man. Int. J. Cancer 4, 93-112.

Corley, R. A., Mendrala, A. M., Gargas, M. L., Andersen, M. E., Conolly, R. B., Staats, D., and Reitz, R. H. (1990): Development of a physiologically based pharmacokinetic based model for chloroform. Toxicol. Appl. Pharmacol. 103, 512-527.

Cox, L. A., and Ricci, P. F. (1992): Reassessing benzene cancer risks using internal doses. Risk Anal. 12, 401-410.

Cox, D.R. and Miller, H.D. (1972): The theory of stochastic processes. Chapman and Hall Ltd..

Crump, K. and Howe, R. (1984): The multistage model with a time-dependent dose pattern: Application to carcinogenic risk assessment. Risk Analysis 4, 163-176.

Davidson, I. W. F., Parker, J. C., and Beliles, R. P. (1986): Biological basis for extrapolation across mammalian species. Regul. Toxicol. Pharmacol. 6, 211-237.

Davies, B. D., and Morris, T. (1993): Physiological parameters in laboratory animals and humans. Pharmaceut. Res. 10, 1093-1095.

Day, N. and Brown, C. (1980): Multistage models and primary prevention of cancer. J. Natl. Cancer Inst. 64, 977-989.

Dedrick, R. L. (1973): Animal scale-up. J. Pharmacok. Biopharm. 1, 435-461.

De Gunst, M.C.M. and Luebeck, E.G. (1994): Quantitative Analysis of Two-Dimensional Clones in the Presence or Absence of Malignant Tumors. Math. Biosci. 119, 5-34.

Dewanji, A., Venzon, D.J. and Moolgavkar, S.H. (1989): A stochastic two-stage model for cancer risk assessment. II. The number and size of premalignant clones. Risk Analysis 9, 179-187.

Dewanji, A., Moolgavkar, S.H. and Luebeck, E.G. (1991): Two-mutation model for carcinogenesis: Joint analysis of premalignant and malignant lesions. Math. Biosc. 104: 97-109.

Edwards, N. A. (1975): Scaling of renal functions in mammals. Comp. Biochem. Physiol. 52A, 63-66.

Ellwein, L.B. and Cohen, S.M. (1992): Simulation modeling of carcinogenesis. Toxicol. Appl. Pharmacol. 113, 98-108.

Emmelot, P. and Scherer, E. (1980): The first relevant cell stage in rat liver carcinogenesis: A quantitative approach. Biochemica et Biophysica Acta 605, 247-304.

Farber, E. and Cameron, R. (1980): The sequential analysis of cancer development. Adv. Cancer Res. 31, 125-226.

Fearon, E.R. and Vogelstein, B. (1990): Cell **61**, 759-7676.

Fiserova-Bergerova, V. (1983): Gases and their solubility: A review of fundamentals. In Modeling of Inhalation Exposure to Vapors: Uptake, Distribution, and Elimination, Vol. 1 (V. Fiserova-Bergerova, Ed.), pp. 3-28. CRC Press, Boca Raton.

Fiserova-Bergerova, V., and Diaz, M. L. (1986): Determination and prediction of tissue-gas partition coefficients. Int. Arch. Occup. Environ. Health 58, 75-87.

Fiserova-Bergerova, V., and Hughes, H. C. (1983): Species differences on bioavailability of inhaled vapors and gases. In Modeling of Inhalation Exposure to Vapors: Uptake, Distribution, and Elimination, Vol. II (V. Fiserova-Bergerova, Ed.), pp. 97-106. CRC Press, Boca Raton.

Fiserova-Bergerova, V., Tichy, M., and Di Carlo, F. J. (1984): Effects of biosolubility on pulmonary uptake and disposition of gases and vapors of lipophilic chemicals. Drug Metab. Rev. 15, 1033-1070.

Fisher, J. W., and Allen, B. C. (1993): Evaluating the risk of liver cancer in humans exposed to trichloroethylene using physiological models. Risk Anal. 13, 87-95.

Fisher, J. W., Gargas, M. L., Allen, B. C., and Andersen, M. E. (1991): Physiologically based pharmacokinetic modeling with trichloroethylene and its metabolite, trichloroacetic acid, in the rat and mouse. Toxicol. Appl. Pharmacol. 109, 183-195.

Frederick, C. B., Potter, D. W., Chang-Mateu, M. I., and Andersen, M. E. (1992): A physiologically based pharmacokinetic and pharmacodynamic model to describe the oral dosing of rats with ethyl acrylate and its implications for risk assessment. Toxicol. Appl. Pharmacol. 114, 246-260.

Freedman, D.A. and Navidi W. (1989): Multistage models for carcinogenesis. Environ. Health Persp. 81, 169-188.

Goldfarb, S. and Pugh, T.D. (1981): Enzyme histochemical phenotypes in primary hepatocellular carcinomas. Cancer Research 41, 2092-2095.

Goldsworthy, T.L., Hanigan, M.H., and Pitot, H.C. (1986): Models of hepatocarcinogenesis in the rat – contrasts and comparisons. CRC Critical Review of Toxicology 17, 61-89.

Günther, B. (1975): Dimensional analysis and theory of biological similarity. Physiological Rev. 55, 659-699.

Günther, B., and Leon de la Barra, B. (1966): On the space-time continuum in biology. Acta Physiol. Latin Am. 16, 221-231.

Guyton, A. C. (1986): Textbook of Medical Physiology (7th ed.). W.B. Saunders, Philadelphia.

Hayssen, V., and Lacy, R. C. (1985): Basal metabolic rates in mammals: taxonomic differences in the allometry of BMR and body mass. Comp. Biochem. Physiol. 81, 741-754.

Heidenreich, W. (1996): On the parameters of the clonal expansion model, submitted to Radiation and Environmental Biophysics.

Hill, A. V. (1950): The dimensions of animals and their muscular dynamics. Proc. R. Inst. Great Britain 34, 450-471.

Hollstein, M., Sidransky, D., Vogelstein, B., and Harris, C.C. (1991): p53 mutations in human cancers. Science, 253, 49-53.

IARC (1992): Mechanisms of Carcinogenesis in Risk Identification, Vainio, H., Magee, P., McGregor, D and McMichael A.J., eds., IARC Scientific Publications No. 116, Lyon.

Jansky, L. (1961): Total cytochrome oxidase activity and its relation to basal and maximal metabolism. Nature 189, 921-922.

Jansky, L. (1963): Body organ cytochrome oxidase activity in cold-and-warm acclimated rats. Can. J. Biochem. Physiol. 41, 1847-1854.

Kendall, D.G. (1960): Birth-and-death processes, and the theory of carcinogenesis. Biometrika 47, 13-21.

Kleiber, M. (1932): Body size and metabolism. Hilgardia 6, 315-353.

Knudson, A.G. (1971): Mutation and Cancer: Statistical study of retinoblastoma. Proc. Nat. Acad. Sci., USA, 68, 820-823.

Kopp-Schneider, A. and Portier, C.J. (1992): Birth and death/differentiation rates of papillomas in mouse skin. Carcinogenesis 13, 973-978.

Kopp-Schneider, A. (1992): Birth-death processes with piecewise constant rates. Statistics and Probability Letters 13, 121-127.

Kunkel, H. O., Spalding, J. F., De Franciscis, G., and Futrell, M. F. (1956): Cytochrome oxidase activity and body weight in rats and in three species of large animals. Am. J. Physiol. 186, 203-206.

Kunz, W., Schaude, G., Schwarz, M., and Tennekes, H. (1982): Quantitative Aspects of Drug-Mediated Tumor Promotion in Liver and Its Toxicological Implications. Carcinogenesis 7, 111-125.

Land, H., Parada, L.F., and Weinberg, R.A. (1983): Cellular oncogenes and multistep carcinogenesis. Science 222, 771-778.

Leung, H., and Paustenbach, D. J. (1990): Cancer risk assessment for dioxane based upon a physiologically-based pharmacokinetic approach. Toxicol. Lett. 51, 147-162.

Levine A.J., Momand J., and Finlay C.A. (1991): The p53 tumour suppressor gene. Nature 351, 453-456.

Lindstedt, S. L. (1987): Allometry: body size constraints in animal design. In Drinking Water and Health. Pharmacokinetics in Risk Assessment, Vol. 8. National Academy Press, Washington, D.C.

Lindstedt, S. L., and Calder, W. A. (1981): Body size and physiological time, and longevity of homeothermic animals. Q. Rev. Biol. 56, 1-16.

Liu, S. H. (1990): Application of a Two Mutation Oncogenic Model to Quantitative Risk Analysis, Ph.D. dissertation, Northwestern University.

Luebeck, E.G. and Moolgavkar, S.H. (1991): Stochastic analysis of intermediate lesions in carcinogenesis experiments. Risk Analysis 11, 149-157.

Luebeck, E.G., Moolgavkar, S.H., Buchmann, A., and Schwarz, M. (1991): Effects of polychlorinated biphenyls in rat liver: Quantitative analysis of enzyme-altered foci. Toxicol. Appl. Pharmacol. 111, 469-484.

Luebeck, E.G. and Moolgavkar, S.H. (1994): Simulating the process of malignant transformation. Math. Biosci. 123, 127-146.

Luebeck, E.G., Grasl-Kraupp, B., Timmermann-Trosiener, I., Bursch, W., Schulte-Hermann, R., and Moolgavkar, S.H (1995): Growth kinetics of enzyme altered liver foci in rats treated with Phenobarbital or α-hexachlorocyclohexane. Toxicol. Appl. Pharmacol. 130, 304-315.

Mathieu, O., Krauer, R., Hoppeler, H., Gehr, P., Lindstedt, S. L., Alexander, R., Taylor, C. R., and Weibel, E. R. (1981): Design of the mammalian respiratory system. VII. Scaling mitochondrial volume in skeletal muscle to body mass. Resp. Physiol. 44, 113-128.

McMahon, T. (1973): Size and shape in biology. Science 179, 1201-1204.

Medinsky, M. A., Sabourin, P. J., Lucier, G., Birnbaum, L. S., and Henderson, R. F. (1989): A physiological model for simulation of benzene metabolism by rats and mice. Toxicol. Appl. Pharmacol. 99, 193-206.

Mills, J. J., and Andersen, M. E. (1993): Dioxin hepatic carcinogenesis: biologically motivated modeling and risk assessment. Toxicol. Lett. 68, 177-189.

Moolgavkar, S.H. (1978): The multistage theory of carcinogenesis and the age distribution of cancer in man. J. Natl. Cancer Inst. 61, 49-52.

Moolgavkar, S.H. and Knudson, A. (1981): Mutation and Cancer: A Model for Human Carcinogenesis. Journal of the National Cancer Institute 66, 1037-1052.

Moolgavkar, S. H. (1983): Model for human carcinogenesis: Action of environmental agents. Environ. Health Perspect. 50, 285-291.

Moolgavkar, S.H., Dewanji, A., and Venzon, D.J. (1988): A stochastic two-stage model for cancer risk assessment. I. The hazard function and the probability of tumor. Risk Analysis 8, 383-392.

Moolgavkar, S.H., Dewanji, A., and Luebeck, G. (1989): Cigarette smoking and lung cancer: reanalysis of the British doctors' data. J Natl Cancer Inst 81, 415-420.

Moolgavkar, S.H. and Luebeck, E.G. (1990): Two-event model for carcinogenesis: Biological, mathematical and statistical considerations. Risk Analysis 10, 323-341.

Moolgavkar, S.H., Luebeck, E.G., de Gunst, M., Port, R.E., and Schwarz, M. (1990a): Quantitative analysis of enzyme-altered foci in rat hepatocarcinogenesis experiments I: Single agent regimen. Carcinogenesis 11, 8, 1271-1278.

Moolgavkar, S.H, Cross, F.T., Luebeck, E.G., and Dagle, G.E. (1990b): A two-mutation model for radon-induced lung tumors in rats. Radiation Research 121, 28-37.

Moolgavkar, S.H. (1991): Stochastic models of carcinogenesis. C.R. Rao and R. Chakraborty, eds., Handbook of Statistics, Vol. 8, Elsevier Science Publishers B.V., 373-393.

Moolgavkar, S.H. and Luebeck, E.G. (1992): Multistage carcinogenesis: Population-based model for colon cancer. J. Natl. Cancer Inst. 84, 610-618.

Moolgavkar, S.H., Luebeck, E.G., Krewski, D., and Zielinski, J.M. (1993): Radon, Cigarette Smoke, and Lung Cancer: A Reanalysis of the Colorado Plateau Uranium Miners' Data. American Journal of Epidemiology, Vol. 4, no.3, 204-217.

Mordenti, J. (1986): Man versus beast: pharmacokinetic scaling in mammals. J. Pharm. Sci. 75, 1028-1040.

Muller, H.J. (1951): Radiation damage to the genetic material. Science Progress 7, 93-493.

National Research Council (1986): Drinking Water and Health, Vol. 6. National Academy Press, Washington D.C.

National Research Council (1987): Drinking Water and Health. Pharmacokinetics in Risk Assessment, Vol. 8. National Academy Press, Washington, D.C.

Neyman, J. and Scott, E. (1967): Statistical aspects of the problem of carcinogenesis. Fifth Berkeley Symposium on Mathematical Statistics and Probability, University of California Press, Berkeley, CA, 745-776.

Nordling, C.O. (1953): A new theory of the cancer inducing mechanism. Br. J. Cancer 7, 68-72.

Paustenbach, D. J., Clewell III, H. J., Gargas, M. L., and Andersen, M. E. (1988): A physiologically based pharmacokinetic model for inhaled carbon tetrachloride. Toxicol. Appl. Pharmacol. 96, 191-211.

Perbellini, L., Brugnone, F., Caretta, D., and Maranelli, G. (1985): Partition coefficients of some industrial aliphatic hydrocarbons (C5-C7) in blood and human tissues. Brit. J. Ind. Med. 42, 162-167.

Pitot, H.C., Goldsworthy, T.L., Moran, S., Kennan, W., Glauert, H.P., Maronpot, R.R., and Campbell, H.A. (1987): A method to quantitate the relative initiating and promoting potencies of hepatocarcinogenic agents in their dose-response relationships to altered hepatic foci. Carcinogenesis 8, 10, 1491-1499.

Portier, C. and Kopp-Schneider, A. (1991): A multistage model of carcinogenesis incorporating DNA damage and repair. Risk Analysis 11, 535-543.

Press, W.H., Flannery, B.P., Teukolsky, S.A. and Vetterling, W.T. (1986): Numerical Recipes: The Art of Scientific Computing. Cambridge University Press.

Prothero, O. (1979): Heart weight as a function of body weight in mammals. Growth 43, 139-150.

Ramsey, J. C., and Andersen, M. (1984): A physiologically based description of the inhalation pharmacokinetics of styrene in rats and humans. Toxicol. Appl. Pharmacol. 73, 159-175.

Renan, M.J. (1993): How many mutations are required for tumorigenesis? Implications for human cancer data. Molecular Carcinogenesis 7, 139-146.

Reitz, R. H., McCroskey, P. S., Park, C. N., Andersen, M. E., and Gargas, M. L. (1990a): Development of a physiologically based pharmacokinetic model for risk assessment with 1,4-dioxane. Toxicol. Appl. Pharmacol. 105, 37-54.

Reitz, R. H., Mendrala, A. L., Corley, R. A., Quast, J. F., Gargas, M. L., Andersen, M. E., Staats, D. A., and Conolly, R. B. (1990b): Estimating the risk of liver cancer associated with human exposures to chloroform using physiologically based pharmacokinetic modeling. Toxicol. Appl. Pharmacol. 105, 443-459.

Satoh, K., Hatayama, I., Tateoka, N., Tamai, K., Shimizu, T., Tatematsu, M., Ito, N., and Sato, K. (1989): Transient induction of single GST-P positive hepatocytes by DEN. Carcinogenesis 10, 11, 2107-2111.

Schmidt-Nielsen, K. (1970): Energy metabolism, body size and problems of scaling. Fed. Proc. 29, 1524-1532.

Schmidt-Nielsen, K. (1984): Scaling: Why is animal size so important? Cambridge University Press, Cambridge.

Schulte-Hermann, R., Timmermann-Trosiener, I., Barthel, G., and Bursch, W. (1990): DNA synthesis, apoptosis and phenotypic expression as determinants of growth of altered foci in rat liver during phenobarbital promotion. Cancer Research 50, 5127-5135.

Schumann, A. M., Quast, J. F., and Watanabe, P. G. (1980): The pharmacokinetics and macromolecular interactions of perchloroethylene in mice and rats as related to oncogenicity. Toxicol. Appl. Pharmacol. 55, 207-219.

Smith, R. E. (1956): Quantitative relations between liver mitochondria metabolism and total body weight in mammals. Ann. NY Acad. Sci. 62, 403-422.

Spear, R. C., Bois, F. Y., Woodruff, T., Auslander, D., Parker, J., and Selvin, S. (1991): Modeling benzene pharmacokinetics across three sets of animal data: parametric sensitivity and risk implications. Risk Anal. 11, 641-654.

Stahl, W. R. (1965): Organ weights in primate and other mammals. Science 150, 1039-1042.

Stahl, W. R. (1967): Scaling of respiratory variables in mammals. J. Appl. Physiol. 48, 1052-1059.

Tan, W.Y. (1986): A stochastic Gompertz birth-death process. Statistics & Probability Letters 4, 25-28.

Tan, W.Y. (1991): Stochastic Models of Carcinogenesis. STATISTICS: textbooks and monographs, volume 116, Marcel Dekker, Inc.

Tiwari, J. L., and Hobbie, J. E. (1976): Random differential equations as models of ecosystems P II. Initial condition and parameter specifications in terms of maximum entropy distributions. Math. Biosci. 31, 37-53.

Travis, C. C., Quillen, J. L., and Arms, A. (1990a): Pharmacokinetics of benzene. Toxicol. Appl. Pharmacol. 102, 400-420.

Travis, C. C., White, R. K., and Arms, A. D. (1989): A physiologically based pharmacokinetic approach for assessing the cancer risk of tetrachloroethylene. In The Risk Assessment of Environmental and Human Health Hazards: A Textbook of Case Studies (D. J. Paustenbach, Ed.), pp. 769-796. John Wiley & Sons, New York.

Travis, C. C., White, R. K., and Ward, R. C. (1990b): Interspecies extrapolation of pharmacokinetics. J. Theor. Biol. 142, 285-304.

U.S. Environmental Protection Agency (1986): Guidelines for carcinogen risk assessment. Fed. Regist. 51, 33992-34003.

Venzon, D.J. and Moolgavkar, S.H. (1988): A method for computing profile-likelihood-based confidence intervals. Appl. Statist. 37 no.1, 87-94.

Ward, R. C., Travis, C. C., Hetrick, D. M., Andersen, M. E., and Gargas, M. L. (1988): Pharmacokinetics of tetrachloroethylene. Toxicol. Appl. Pharmacol. 93, 108-117.

Watanabe, K. H. (1993): Mathematical Modeling of Benzene Disposition: A Population Perspective, Ph.D. dissertation, University of California, Berkeley.

Weiss, M., Sziegoleit, W., and Forster, W. (1977): Dependence of pharmacokinetic parameters on body weight. Int. J. Clin. Pharmacol. 15, 572-575.

Whittemore, A.S. (1977): The age distribution of human cancer for carcinogenic exposures of varying intensity. Am. J. Epidemiol. 106, 418-432.

Wicksell, D.S. (1925): The Corpuscle Problem, Part I. Biometrika 17, 87-97.

Woodruff, T. J., Bois, F. Y., Auslander, D., and Spear, R. (1992): Structure and parametrization of pharmacokinetic models: Their impact on model predictions. Risk Anal. 12, 189-201.

Yates, F. E., and Kugler, P. N. (1986): Similarity principles and intrinsic geometrics: contrasting approaches to interspecies scaling. J. Pharm. Sci. 75, 1019-1027.

Chapter 7

STATISTICAL ISSUES IN THE APPLICATION OF MULTISTAGE AND BIOLOGICALLY BASED MODELS

W. Wosniok[1], C. Kitsos[2], and K. Watanabe[3]

[1]Institute of Statistics, University of Bremen, Bremen, Germany
[2]Department of Statistics, Athens University of Economics and Business, Athens, Greece
[3]Tulane University Medical Center, New Orleans, USA

7.1. INTRODUCTION

The preceding chapters provided the background to formulate mathematical models which reflect to a large extent current knowledge or hypotheses concerning the process of carcinogenesis. Also, the class of models which presently serves as a kind of standard in interpreting carcinogenesis data has been introduced. In the present chapter we will deal with the step from model building to model application in practical routine situations. Characteristic for these is that model parameters like rates or other coefficients are usually unknown and must be inferred from empirical data. The amount of available information to do so tends to be limited in several ways: the total number of observations is relatively small, the range of observed response proportions might cover only a small part of the possible range from 0 to 100%, varying dose-time patterns and censoring may play an important role. If data results from epidemiological studies on human cancer, further complications may arise from the fact that the dose of the carcinogen under study has not been under the investigator's control.

But estimating parameters within a given mathematical model is not the only task to accomplish. As outlined in previous chapters, there is a wealth of mathematical models for carcinogenesis, from which a particular one has to be selected in a specific situation. Only lucky circumstances will allow a clear-cut theoretical decision in favour

Perspectives on Biologically Based Cancer Risk Assessment, edited by Cogliano *et al.*
Kluwer Academic/Plenum Publishers, New York, 1999.

of one and only one mathematical model to analyse a given data set. So we have to face two possible kinds of errors which may occur when drawing conclusions from empirical data: errors due to sampling fluctuations and errors due to improper model choice.

Sampling errors are those errors which arise as a consequence of considering a sample, not the whole universe under study. They generally decrease with increasing sample size (assuming that some mild regularity conditions hold). However, as mentioned previously, sample size in practice is clearly limited and hence sampling errors are to be anticipated. There are statistical approaches to quantify the size of these errors, but these approaches again involve in most cases asymptotic arguments and it is not obvious to what extent asymptotic theory leads to correct conclusions in an actual non-asymptotic situation.

The choice of an inappropriate model to analyse a data set has at least two consequences. First, the interpretation of a parameter may loose its meaning, e.g. if the true biological process described by a parameter is different from the one assumed in the model. Second, estimated values, variances and covariances of parameters may be wrong. There is no general way to quantify such model selection errors. Only for well defined alternatives there is a chance to describe numerically the effect of having chosen an inappropriate model.

Frequently the main interest of a study does not focus on model parameters per se, but on derived quantities like the baseline risk, the unit risk or the dose required to generate a certain additional risk. Sampling errors and errors due to the choice of an inappropriate model carry over to derived quantities, often in a non-trivial way, and hence an estimate for the precision of these is required as well.

One could feel tempted to escape the problem of a possibly inappropriate model choice by using a very detailed model, containing parameters for all biologically founded hypotheses at the same time. Though this might avoid an oversimplification, it is not a realistic solution of the problem, mainly because it will hardly be possible to formulate a model which absorbs really all biologically based hypotheses. But even if we think only of a very large (but not universal) model, we will soon reach practical limits. More elaborated models usually require the estimation of more parameters, hence more effort in data collection and processing. Also the precision of estimates is affected by employing a larger model. It must be assumed that if many parameters are to be estimated from a data set, then a single of these will have higher variance (imprecision) than in an alternative case, in which only few parameters are extracted. Besides all these limitations it is not sure that dose-time-response relations derived from detailed models will differ markedly from relations based on simpler models. Consequently, even if strong theoretical arguments favour the use of a more sophisticated model, conclusions from a simple model might be similar to those drawn from a complicated one.

In order to throw some light on the issue of how much model choice matters in practice we will pick two representative members from the previously discussed set of carcinogenesis models and compare them with respect to their behaviour particularly when applied to assess low-dose effects. The models under consideration are the generalized multistage (GMS) model, which generalizes the Armitage-Doll model, and the Moolgavkar-Venzon-Knudson (MVK) model. Both have been introduced in chapters

5 and 6 (cf. Armitage and Doll 1954, Moolgavkar and Venzon 1979, Moolgavkar and Knudson 1981) and seem to be the most important alternatives at present: the first represents the "standard" way of dose-response assessment, the other one is the most prominent member of the class of biologically based models. It should be noted that "biologically based" is not a very clear characterization, since also the GMS model has a certain biological background, but we will as in the previous chapters follow the usual terminology.

7.2. CHARACTERIZATION OF MODELS

The GMS and the MVK model share the assumptions that (i) carcinogenesis is a stochastic multi-stage process on cell level and that (ii) transition between stages is caused by an external carcinogen, but may also, though to a smaller extent, occur spontaneously.

Both models differ with respect to the number of stages involved (three in the MVK model, two or more in the GMS model). However, the more important difference from the point of modeling lies in the incorporation of cell dynamics. While cell death and division are not explicitly modeled in the GMS model, they play a central role in the MVK model. This distinction is surely important as an aspect of modeling philosophy. Before discussing the practical relevance of this difference we will briefly review relevant model characteristics.

To describe the distribution of cancer occurrence in dependence of dose and time it is necessary to define "cancer occurrence" in terms of each model. The most common definition is to declare that cancer has irreversibly occurred, as soon as the first cell has reached the final stage. This definition needs reviewing and modification if a considerable cell dynamic is present, as there is no sense in declaring cancer to be present, if all malignant cells have become extinct due to cell dynamics and the tissue as a whole is still alive. However, for the present purpose of comparing model properties we will as before in chapters 5 and 6 maintain this preliminary definition of cancer occurrence. The MVK model allows a more detailed definition, which accounts for the fact that in reality a cancer (or tumor) can be seen only if it exceeds a certain size. Chapter 6 contains extensions of the basic MVK model which refer explicitly to the size of the final tumor.

7.2.1. Model Components

In chapter 5 we saw that the central quantity in the GMS model, the probability of cancer development until time t under constant dose d, is given by $P(t,d) = 1 - \exp(-\sum_{i=0}^{k} q_i d^i t^k)$, or equivalently by the survival distribution $S(t,d) = 1 - P(t,d)$. If the dose dependency is omitted, the model simplifies to $P(t) = 1 - \exp(-ct^k)$, which is the cumulative distribution function of a Weibull distribution. The parameters q_i are subject to the condition $q_i \geq 0$ for $i = 0, 1, \ldots, k$, not the stronger conditions of the original Armitage-Doll model. Particularly for low-dose problems the generalized

GMS model is frequently simplified to the linearized multistage (LMS) model. Here special emphasis is put on the linear term q_1, which is the most important one for low-dose extrapolation, and the objective is to not underestimate this term. To this end a strategy is employed that increases q_1 to a value q_1^* by concentrating the estimation variance essentially on q_1. Chapter 5 and Section 7.3.3.2provide detailed information on how to estimate q_1^*.

In the MVK model, $X(t), Y(t), Z(t)$ are the numbers of normal, intermediate and malignant cells, respectively, at time t. Intermediate cells arise from normal cells acccording to a Poisson process with rate $\nu(t)X(t)$. A single intermediate cell may die with rate $\beta(t)$, divide into two intermediate cells with rate $\alpha(t)$, or divide into one intermediate and one malignant cell with rate $\mu(t)$. The structure of this model is shown in Fig. 5.1. Dose may in principle act on each of the rates, giving rise to processes like initiation, promotion and progression, which are very different from the biological point of view. Process rates may depend on time in an arbitrary manner, however, in most practical applications rates are treated as being piecewise constant. This is a severe formal restriction, but it will hardly be a practical one. In a real application it should nearly always be possible to approximate a time dependent rate by a piecewise constant function in a sufficiently precise manner. Further, due to the assumption that the number $X(t)$ of normal cells in a tissue is large, while the transition rate $\nu(t)$ is small and does not show large fluctuations over time, the product $\nu(t)X(t)$ is approximated by a piecewise constant function as well. The essential quantity, the *survival distribution* $S(t)$, also called the *survivor function*, has been given under these assumptions by equations (6.9) – (6.11). For the present purpose of comparing properties of the GMS and the MVK model, we will make one more simplifying step by assuming that all rates are completely constant over time. Further, as a technical detail to facilitate parameter estimation, we will use the ratio $\gamma = \beta/\alpha$ instead of the absolute rate β. With these assumptions and definitions we can calculate the survivor function $S(t)$ in the following way:

$$A, B = \frac{1}{2}\left(1+\gamma+\frac{\mu}{\alpha} \mp \sqrt{\left(1+\gamma+\frac{\mu}{\alpha}\right)^2 - 4\gamma}\right) \quad (7.1)$$

$$\delta = \alpha(A-B) \quad (7.2)$$

$$G(t) = (1-A)\exp[\delta t] + B - 1 \quad (7.3)$$

$$H(t) = \nu X\left[(1-A)t - \frac{1}{\alpha}\ln(B-A) + \frac{1}{\alpha}\ln G(t)\right] \quad (7.4)$$

$$S(t) = \exp[-H(t)]\ . \quad (7.5)$$

In this case of constant rates we can express $S(t)$ in closed form. The more general case of piecewise constant rates requires some more bookkeeping during the computation of $y(u,t)$ which is contained in the original $H(t)$ from equation (6.10). The characteristic $y(u,t)$ is chosen from the set of all characteristics as that curve for which $y(t,t) = 1$ holds. From this condition and eq. (5.8) we obtain $y(t_{n-1}, t_n)$, noting that $t_n = t$. This is used as the initial value $y(t_{n-1}, t)$ for the computation of $y(u,t)$ in the adjacent subinterval $[t_{n-2}, t_{n-1})$. Proceeding in this way through the intervals down to

$[t_1, t_0), t_0 = 0$, we obtain the remaining components of H_i and hence $S(t)$.

A dose d of a carcinogenic substance enters the GMS model as part of the polynomial $\sum_{i=0}^{k} q_i d^i$ in the exponent of $S(t, d)$. This form of dose dependency is derived from the Armitage-Doll model, which describes the relation between dose and the rate μ_i of transition from stage $i-1$ to stage i by $\mu_i = a_i + b_i d,\ a_i, b_i \geq 0$. Combining all transitions leads to a total transition rate of $\prod_{i=1}^{k}(a_i + b_i d)$, a k-th order polynomial in d. This is generalized to the GMS model by allowing arbitrary nonnegative values q_i for the polynomial coefficients, not only those which can be represented as coefficients of $\prod_{i=1}^{k}(a_i + b_i d)$. A component $q_i d^i$ cannot be related to a particular biological event, hence there is no interpretation of a q_i parameter in the GMS model.

The situation is different in the MVK model, where each rate has a biological interpretation. A dose-dependent ν means that the chemical under study acts as an *initiator*, while a dose dependent α or β characterizes *promotion* or *anti-promotion.* Further types of chemical actions have been described in Chapter 6.4. Unless there is better knowledge, the standard assumption for the relation between parameter and (external) dose is linearity: parameters in the MVK model have the form $\theta(d) = \theta_0 + \theta_1 d$, where θ replaces ν, μ, α, γ, as far as these parameters are assumed to depend on dose. The θ_0-coefficients are responsible for dose-independent, spontaneous events, while the θ_1-coefficients describe the degree of dose dependency.

The value d of dose by itself is subject to specific considerations in either model. Dose is not necessarily to be understood as the (external) dose applied to an experimental unit. It might be much more appropriate to account for transport mechanisms, metabolic activities or more general pharmacokinetics of a carcinogen in order to quantify the dose value effective at the site of its biological action. Approaches in this direction have been introduced in previous chapters and will again be addressed in section 7.5.

Until here it was assumed that dose is constant over time. This assumption was a construction principle of the Armitage-Doll model and carries over to the GMS model. For the expressed incorporation of time dependent dose an extension of the GMS model is needed (cf. Crump and Howe 1984). The MVK model, however, is designed to incorporate time dependent rates directly. If, as in most cases, piecewise constant rates are assumed, then truly time dependent rates need a careful approximation by an appropriately selected set of constants. If such an approximation is found to be unsatisfactory, then $S(t)$ should be computed not via eq. (6.9) – (6.11), but by integrating the partial differential equation for $\psi(y, z; t)$ from chap. 6 along characteristics by numerical methods. This will be time consuming and is therefore not recommended as a general procedure, but it will be possible where model specification or data peculiarities require the treatment of strongly time dependent rates.

7.2.2. Model Comparison

Each combination of a model structure (GMS or MVK) and a set of parameter values (for q_i, k or $\alpha, \gamma, \nu X, \mu$, respectively) leads to a specific survival distribution $S(t, d)$, where the argument d is introduced to make the dose dependency of S explicit. However, the difference between a survival function from a MVK model and one derived from a GMS model is not necessarily large.

This means that it could be a problem to solve the inverse problem, namely having only a set of numerically given survival probabilities available, to identify the model structure which generated them. Such a task is typical for practical failure time or dose reponse analysis, where only a set of failure time curves for a moderate number of doses has been observed.

Figure 7.1 shows a set of failure time curves derived from an MVK promotion model, an MVK initiation model and from a GMS model, each for various dose values. The parameters used for the MVK models are given in Table 7.2, and for the GMS model the values $k = 2, q_0 = 1.35 \times 10^{-6}, q_1 = 1.87 \times 10^{-7}, q_2 = 3.17 \times 10^{-9}$ were used. Parameter values for the initiation model have been chosen such that the survival distribution $S(t, d)$ covers most of the range [0,1] at least for one dose value and that there also is a reasonable dose-response relation within the dose range covered if the data were considered only at $t = 600$, the end of the observation time. The parameters for the promotion and the GMS model were chosen in way which results in survival distributions "as close as possible" to the initiation model distribution. Details on what is meant by "close" will be given in the next sections.

An inspection of the various failure time curves shows that in most cases and in particular for the dose values 0,1,2 there is no large difference in the survival probabilities $S(t, d)$ corresponding to the various models. It must be emphasized that the curves shown are the theoretical ones, derived from the known distribution functions. These functions are not observable in practice. They can well be approximated by empirical distributions obtained from large samples. But in most cases, sample size is not large and empirical survivor functions are step functions with a moderate number of steps. Differences between the underlying theoretical curves must then be set in relation to the jumps in the empirical survivor function estimated from a real experiment: if an experimental group consists of 50 units, then each event (e.g. appearance of a tumor) produces a decrease of $1/50 = 0.02$ in the empirical survivor distribution, if no censoring occurs. If censoring takes place, the jumps may even be larger. Consequently, if there is a true difference between two theoretical survivor functions at a certain time point t, then this difference could only be detected if it were larger than the jump size of the empirical functions at that time point. But this is of course an optimistic statement, as there can always be a considerable amount of random deviation between theoretical and empirical survivor function. Figure 7.1(F) shows the ranges, obtained by simulation, in which 90% of all empirical distribution functions will lie, if the data generation follows either the MVK promotion or the GMS model, given the MVK parameters from Table 7.2, the GMS parameters mentioned above, and a constant dose of $d = 8$. The simultaneous confidence bands for the doses 0,1,2,4, for which the underlying survival functions are given in Figures (A) to (E), have a width similar to the one for $d = 8$ shown in (F). This means that, if only doses smaller than 8 were available, a proper discrimination between the model structures under discussion were possible only under lucky circumstances.

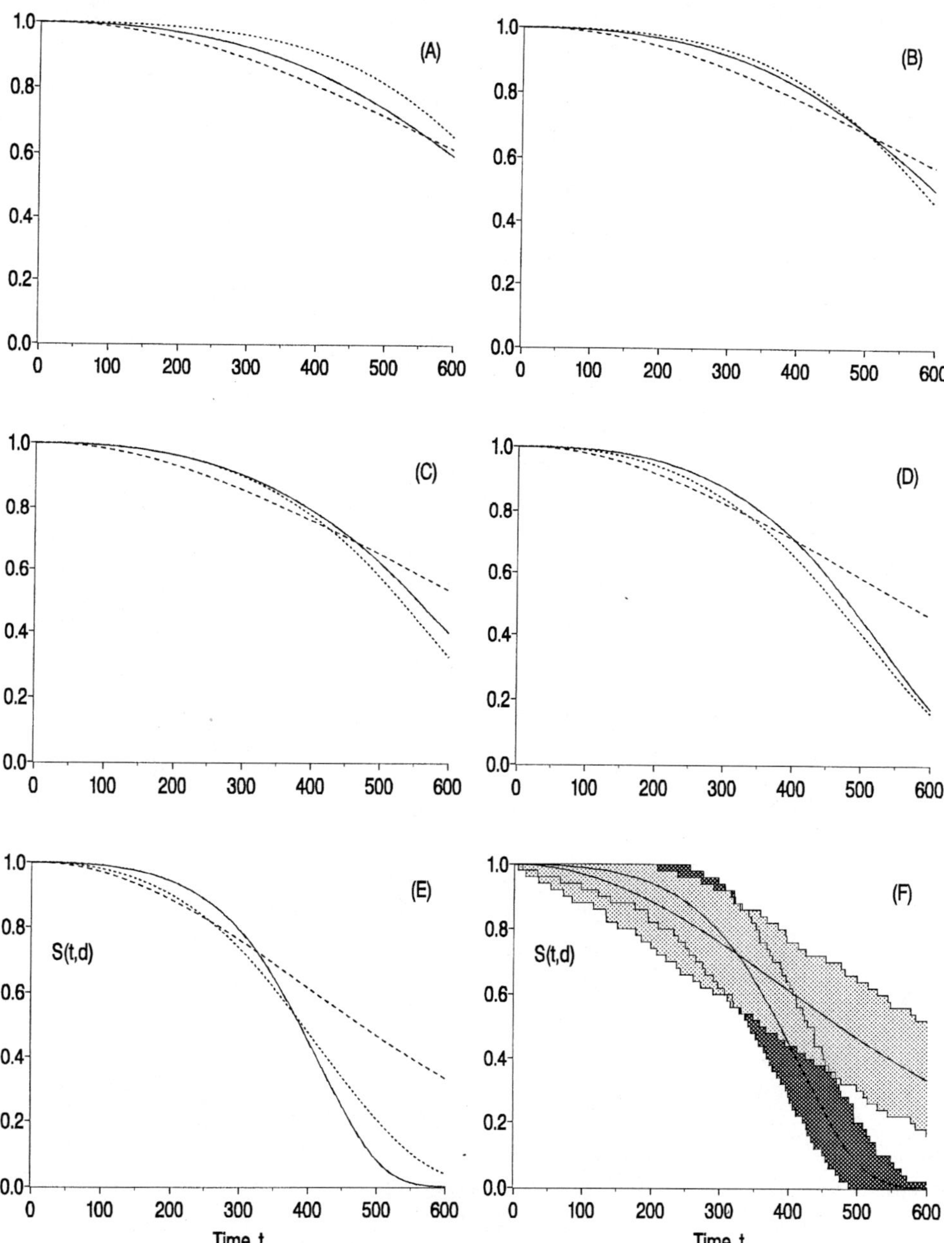

Figure 7.1: *Failure time distributions arising for dose $d = 0$ (A) $d = 1$ (B) $d = 2$ (C) $d = 4$ (D) $d = 8$ (E) from the MVK promotion model (solid curve), the MVK initiation model (dotted) and the GMS model (dashed). Underlying parameters are given in the text. Figure (F) shows the simulated simultaneous 90% confidence bands corresponding to the expected promotion and GMS curves given in (E), assuming that observations are made in groups of 50 units each.*

In summarizing it must be stated that the discrete nature of the events under study, together with the considerable random fluctuation to be expected in samples of typical size could be a source for not properly identifying the model structure that has generated a given data set.

Hence, also the attempt to identify the biological "truth" by looking for the theoretical model with the best fit to an empirical dataset cannot be expected to be successful in general. In section 7.3. we will address the problem of discriminating between model structures when the basis for discrimination is empirical data, with explicit reference to the consequences of erroneous conclusions in the field of low-dose assessment.

Besides comparing complete survival distributions which depend on dose and time jointly, it is sometimes necessary to compare survival probabilities at a fixed time t_0. If the effect of a life-long exposure is of interest, then the expected length of life would be inserted for t_0.

The comparison of model behaviour for fixed time and time-constant dose can be performed using various criteria. In Chapter 5 we have already defined the *extra risk*, or *risk above background* as $E(d) = [P(d) - P(0)]/[1 - P(0)]$, where $P(d)$ is related to the survivor function $S(t, d)$ by $P(d) = 1 - S(t_0, d)$ for some fixed time t_0. Another way to describe behaviour at fixed time is to use the difference $A(d) = P(d) - P(0) = S(t_0, 0) - S(t_0, d)$, the *additional risk*, directly. This criterion has an immediate interpretation as the proportion of the universe under study which will experience a tumor due to the dose d. Both criteria can be transformed from one to the other, as long as the base risk $BR = P(0) = 1 - S(t_0, 0)$ is given. In the comparisons to follow in the next section we will concentrate on the additional risk $A(d)$, as it is of direct interest for regulatory purposes. In connection with regulation, sometimes the term "virtually safe dose" (VSD) is used for $d(A)$, if A is sufficiently small. The meaning of "sufficiently small" depends on the problem under study, in particular on the size of the population, which is exposed to the risk. The basic concept is to determine a dose so small that the associated number of responses in the whole population is neglectably small, preferably smaller than one. Practically, most of the A values considered lie in the range 10^{-3} to 10^{-6}.

7.2.3. Low Dose

A major application of mathematical models in carcinogenesis lies in the assessment of cancer risk at low dose. This situation occurs frequently when the carcinogenic potency of a chemical present in the environment is to be evaluated. A characteristic feature then is a large exposed population, making risk quantification important, but the individual dose and risk are small, making direct empirical quantification impossible in many cases. Here empirical evidence must be supported by extrapolation based on a mathematical model, and the choice of a particular model might be an important decision. The theoretical justification to employ a particular mathematical model has special weight in the low-dose problem, because the other central criterion, the goodness of fit of a model-based prediction to empirical data, can hardly be applied.

If dose is small, then most dose-response relations can be approximated quite well by a linear expression of the form $1 - S(t_0, d) = P(d) = \theta_0 + \theta_1 d$. This is an immediate property of the Taylor expansion of $P(d)$. An n-th order Taylor expansion of $P(d)$ around d_0 in an open interval I ($d_0 \in I$) is available if $P(d)$ has inside I at least $n+1$ derivatives with respect to d. The expansion represents $P(d)$ by a weighted sum of polynomials and a remainder term:

$$P(d) = \sum_{k=0}^{n} \frac{\mathrm{d}^k P}{\mathrm{d}d^k|_{d=d_0}} (d - d_0)^k + R(d),$$

where the remainder term R tends to zero if d tends towards d_0. Setting $n = 1$ and neglecting the remainder term leads to the linear form mentioned before. In this linear approximation the properties of the specific model used for $P(d)$ is now summarized in θ_0 and θ_1: $\theta_0 = P(d_0) - P'(d_0)d_0$, $\theta_1 = P'(d_0)d$.

In section 5.4 we have already seen that the first order low-dose approximation for the GMS model is ($t_0 > 0$ fixed, $d_0 = 0$)

$$P(d) \approx 1 - \exp(q_0 t_0^k) + \exp(q_0 t_0^k)\, q_1 t_0^k d,$$

leading to

$$\begin{aligned} E(d) &\approx q_1 t_0^k d \\ A(d) &\approx \exp(q_0 t_0^k)\, q_1 t_0^k d. \end{aligned}$$

There is no such simple representation for the general low-dose behaviour of the MVK model, due to the more complicated form of $S(t, d)$. An exception is the initiation case, where $\nu(d)$ is the only term which depends on dose. Here we have

$$\begin{aligned} H(t) &= \nu(d) X \left[(1 - A)t - \frac{1}{\alpha} \ln(B - A) + \frac{1}{\alpha} \ln G(t) \right] \\ &= \nu(d) X\, h(t) \\ S(t, d) &= \exp\left[-\nu(d) X\, h(t)\right] \\ \frac{\partial S(t, d)}{\partial d} &= -\exp\left[-\nu(d) X\, h(t)\right] \frac{\partial \nu}{\partial d}\, h(t) \\ &= -S(t, d) \frac{\partial \nu}{\partial d}\, h(t) \end{aligned}$$

For fixed t_0, d sufficiently small and $\nu(d) = a_\nu + b_\nu d$ we can approximate $P(d)$ by

$$P(d) = 1 - S(t_0, d) \approx 1 - S(t_0, 0)[1 - b_\nu h(t_0) d], \tag{7.6}$$

which is linear in d. Extra risk and additional risk then have the forms

$$\begin{aligned} E(d) &\approx b_\nu h(t_0)\, d \\ A(d) &\approx S(t_0, 0) b_\nu h(t_0)\, d. \end{aligned}$$

The MVK promotion model has the same general linear approximation of $P(d)$ as the initiation model. However, as the derivatives of $S(t, d)$ with respect to d involve lengthy formulae and do not lead to simple coefficients within the linear expression, we will not show them here.

dose group l	time of event x_{jl}	type of event: malig. clone ($\delta_{jl} = 1$) censoring ($\delta_{jl} = 0$) δ_{jl}	no of units at risk before x_{jl} n_{jl}
1	x_{11}	δ_{11}	$n_{11} = m_1$
$\vdots$	$\vdots$	$\vdots$	$\vdots$
1	x_{j1}	δ_{j1}	$n_{j1} = \sum_{s<j} \delta_{s1}$
$\vdots$	$\vdots$	$\vdots$	$\vdots$
1	$x_{m_1 1}$	$\delta_{m_1 1}$	$n_{m_1 1}$
$\vdots$	$\vdots$	$\vdots$	$\vdots$
l	x_{jl}	δ_{jl}	$n_{jl} = \sum_{s<j} \delta_{sl}$
$\vdots$	$\vdots$	$\vdots$	$\vdots$
g	$x_{m_g l}$	$\delta_{m_g l}$	$n_{m_g l} = \sum_{s<m_g} \delta_{sm_g}$

Table 7.1: *The data structure in a failure time experiment with censoring. There are g dose groups with $m_l, l = 1, 2, \ldots, g$ units in group l. All members of group l have been exposed to the constant dose d_l. Event times x_{jl} are recorded individually for each unit j and sorted in increasing order within each group.*

It must be emphasized that in the derivations above linearity in the low-dose region is due to the investigator's decision to *approximate* $P(d)$ by a linear function. The full GMS and MVK model both are not linear in the low-dose region, but it is a property of these models to allow a linear approximation (not every dose-response relation has a reasonable linear approximation). The linearity is used here as a tool to facilitate calculations. It is not a component of model definition like, e.g., in the Mantel-Bryan model (cf. section 5.2).

The use of different models for $P(d)$ may lead to considerable differences in the resulting low-dose behaviour (cf. Drescher, Timm, Wosniok 1983). We will in the following section provide some simulation results to illustrate the model effect when the choice is between the GMS and the MVK model.

7.3. STATISTICAL INFERENCE

7.3.1. Available Data and Parameter Estimation

Basic events like transition, division, and death in the stochastic process which is the background of either model cannot normally be observed in reality. Typically, the only observable event is the appearance of a malignant clone, and this will happen only if the clone has reached a certain size. The technical aspects of detecting real clones based on two dimensional sections of a tissue has been dealt with in chapter 6. Simplifying like in the previous chapter we will assume here too that already a clone consisting of only one cell will be detected in an experiment. An experiment, organized in g groups with $m_l, l = 1, 2, \ldots, g$ units in group l, would then lead to observed data with a structure as shown in Table 7.1.

The number of units with malignant clone observed in group l is equal to $\sum_{j=1}^{m_l} \delta_{jl}$. This usually is not equal to the number of units m_l in that group, because some units may have been censored due to death without tumor or other type of withdrawal. Units that are still at risk at the end of the experiment are treated as being censored at closing time.

The estimation of unknown model parameters can be performed by a maximum likelihood (ML) procedure. An experimental unit j in group l contributes to the total likelihood function either by $L_{jl} = \log(-S'(x_{jl})) = \log f(x_{jl})$, if a malignant clone was observed at time x_{jl}, or by $L_{jl} = \log S(x_{jl})$, if the unit was censored at time x_{jl}. Contributions from different units are assumed to be independent. Then the total likelihood function has the structure

$$L = \sum_{l=1}^{g} \sum_{j=1}^{m_l} L_{jl} = \sum_{l=1}^{g} \sum_{j=1}^{m_l} \log\left[\delta_{jl} f(x_{jl}, \theta) + (1 - \delta_{jl}) S(x_{jl}, \theta)\right], \tag{7.7}$$

which has to be maximized over the admissible values of q_i in the GMS model or ν, μ, α, γ in the MVK model, leading to estimates $\hat{q}_i$ and $\hat{\nu}, \hat{\mu}, \hat{\alpha}, \hat{\gamma}$, respectively, for the unknown true values. Only these estimates are available in a practical application, so that conclusions based on either model always are subject to error due to errors in the parameter estimates. This remains true also if a parameter value (e.g. $\gamma = \beta/\alpha$) is taken from earlier experience or from theoretical considerations and implanted into the model, instead of being estimated from the actual data set. Only the source of the error and its size might be modified.

General maximum likelihood theory provides statements about the distribution of parameter estimates in the large sample case, with the number of units per dose group tending to infinity. Complications in the use of this theory can arise, when a parameter has a finite domain and the true value lies on the boundary. Such a situation occurs if, e.g. in the GMS model, a true q_i is zero, and its value is estimated from the data.

The boundedness of model parameters $(q_i, \alpha, \gamma, \mu, \nu \in [0, \infty) \subset \mathbb{R})$ could be removed by a transformation, e.g. by using $u_i = \log q_i$ instead of q_i. This, however, transforms a true value of zero to minus infinity, which makes theoretical investigations difficult. So, special considerations are necessary to derive the asymptotic distribution of the parameter estimates in all those cases where parameters could lie on the boundary of a limited domain. Portier and Hoel (1983) gave the asymptotic distribution of the q_i estimates within the GMS framework for various constellations of true q_i values. They also investigated the appropriateness of asymptotic approximations to small sample situations, where they used $\log d(A)$, the logarithm of the dose which generates the additional risk A, as target variable, instead of the model parameter estimates. Their conclusion was that "for the typical bioassy of 150 animals, the distribution of the VSD [Virtually Safe Dose, here VSD $= d(10^{-3})$] resulting from the use of the asymptotic theory differed dramatically from what was observed in the simulations". An acceptable agreement of simulated and asymptotic distributions was achieved only when the sample size was increased considerably, which could mean that, depending on the underlying true model, even with as many as 100,000 animals a clear deviation between simulated result and asymptotic theory remained. As such sample sizes are far from realistic in practice, it is necessary to investigate explicitly the small sample distributions of, e.g., the dose $d(A)$, when estimated from the GMS or the MVK model fitted to small sample data.

7.3.2. Comparing Low-Dose Extrapolations from Different Models: A Simulation Study

Assuming that the problem is to determine the value of $d(A)$, the dose which generates a certain additional risk A, given a set of failure time data, then obviously the best thing to do would be to (i) identify the correct model underlying the data, (ii) to estimate unknown parameter values by an appropriate method like maximum likelihood estimation, and (iii) finally to compute $d(A)$ using the previously identified model and the estimated parameter values. This straightforward approach will fail already in the first step, as it will never be possible to identify the "correct" model. All what can be hoped is that a model can be found, which provides a satisfactory approximation to the true process. In this sense it is possible that two different models could behave quite similarly by leading to similar approximations, though having different construction principles.

In order to compare the behaviour of the GMS and the MVK model in their function to approximate a true process, represented by a set of failure time data, it is necessary to define a measure by which both approaches may be compared. Goodness-of-fit measures can lead to relative statements like "model A fits better than model B", but they cannot be used for significance statements, as none of the models is nested in the other. The paper by Kopp-Schneider and Portier (1991) shows a way to circumvent the problem at least partially and provides also some results concerning the possibility to discriminate generally between GMS and MVK generated data. In this section we will concentrate not on general discrimination between models, but compare the approaches with respect to their behaviour when the aim is low-dose extrapolation to calculate $d(A)$, starting from a data set of realistic size and structure.

More specific, the question to be answered is: *Which difference, if any, is to be expected between the low-dose extrapolation based on the GMS/LMS model and the low-dose extrapolation based on the MVK model, all derived from the same dataset?* If there were no relevant differences between both extrapolations, then the choice of a model for analysis would obviously be an uncritical decision. However, if there were differences, then further considerations would become necessary, as the decision for one of the models would mean to either overestimate or to underestimate the true risk.

A simulation study with special emphasis on using realistic conditions was carried out in order to answer the question formulated above. The particular aim of the study was to provide estimates and error bands for $d(A)$ derived from each of the models, together with auxiliary information for model choice.

Data set	Type of data generation	Parameters α_0	α_1	γ_0	γ_1	μ_0	μ_1	ν_0	ν_1
I	MVK, initiation	0.07500	0	0.9000	0	10^{-8}	0	10	40
II	MVK, promotion	0.03837	0.01001	0.9059	0	10^{-8}	0	121.9	0

Table 7.2: *Parameters used to simulate failure time data.*

7.3.3. Design of the Simulation Study

7.3.3.1. Data Generation The basic component of the simulation study was one *experiment.* It summarizes the simulated outcome of an animal experiment in which groups of m_l animals were exposed to a dose d_l of a (potential) carcinogen. If animal j in dose group l developed a tumor, the time of its detection was recorded as the failure time x_{jl} associated with the animal, and its failure indicator was set to 1 ($\delta_{jl} = 1$). If no tumor was detected until the end of the study (or as long as the animal participated in the study), the failure time was set equal to the length of the observation interval and the failure indicator was set to 0 ($\delta_{jl} = 0$). The data structure arising in this way for one experiment is the one shown in Table 7.1.

Two data sets were used in the study: in the first one an MVK initiation model served as the "truth", meaning that sample "experiments" were generated according to this model. In the second data set an MVK promotion model was used as the generating model. The parameters involved are given in Table 7.2.

As mentioned before, the parameter values of the "true" initiation model were chosen such that a reasonable number of responses was expected to "occur" for dose values in [0,8] and time values in [0,600]. Dose and time are given in arbitrary units, however, the time range was chosen similar to the range (in days) as observed in real animal experiments.

In each dose group l there were $m_l = 50$ units. One experiment had 5 dose groups: $d = 0$ (control), 1, 2, 4, 8. Dose was defined to be constant over time. The dose-rate relation was linear: $\theta = \theta_0 + \theta_1 d$, where θ has to be replaced by ν or γ, depending on the type of model.

A response time x_{jl} was generated according to the "true" model (the initiation model in data set I) for each experimental unit ("animal") by generating uniform random numbers on [0,1] and transforming them via the inverse distribution function of the underlying model. Endpoint censoring took place at $x = 600$. Intermediate censoring was not considered.

Following this procedure, 1000 experiments were simulated based on the MVK initiation model as the "true" model. To each of these, a MVK promotion model was fitted by the iterative procedure described below. The arithmetic means of the estimated parameters $(\alpha_0, \alpha_1, \gamma_0, \nu_0)$ served as parameter values for the generation of MVK promotion data used in study data set II. They are given in Table 7.2; some failure time curves derived from these models and parameters are shown in Figure 7.1. As in the initiation case, 1000 experiments were simulated for the promotion model. This way to select parameter values for the data generation made sure that the theoretical survival distributions underlying the two study data sets were close together. It would

Type of	Parameters													
fitted model	α_0	α_1	γ_0	γ_1	μ_0	μ_1	ν_0	ν_1	k	q_0	q_1	q_2	q_3	q_4
MVK, initiation	e	0	e	0	10^{-8}	0	e	e						
MVK, promotion	e	e	e	0	10^{-8}	0	e	0						
GMS and LMS									1	e	e			
GMS and LMS									2	e	e	e		
GMS and LMS									3	e	e	e	e	
GMS and LMS									4	e	e	e	e	e

Table 7.3: *List of models which were fitted to each experiment in each of the two study data sets. Numerical values are those of fixed parameters, an 'e' indicates a parameter to be estimated.*

not have been useful to employ theoretical distributions which were in every respect far apart from another. If the GMS model were fitted to data from extremely different underlying true distributions and would then show a very variable behaviour, then this effect could be due merely to the differences in the basic data. If, however, the basic data were similar in both study parts, then no large variation should be expected in the behaviour of the fitted GMS model. Large variation could then be interpreted as a kind of instability arising from fitting the wrong model.

7.3.3.2. Estimation of Parameters The question formulated in section 7.3.2. required that various models had to be fitted to the generated data. First, to get an impression about the variability of additional risk estimates derived from a moderate-sized sample without model misspecification error, it was necessary to fit the correct type of model to each of the study data sets. Second, to provide insight into the effect of model misspecification, models were fitted crosswise to the data sets, so that finally 10 models, listed in Table 7.3, were fitted to each experiment in each study data set.

Table 7.3 shows that four parameters were estimated for each MVK model, while for the GMS/LMS structure a series of four models was fitted with between two and five parameters to be estimated. The reason is that there are several motivations to use the GMS model, depending on the assumptions the investigator makes. If the GMS model is used under the assumption that there is a certain (known) number k of stages in the carcinogenesis process, but that details on the cell level do not play an important role, then the GMS model should be used with the number of stages fixed at this k value. In view of the conditions of the present study this would mean to set $k = 2$, since two stages were involved in the data generation. Another motivation to use the GMS model is that of curve-fitting: varying the number of stages and using a dose polynomial with variable degree k gives a high flexibility to describe empirical dose-time-failure relations. As long as k is restricted to be a natural number and the q_i to be nonnegative, as it was the case here, there is still a certain biological interpretation of the model components. When following a curve-fitting approach, the parameter k is varied and the decision for a certain k is made on the basis of some goodness-of-fit measure. The range of reasonable k values is limited by the data: if the dose affects k transitions between stages, then the proper GMS model contains a polynomial of degree k, which in turn has $k+1$ coefficients. To estimate these, at least $k+1$ dose groups are necessary. For the present case with five dose groups this means that k values between 1 and 4 can be (and were) considered.

All model fitting was performed by maximizing the likelihood function (7.7) with respect to the model parameters, with the proper functions for f and S inserted. The maximization was done numerically by a modified Newton-Raphson iterative procedure using the Broyden-Fletcher-Goldfarb-Shanno approach to approximate the matrix of second derivatives (cf. Kennedy and Gentle 1980 – note that a transpose sign must be inserted in their equation 10.24). The gradient was calculated exactly. A golden section search was used to determine the parameter q_1^* of the LMS model. Starting from the estimates q_i, $i = 1, 2, \ldots, k$, obtained by the GMS approach and their associated likelihood function value ℓ, the q_1 estimate was increased iteratively according to the golden section principle in order to derive an upper bound for q_1. For each modification of q_1, the remaining parameters q_i, $i \neq 1$, were re-estimated by maximizing (7.7) with respect to q_i, $i \neq 1$, while keeping q_1 at its actual modified value. The procedure stopped when the likelihood function corresponding to the modified q_1 and the re-estimated q_i had a value of $\ell^* = \ell + \chi^2_{1,0.10} = \ell + 2.706$. In this way the estimate q_1 from the original GMS model had been increased so far that in a comparison of the original GMS model (all $k+1$ parameter estimated by the maximum likelihood principle) and the modified version (q_1 replaced by q_1^*, q_i, $i \neq 1$, re-estimated), the modified version would be on the border to show a significantly worse fit. This means that all admissible variation in the parameter estimates had been used to increase q_1, thus leading to an upper bound for q_1.

For each fitted model the dose $d(A)$ corresponding to an additional risk of $A = S(600, 0) - S(600, d) = 10^{-6}$ was determined. Also, the Kolmogorov-Smirnov goodness-of-fit statistic

$$D = \max_{\substack{0 \leq t \leq 600 \\ l=1,2,\ldots,5}} |S(t, d_l, \hat{\theta}) - \hat{S}(t, d_l)| \tag{7.8}$$

was calculated, where $S(t, d_l, \hat{\theta})$ is the theoretical survival distribution derived from the fitted model, using the estimated parameter vector $\hat{\theta}$, and

$$\hat{S}(t, d_l) = \prod_{x_{jl} \leq t} \left(1 - \frac{\delta_{jl}}{n_{jl}}\right)$$

is the nonparametric Kaplan-Meier estimator for the empirical survival distribution.

7.3.4. Simulation Results

As always in a simulation study, also the results described here are conclusions drawn from a particular set of data. Though efforts were made to choose simulation conditions which do not show peculiarities, all generalizations should be made with care.

To begin with a general statement, the simulation has shown that the three models under study, namely the MVK initiation model, the MVK promotion model and the GMS model have their specific characteristics. These models are not interchangeable in the sense that conclusions concerning additional risks are independent from the true model or from the model used for estimation. To express it from the investigator's viewpoint: conclusions are not robust against model misspecification.

7.3.4.1. Parameter Estimates Before turning to the comparison of estimated additional risks $d(A)$, we shall first inspect the estimated model parameters (q_i and α_0, α_1, γ_0, γ_1, ν_0, ν_1). Here we have to distinguish between two levels of assessment: the first level refers to the properties of estimates from one experiment, the second level to the properties of the total set of estimates from the whole study. The first level is important mainly for the design of experiments, or retrospectively to assess the accuracy of estimates from one experiment, while the second one serves to check the quality of the simulation study as a whole.

Referring to the first level, we know from maximum likelihood (ML) theory that ML parameter estimates are consistent (given some regularity conditions), which means that they tend to the true value (the population value), when the sample size tends to infinity. Further, the estimates, being random quantities because they are derived from random quantities, are asymptotically normally distributed with a variance which can be estimated from the second derivative of the likelihood function. These asymptotic properties are often sufficiently accurately approximated by the distribution found in a finite sample, so that asymptotic results then can be used to calculate confidence regions for estimated parameters. This, however, is a vague statement, as 'finite' can still mean 'huge', and it is not generally possible to decide whether asymptotic conditions do already hold for a finite sample. On the other hand, ML estimates derived from small finite samples may be biassed, which means that if we calculate an estimate from a finite sample, then the expected value of the estimate is not necessarily the true (population) value. Also the distribution of estimates derived from small samples is not necessarily close to the asymptotic distribution.

In the present study the basic sample size was 250 units, which is clearly not infinitely large, but statistical experience suggests that this size could be sufficient to use asymptotic properties. However, it was not the purpose of this study to provide an assessment of this problem, and so it will not followed further here. A study of this aspect could be done by using resampling methods like the bootstrap approach to derive e.g. confidence intervals, and by then comparing these results with those obtained from asymptotics based intervals.

The second level of assessment addresses the distributional properties of the $w = 1000$ replications of parameter estimates per study data set. Here we can make use of the law of large numbers, which states that the arithmetic mean of such replications tends to its expected value. But, as indicated above, this expected value is not necessarily the true population value of the parameter. If the ML estimates are biassed due to a particular model structure and the use of finite samples, then the limit of the mean parameter estimate and the true value do not coincide. So, in order to obtain an impression about a possible bias, the mean of the estimated parameters should be compared with the values from Table 7.2, which are the true population values. It is, of course, impossible to prove (in the mathematical sense) a statement about an asymptotic property like biasedness from a simulation, but a numerical comparison can be made in a case like the present, where true values are known.

Another problem to consider is whether the number of replications in the simulation study is large enough to allow general conclusions. This question is always difficult to answer, but a minimum requirement is that effects from single samples within the simulation data should not dominate the overall results from the study. As an auxiliary way to check this we use the central limit theorem to predict confidence intervals for the estimated parameters and compare these with the empirical intervals of the study. Roughly spoken, one condition for the validity of the central limit theorem is that none of the underlying random variables dominates the others. So, if this condition is violated, then the confidence interval derived via the central limit theorem should be different from the empirical interval. Similar intervals indicate that no dominating effects of single estimates are present.

It should be noted, however, that it cannot be expected that both versions of confidence intervals are completely identical, as slightly different basic assumptions beyond the validity of asymptotic properties are involved. While the first version is nonparametric in the sense that it is based only on the assumption that the density of $\hat{\theta}_i$ has a smooth form, without making a distributional assumption, the second version specialises the smoothness assumption to the parametric assumption of normality, and it is also assumed that the found values of $\bar{t}$ and s_t are correct. Errors in this respect are transferred to errors in the derived interval limits. Hence, the comparison of confidence intervals should be understood as a clearly approximative check.

Table 7.4 contains descriptive statistics for the estimated parameters. Technically not the original parameters, but instead their logarithms were estimated, in order to obtain nonnegative values on the originally scale. In the table, however, all quantities are transformed to the original scale for easier interpretation and to facilitate the comparison with the values used for data generation (Table 7.2).

Let θ denote one model parameter ($\theta \in \{\alpha_0, \alpha_1, \gamma_0, \gamma_1, \nu_0, \nu_1\}$) and let $t = \log\theta$. Then we define

$$\begin{aligned} \bar{u} &= \sum_{i=1}^{w} \hat{u}_i/w, \qquad \bar{\theta} = \exp(\bar{u}) \\ s_u^2 &= \sum_{i=1}^{w} (\hat{u}_i - \bar{u})^2/(w-1), \end{aligned}$$

where w is the number of simulated experiments and $\hat{u}_i$ represents the estimate for $\log\theta$ in experiment number i. Table 7.4 also gives two versions of 90% confidence intervals for the estimates. The first version is the empirical interval, calculated by a linear interpolation of the empirical distribution function of the $\hat{u}_i$ values and back transformation to the original scale. The second version bases on the central limit theorem and is calculated by $\theta_{\text{low,high}} = \exp(\bar{u} \mp 1.64 \cdot s_u)$, according to the central limit theorem. These intervals describe the range in which 90% of all estimates for θ are expected to lie, when each estimate is calculated from a sample of size 250.

Mean values of estimated parameters, as shown in the third column of Table 7.4, lie close to the true values (Table 7.2 which were used to generate the data sets of the simulation study. Both versions of confidence intervals include the true parameter values for each θ, so that there is no indication of a biassed estimate.

Comparing the two versions of confidence intervals in Table 7.4, we see that there are certain differences. Most of them are small, compared with the empirical variation

Model for data generation and parameter estimation	parameter θ	mean estimate $\bar{\theta}$	empirical 90% c.i.	large sample 90% c.i.
MVK, initiation	α_0	0.07474	(0.06616, 0.07860)	(0.06819, 0.08191)
	γ_0	0.9002	(0.8898 , 0.9087)	(0.8910 , 0.9096)
	ν_0	9.304	(3.129 , 19.27)	(3.034 , 28.53)
	ν_1	39.95	(24.89 , 56.53)	(26.89 , 59.34)
MVK, promotion	α_0	0.03735	(0.02163, 0.05034)	(0.02108, 0.06616)
	α_1	0.01026	(0.00765, 0.01226)	(0.00654, 0.01610)
	γ_0	0.9067	(0.8955 , 0.9170)	(0.8934 , 0.9203)
	ν_0	122.1	(73.82 , 173.7)	(80.62 , 184.9)

Table 7.4: *Parameter estimates and the two versions of 90% confidence intervals.*

of the estimates. Only the upper limits of the intervals for ν_0 in the initiation case differ by a considerable amount. This is mainly due to one extremely outlying value of $\hat{\nu}$, which increases the estimated standard deviation s_t excessively.

In the light of the previously mentioned difference in the underlying assumptions, the differences between the two confidence interval versions seem negligible. This shall be interpreted as an indicator that, as desired, the size of the simulation study is large enough to prevent dominating effects of single random fluctuations.

7.3.4.2. Estimates of Additional Risk Table 7.5 gives a summary of the estimated doses associated with an additional risk of 10^{-6}. Individual values together with 5% and 95% quantiles and kernel estimates of their densities are displayed graphically in Figures 7.2 and 7.3.

The inspection of Table 7.5 shows that there were considerable differences between $d(10^{-6})$ estimates based on the correct model, compared with those derived from other models, and also among the other, non-correct models. Even in those cases where means or medians were close together, large differences could exist between the distribution of the estimates, so that an assessment of model behaviours can not be reduced to a comparison of the average estimates. For the interpretation of differences between $d(10^{-6})$ values it is important to note that an estimate larger than the correct model based value suggests that a higher dose is necessary to generate an additional risk of 10^{-6}. Accepting this dose estimate means to underestimate the correctly estimated risk. Correspondingly, a value smaller than the correct model based value means an overestimation. To avoid confusion in the usage of "underestimation/ overestimation", we will always use these when referring to a risk, not to a dose. Another point to clarify is the distinction between the *true* value of $d(A)$ and the $d(A)$ *estimate based on the correct model.* The first one is obtained by solving $A = S(t_0, 0; \theta) - S(t_0, d(A); \theta)$ for $d(A)$, where $S(t, d; \theta)$ is the true survivor distribution from which the data was generated and θ is the true parameter vector. Such a value is obviously accessible only in a simulation study. The second quantity is also based on the true survivor function, but the true parameter vector θ is replaced by an estimate $\hat{\theta}$, calculated from empirical

Model for data generation	Model for parameter estimation	Estimated dose for an additional risk of 10^{-6} mean	median	90% c.i.
MVK, initiation	MVK, initiation	1.96	1.92	(1.57, 2.78)
	MVK, promotion	12.10	12.06	(10.41, 13.93)
	GMS, $k = 2$	3.47	3.42	(2.77, 4.33)
	LMS $k = 2$	2.58	2.56	(2.15, 3.10)
	GMS, $k = k_{\text{opt}}$	2.26	2.19	(1.69, 3.04)
	LMS $k = k_{\text{opt}}$	1.70	1.66	(1.35, 2.13)
MVK, promotion	MVK, promotion	12.40	12.38	(10.96, 13.95)
	MVK, initiation	4.42	4.35	(3.25, 5.89)
	GMS, $k = 2$	217.70	11.24	(5.80, 76.63)
	LMS $k = 2$	5.04	4.84	(3.82, 6.83)
	GMS, $k = k_{\text{opt}}$	763.58	12.00	(4.77, 4599.98)
	LMS $k = k_{\text{opt}}$	4.33	4.03	(2.68, 7.00)

Table 7.5: *Estimated doses for an additional risk of* 10^{-6} *(arithmetic mean, median, 90% confidence interval defined by the empirical 5% and 95% quantiles). The parameter* k_{opt} *refers to the* k *value associated with the best fitting GMS model. All values have been multiplied by* 10^6.

data. This is the best situation one could achieve in real life. But as it is clear that parameter estimates are subject to random errors, there will also be a random error in the estimate of $d(A)$, however, for unbiassed estimations, this error tends to zero in the long run. In both parts of the present simulation study the difference between the true $d(A;\theta)$ and the mean of the $d(A;\hat{\theta})$ estimates based on the correct model was much smaller than the differences caused by using a wrong model for the estimation of $d(A)$. As the present study has the purpose to elucidate the effects of using different models for risk assessment under realistic conditions, we cannot exploit our knowledge about true parameters, as they are never known in practice. Hence, for the model comparisons to perform here, the $d(A)$ estimates based on the correct model serve as reference values, not the true values.

Figure 7.2 shows that in the first study data set, with an initiation model used to generate the data, the ranges of estimates based on the GMS or LMS approach (panels C – F) overlapped more or less those from the correct model (A). Estimates based on the promotion model (B) were clearly different, as all of them underestimated the true risk. The deviation between average initiation-based estimates and promotion-based estimates was about one order of magnitude. All distributions were unimodal and nearly symmetric, as can be seen by inspection of the densities and from the fact that means and medians were close together. The GMS model with k fixed at $k = 2$ (C) had a tendency to lead to $d(10^{-6})$ estimates which were too large by a factor of $3.42/1.92 = 1.8$, but this is moderate compared with the fact that the endpoints of the 90% confidence interval for estimates based on the correct model already varied by a factor of $2.47/1.57 = 1.6$. Using the corresponding LMS (D) instead of the GMS model reduced the ratio between medians to a value of $2.56/1.92 = 1.3$, which means that a correction had taken place in the desired direction, but the amount of correction was

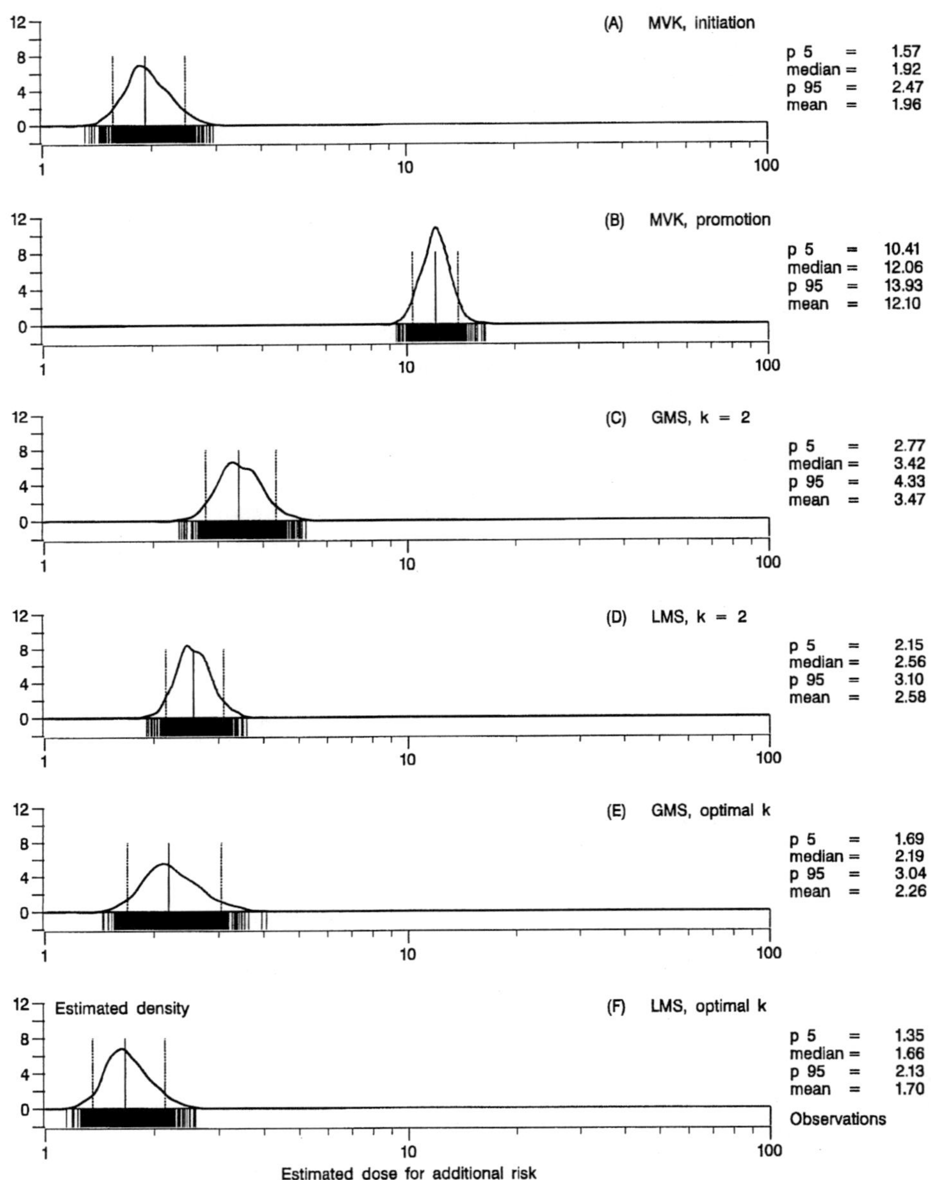

Figure 7.2: *Estimates of the dose which increases the risk of failure by 10^{-6} above the background risk. Data was simulated according to the MVK initiation model with parameters given in Table 7.2, simulation details are given in section 7.3.3. The dose for the additional risk was estimated from each of the simulated experiments by fitting an MVK initiation model (A), an MVK promotion model (B), a GMS (C) and an LMS model (D) with $k = 2$. Further, for each experiment the GMS model with the optimal $k \in \{1, 2, 3, 4\}$ was determined, where "optimal" refers to the minimal Kolmogorov-Smirnov goodness-of-fit statistic. Estimates from the corresponding models are shown in (E), (F). Each vertical bar in (A)-(F) represents the estimate for one experiment.*

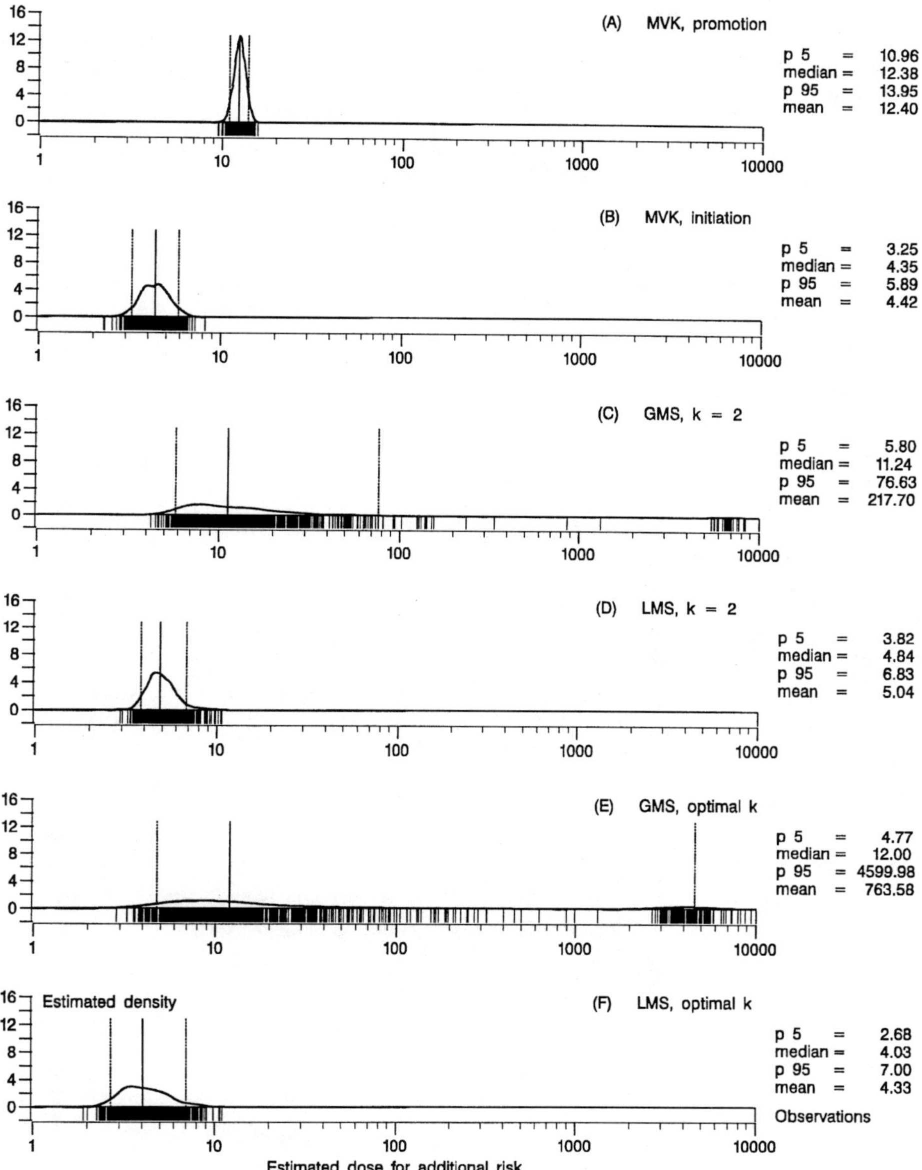

Figure 7.3: *Estimates of the dose which increases the risk of failure by 10^{-6} above the background risk. Data was simulated according to the MVK promotion model with parameters given in Table 7.2. The dose for the additional risk was estimated from each of the simulated experiments by fitting an MVK promotion model (A), an MVK initiation model (B), a GMS (C) and an LMS model (D) with $k = 2$. Further, for each experiment the GMS model with the optimal $k \in \{1,2,3,4\}$ was determined, where "optimal" refers to the minimal Kolmogorov-Smirnov goodness-of-fit statistic. Estimates from the corresponding models are shown in (E), (F). Each vertical bar in (A)-(F) represents the estimate for one experiment. 9 values greater than 10000 were clipped from (E).*

not yet large enough. Following the curve-fitting approach by selecting among the GMS models for each simulated experiment the one with the smallest Kolmogorov-Smirnov statistic D, led to improved $d(10^{-6})$ estimates, but showed a tendency to underestimate the risk, if the GMS model class was maintained. Only the LMS version produced a (slight) overestimate of the additional risk. It should be mentioned that in the curve-fitting approach the optimal k value was either 3 (in 26.7% of all experiments) or 4 (73.3%). Hence one would have been led on the wrong path, if one had inferred the correct number of stages from the degree of the best fitting GMS model.

The situation is a little more complicated for the second study data set, which was generated on the basis of a MVK promotion model. Here the initiation model (Figure 7.3 B) led to an overestimate of the true risk (Figure 7.3 B) by a factor of $12.38/4.35 = 2.8$, and the LMS models in either versions (D, F) behaved similar. In all cases there was a nearly perfect separation between the distribution of estimates based on the true model on one side and the initiation or LMS model versions on the other (lower) side. This means especially for both versions of the LMS model (D, F), that the purpose of their construction, namely to provide a cautious estimate of risk, had been attained here. The GMS model (C, E), however, showed a very particular behaviour in two respects: first, the spread of values was enormous, compared with all other models, and second, the distribution of estimates was bimodal with a factor of about 375 between the modes. Interestingly, the mean values of the GMS-based estimates were closest to the mean of the true (promotion-based) estimates. Hence, we have the result that the mean of the GMS-based $d(10^{-6})$ estimates was nearest to the mean of the true-model based values, but at the same time the individual GMS estimates were by far the most imprecise ones. The limits of the 90% confidence interval showed a variation of 1:1.3 in the promotion case, but a ratio of 1:13 in the GMS case with $k = 2$ and even a ratio of 1:964 in the case when the optimal k was used. Here the optimal k was either 3 (17.7%) or 4 (82.3%), so that, similar to the results from the first study data set, a conclusion about the number of stages in the biological process would have been misleading, had it been drawn from searching for the best fitting GMS model.

The bimodality of the $d(10^{-6})$ distribution shown in Figures 7.3 (C,E) seems surprising at first sight. One might expect that $d(10^{-6})$, calculated on the basis of maximum likelihood estimates $\hat{q}_i$ of the GMS model, should show a unimodal, perhaps skewed distribution, because the estimates should have an approximate normal distribution and the function $d(A) = d(A; \hat{q}_i)$ has no strong curvature for small A. However, the standard normal theory for the asymptotic properties of ML estimates does not apply here, as the fitted model (GMS) is not the model which generated the data (MVK). Besides that, there is another explanation for the bimodal distribution of the d values. An inspection of the estimated $\hat{q}_i$ showed that large values of $d(10^{-6})$, lying in the right mode of Figures 7.3 (C,E), are associated with small values of $\hat{q}_1$, while small values of $d(10^{-6})$ coincide with large $\hat{q}_1$. Large or small $\hat{q}_1$ are a consequence of the random constellation of the data available for parameter estimation. It should be recalled that the underlying data gives information about relatively few dose points, and all of these, except the control group, belong to doses much higher than $d(10^{-6})$. So here we actually have a "small sample effect" of the form that the parameter estimates are mainly determined by data points which are only partially relevant for risks in the low-dose region. For the example of fitting a GMS model to the promotion data this means to underestimate drastically the true risk, whenever the fitting procedure found it appropriate to end with a small $\hat{q}_1$ value. In all these cases there is nearly no effect of $\hat{q}_1 d$ for small dose d, because both $\hat{q}_1$ and d are small, and similarly there is nearly no effect of $\hat{q}_2 d^2$, because d^2 is very small. A comparison of Figure 7.3 (C) with (E) shows that this effect is even amplified, if a good model fit is the principal criterion to select a model. The requirement to have a well-fitting GMS model leads automatically to a high order dose polynomial in the GMS model, which in turn leads to an even stronger underestimation in the low-dose region. Similar effects have been observed earlier by Portier and Hoel (1983), who compared the behaviour of various GMS model versions.

7.3.4.3. The Direction of Error So far, the various models have mainly been discussed by referring to summarizing statistics which characterized the distribution of the whole set of $d(10^{-6})$ estimates from each model. A comparison on the level of individual experiments could provide further insight. Table 7.6 shows the effect of employing various models for the $d(10^{-6})$ estimation by comparing for each experiment the reference estimate (based on the true model) with each of the alternative estimates (based on the other models). The difference was calculated as (estimate from true model) - (estimate from alternative model), and again a negative value indicates underestimation of risk. All in all, and not quite unexpectedly, the individual differences exhibit tendencies similar to those which were observed for the summarizing statistics. The estimates from the GMS model again show bimodal distributions of the $d(10^{-6})$ values in the case of promotion-generated data, and in the same cases there is also an extraordinary large dispersion of values. This indicates that particularly the behaviour of the GMS model needs careful attention in the context of low-dose risk estimation.

The last column in Table 7.6 provides information about the direction of the error when using the wrong model. It gives the proportion of experiments, in which the risk was underestimated, compared with the estimate based on the correct model. This amounts to 0% or 100% in those cases, where distributions were completely separate, and to about 50%, where median values nearly coincide. An underestimation rate near to zero, as exhibited essentially by some LMS versions, means that generally the estimated value of $d(10^{-6})$ was smaller than the one which resulted from the application of the correct model. This is desirable from the standpoint of safety, but it might mean that the $d(A)$ estimates are much smaller than necessary, which is undesirable for economic reasons. A large underestimation rate near to 100% will be undesirable in general, as it means that the risk associated with the estimated $d(10^{-6})$ exceeds the tolerated risk in nearly all cases. This situation is found particularly for the initiation data, when the GMS model is fitted, but also for the MVK promotion model. Underestimation rates about 50% indicate coinciding averages of the $d(10^{-6})$ estimates derived from the two model classes, however, the dispersion around the common median can be enormous, and for a single experiment the difference between the estimates can still be large. Hence in these cases an additional look at the confidence intervals is useful.

Model for data generation and reference estimate	Model for alternative estimate	mean	Error in $d(10^{-6})$ median	90% c.i.	% under-estimates
MVK, initiation	MVK, promotion	-10.13	-10.11	(-11.76, -8.69)	100.0
	GMS, $k = 2$	-1.51	-1.49	(-2.05, -1.07)	100.0
	LMS, $k = 2$	-0.62	-0.61	(-0.88, -0.35)	100.0
	GMS, $k = k_{\text{opt}}$	-0.29	-0.24	(-0.75, 0.01)	94.5
	LMS, $k = k_{\text{opt}}$	0.27	0.26	(0.01, 0.53)	3.8
	"global curve fit"	-0.15	0.00	(-0.67, 0.00)	44.6
MVK, promotion	MVK, initiation	7.99	7.99	(6.58, 9.42)	0.0
	GMS, $k = 2$	-205.30	1.11	(-65.89, 6.55)	44.7
	LMS, $k = 2$	7.36	7.44	(5.36, 9.29)	0.0
	GMS, $k = k_{\text{opt}}$	-752.80	0.46	(-4596.63, 7.69)	48.4
	LMS, $k = k_{\text{opt}}$	8.08	8.26	(5.23, 10.23)	0.0
	"global curve fit"	-454.56	0.00	(-3911.91, 8.15)	16.1

Table 7.6: *Comparison of various $d(10^{-6})$ estimates. For each experiment the difference (estimate based on reference model) - (estimate based on alternative model) is computed. Table entries give means, medians and 90% confidence intervals (empirical 5% and 95% quantiles) of these differences. Negative values of these indicate that the risk has been underestimated. All dose values have been multiplied by 10^6. The specification "global curve fit" in the second column refers to selecting the $d(10^{-6})$ estimate from the model with the smallest Kolmogorov-Smirnov goodness-of-fit statistic, where the selection is experimentwise among the initiation, promotion, and GMS ($k = k_{opt}$) model.*

7.3.4.4. Goodness of Fit as a Criterion for Model Choice Until here, we treated the two model classes under study as two alternative components with equal rights in the process of low-dose extrapolation. No biological arguments were considered, and no information was extracted from the data to arrive at a decision in favour of one final model to use for extrapolation. This way to proceed is, of course, somewhat unrealistic. In fact, biological arguments exists, which could be put forward in favour of a certain way of modelling. They have already been discussed in previous chapters, and will be addressed again in the case studies to follow in chapter 8, so that we can confine ourselves here to the discussion of the statistical aspects of model choice. Such a discussion has become necessary, as the previous sections have demonstrated that, although random fluctuations are considerable, the different models actually lead to different low-dose extrapolations, and that the use of an inappropriate model can be desastrous.

The only way to obtain information about the appropriateness of a mathematical model by statistical means is to compare the prediction from the model with what was observed. This can obviously be done only as far as observations exist, and in the low-dose extrapolation problem this means that no comparison can be made in the dose region of interest. Hence, the result of comparing goodness-of-fit statistics from within the observed dose region must be considered as valid also for the not observed low-dose region, or the idea to rely on goodness of fit must be abandoned. Goodness of fit has already been used in some of the previous figures and tables as a criterion for the curve fitting approach, which means nothing else than to decide for a certain

Model for data generation	percentage of experiments with best fit by ...			percentage of experiments with best fit by ...				
	MVK/ I	MVK/ P	GMS, $k = 2$	MVK/ I	MVK/ P	GMS, $k = 2$	GMS, $k = 3$	GMS, $k = 4$
MVK, initiation	99.3	0.2	0.5	53.2	0.1	0.0	13.2	33.5
MVK, promotion	13.0	87.0	0.0	6.4	61.5	0.0	6.3	25.8

Table 7.7: *Model selection on the basis of the Kolmogorov-Smirnov goodness-of-fit statististic D. The middle part of the table shows the proportion of experiments, for which the initiation (MVK/I), the promotion (MVK/P) or the GMS model with $k = 2$ showed the best fit. In the right part of the table, additionally the GMS model with $k = 3$ or $k = 4$ was available for selection.*

extrapolation on the basis of goodness-of-fit within the observed data. Table 7.7 lists, which models would be chosen in the simulation study, if goodness-of-fit, measured by the Kolmogorov-Smirnov distance D (7.8), were the criterion to select a model for low-dose extrapolation.

The selection rates in Table 7.7 demonstrate that, under the given circumstances, goodness of fit is not a safe basis for a conclusion about the structure of the underlying process. In the middle part of the table all model versions describing a biological process with two stages are compared, namely the initiation, the promotion and the GMS model with $k = 2$. In this frame one could conclude that the initiation model was safely identified as such, and the promotion model fairly well. A further consequence of this is that the explicit introduction of cell dynamics, as it was the case in the initiation and the promotion model, led to dose-failure-time relationships which cannot appropriately be described by an approach which assumes balanced dynamics. From a formal viewpoint, however, this result is not surprising, as for the initiation and promotion model four parameters were available to produce a good fit, while for the GMS model there were only three. This is a potential advantage for both MVK models, no matter which biological interpretation the additional parameters have. This unfairness is removed in the extended selection, shown in the right part of the table, where the biologically background was abandoned and instead also the fits of the GMS versions with three or four stages were considered. Here the models with high flexibility in the form of many free parameters exhibit the best fit, as expected. The chance to recognize the underlying model is drastically reduced, though there still is a probability of more than 50% that it is identified correctly. So, if model fit is used to identify model structure, there is a certain chance that the correct structure is found, but there is also a substantial chance that a wrong model is assigned. Additionally it must be recalled that only five selected model versions were considered in the present comparison. An extended investigation with more models to discriminate between could lead to other, more unfavourable results. It must also be noted that model fit can hardly be the only criterion to select a model, as long as low-dose extrapolation is the final aim. If the class of models under considerations were not restricted by biological considerations, one could simply use a smooth function like a spline to obtain a model with an arbitrary good fit. The usefulness of such a well-fitting model for extrapolation is more than doubtful, as the behaviour of such models outside the region of observations is arbitrary.

The problem of model selection was not the central problem of this section. It was discussed only with respect to the possibility to improve the quality of the low-dose risk assessment. The immediate consequence of making model fit the only criterion for model selection and then to use the best fitting model for extrapolation has already been discussed in the preceding sections.

7.4. DESIGN CONSIDERATIONS FOR LOW-DOSE PROBLEMS

In the previous section we discussed the estimation of low-dose risks from experimental data, which was obtained from a general experimental design. Such a design is appropriate to provide insight into the overall dose-time-failure relation, and consequently no special arrangements are made to account for the specific needs of risk assessment at low dose. But if the latter is the principal purpose of the investigation, then something might be gained by using a specific experimental design.

A first, naive, approach to an experimental design suitable for low-dose risk assessment is to use dose values in the presumed relevant range, and to increase the number of experimental units so far that a sufficiently large number of failures can be expected. This would lead to direct empirical evidence in the relevant risk range, and had the advantage to avoid possibly doubtful assumptions about the nature of underlying biological processes. However, such a way to proceed is impossible because of obvious ethical and economical reasons. Millions of experimental units (animals) were necessary to conduct an experiment from which dose-response relations for risks in the range of 10^{-6} can be derived directly. One of the largest carcinogenesis experiments ever carried out (Cairns, 1980, Littlefield, Farmer and Gaylor, 1980, Krewski, Gaylor and Lutz, 1995), the "megamouse" experiment with about 24,000 animals involved had a much smaller size and could have given direct evidence only for risks of order near to 10^{-4}. Actually, the experiment, conducted by the National Center of Toxicological Research, had the purpose to study the low-dose effects of exposure to 2-aetylaminofluorine (2-AAF), particularly to estimate the dose which produced a 1% tumor rate, i.e. $d(10^{-2})$. Hence, in order to estimate a VSD or "safe dose" (Hartley and Sielken, 1977) associated with a small additional risk A, it is necessary to develop effective sample designs under the restriction of moderate sample sizes.

As a first step in the design of an experiment, an optimality criterion has to be fixed, most frequently in the form that a certain error in a test decision should be kept below a certain limit, or that the variance of an estimated parameter should be minimal. In the present setting it is reasonable to require that $d(A)$ should be estimated with minimal variance, where A (or a set of several A's) is fixed in advance by the experimenter. Alternatively one could put emphasis on the precision of model parameters, arguing that $d(A)$ is derived from these. A vast literature exists on the principles of experimental design, though the nonlinearity of the present models makes specific considerations necessary. General references on optimum designs are Silvey (1980), Atkinson (1988), and Pukelsheim (1993). The principle of c-optimal design, which essentially means to mimimize the variance of a linear combination of estimated parameters, has been extended to applications in nonlinear settings by Kitsos, Titterington, and Torsney (1988), Ford, Kitsos, and Titterington (1989). A robust approach was addressed by Kitsos and Müller (1995). Aspects of D-optimum designs have been discussed by Kitsos (1992), Atkinson et al. (1993). For the Probit, Logit and Weibull model, explicit optimal design structures are given by Gart et al. (1986, ch. 3.4). Designs based on an underlying GMS model can be found in Portier and Hoel (1984).

Besides the one-step designs mentioned above one could consider sequential designs (Kitsos 1992). These involve an iterative stochastic approximation procedure to approach the desired value of $d(A)$, which have theoretical merits in the sense of fulfilling formal optimality criteria.

7.5. SENSITIVITY ANALYSIS AND PHYSIOLOGICALLY BASED TOXICOKINETIC MODELING

In the previous sections it has become clear that uncertainties in the selection of models and imprecise estimates of model parameters must be expected. Approaches to quantify the sensitivity of the quantities of interest against these error sources can be helpful in order to assess the usefulness of the investigation which was undertaken.

A wide range of univariate sensitivity analyses have been developed for mathematical models. That is, individual parameters are ranked according to various measures (e.g., their effect on a model output, or the contribution that their variability makes to the total variability in the output). In this section we discuss sensitivity analyses and how they have been applied to physiologically based toxicokinetic (PBTK) models.

7.5.1. Current Methodology

Sensitivity , as defined by Iman and Helton (1988), is the determination of the change in the response of a model to changes in each model parameter. As such, the three sensitivity analysis techniques described by Iman and Helton are univariate in nature. They are response surface replacement, Latin Hypercube sampling, and differential analysis. Response surface replacement uses experimental design (e.g., a fractional factorial experiment) to select input variable combinations. The model output (dependent variable) is then fitted to a general linear model known as the response surface. Latin Hypercube sampling is a modification of the Monte Carlo technique. Because of its probabilistic basis, estimates of the model output cumulative distribution function and variance can be obtained directly. Lastly, differential analysis uses a first order Taylor series expansion about some base parameter vector x_0. It is designed to study small perturbations about this point, so its usefulness in a global sensitivity analysis may be limited. Parameter rankings are obtained for each of the three techniques according to a variety of measures such as normalized coefficients, the percent of variation in the model output due to each parameter, and standardized rank regression coefficients.

The Fourier Amplitude Sensitivity Test or FAST (Cukier et al., 1973; Koda et al., 1979; McRae et al., 1982) is a means of determining local as well as global sensitivity where the parameters are allowed to range over an order of magnitude. One obtains a normalized sensitivity coefficient that is the ratio of the variance due to a parameter to the total variance. This result is also a univariate sensitivity measure. Liepmann (1983; 1985) applied FAST to a mathematical model of an ecosystem. He states that detection of parametric coupling or multivariate effects is easy with FAST. Other applications of FAST have been in the area of chemical kinetics where systems of coupled rate equations are common (Cukier et al., 1973; Koda et al., 1979; McRae et al., 1982). Saltelli and Marivoet (1990) review the use of various nonparametric statistics in sensitivity analysis. They sample the parameter space using a Monte Carlo approach similar in nature to the Latin Hypercube sampling. The distribution of the model output and each of the parameter distributions is analysed statistically. This sensitivity technique is distinct from the Monte Carlo parameterization technique of Spear et al. (1991). Monte Carlo parameterization maps the parameter space into regions that pass and fail the criterion function test. Saltelli and Marivoet sample the parameter region using a Monte Carlo method, but analyse the entire model output distribution without restriction.

7.5.2. Physiologically Based Toxicokinetic Model Sensitivity Analysis

Sensitivity analysis has been performed using a variety of techniques in connection with PBTK models. Cohn (1987) performed an analysis using the PBTK model developed for methylene chloride by Andersen et al. (1987). Without any formal parameterization or goodness-of-fit measure, Cohn found a different set of kinetic parameters which fit the mouse data. Although this was called a sensitivity analysis, it addresses the issue of parameter identifiability (Godfrey and DiStefano, 1987). Cohn showed that the methylene chloride model parameters were not uniquely identifiable given the experimental data.

A second type of sensitivity analysis was performed on a tetrachloroethylene PBTK model (Bois et al., 1990). In this study, the correlation between the predicted rate of metabolite formation and each model parameter was evaluated. Bois et al. used this as a measure of sensitivity with the caveat that a high correlation could also be due to parameter covariance and not exclusively a high sensitivity. This approach is consistent with that reviewed by Saltelli and Marivoet (1990). Hetrick et al. (1991) used Latin Hypercube sampling to perform sensitivity analyses on physiologically based toxicokinetic models of styrene, methylchloroform, and methylene chloride. The sensitivity of venous blood concentration and total metabolite production to changes in metabolic and biochemical parameters was investigated. In a preliminary analysis, all the model parameters were allowed to vary, but seven parameters were found to be the most sensitive and only these were used in the final analysis (blood/air partition coefficient, tissue/air partition coefficients, V_{max} and K_m - the Michaelis-Menten metabolism rate constants). PRISM, a Monte Carlo based computer code, provided a ranking of the model input parameters based on their contribution to the model output variability at each time step. Hetrick et al. found that the sensitive model parameters were time, dose, and species dependent.

Through Monte Carlo simulations, Spear et al. (1991) divide the n-dimensional parameter space of a PBTK model into regions that yield simulations which pass or fail an objective function test (criterion function). Sensitivity analysis in this context involves comparing the distributions of the parameters that produce passing and failing simulations. A sensitive model parameter is one that has a significantly different pass-parameter distribution compared to the fail-parameter distribution. The lack of univariate sensitivity does not preclude the possibility that multiple parameter interactions affect the model behaviour.

Gearhart et al. (1993) investigated the effect of partition coefficient parameter variability on tetrachloroethylene dose surrogates. Partition coefficient measurements were made in mouse and human tissues, then the mean and standard deviations were used to perform Monte Carlo simulations. Pearson correlation coefficients were calculated between three dose surrogates and seven model input parameters (pulmonary ventilation, cardiac output, body weight, liver/air partition coefficient, blood/air partition coefficient, liver volume as % of body weight, and slowly perfused tissue volume as % of body weight). They concluded that partition coefficient uncertainty does not significantly increase the variability in risk assessment when PBTK models are incorporated. Although the terms uncertainty and variability are used, in a broader sense, this investigation is a form a sensitivity analysis.

We described the examples above to provide the reader with a starting point for conducting a sensitivity analysis. Consideration should be given to the model output of interest since this greatly affects the identification of sensitive parameters. Furthermore, the method used may affect the ranking of the model parameters and depends largely on the needs and the resources of the investigator.

7.6. DISCUSSION

It has become clear that the Moolgavkar-Venzon-Knudson model and the generalized multistage model will in many cases lead to different conclusions concerning the dose-time-failure relationship in a carcinogenesis problem. These differences can be large and are present above the random fluctuation which must be expected, when only limited data is available for parameter estimation. The uncertainty due to inferring from small samples can be considerable, but using different models for analysis will still have a clear impact on a quantity like the virtually safe dose (VSD). So, before applying a mathematical model, it will be necessary to obtain as much information as possible about the underlying biological process. This is not a basically mathematical or statistical task, but has to rely on essentially biological findings. Biologically based assumptions and modelling approaches will always play a central role in tasks like low-dose approximations, which can only partially be supported by observational data. Statistical methods will be inevitable to optimize the collection of additional knowledge, e.g. by the development of specialised experimental designs, and they will be necessary to assess the type and amount of still remaining uncertainty.

7.7. REFERENCES

Andersen, M. E., Clewell III, H. J., Gargas, M. L., Smith, F. A., and Reitz, R. H. (1987): Physiologically based pharmacokinetics and the risk assessment process for methylene chloride. Toxicol. Appl. Pharmacol. 87, 185-205.

Armitage, P. and Doll, R. (1954): The age distribution of cancer and a multi-stage theory of carcinogenesis. Brit. J. Cancer 8, 1-12.

Atkinson, A.C. (1988): Recent developments in the methods of optimum and related experimental designs. International Statistical Review 56, 99-115.

Atkinson, A.C., Chaloner, K., Herzberg, A.M., and Juritz, J. (1993): Optimum experimental designs for properties of a compartmental design.

Bois, F. Y., Zeise, L., and Tozer, T. N. (1990): Precision and sensitivity of pharmacokinetic models for cancer risk assessment: Tetrachloroethylene in mice, rats, and humans. Toxicol. Appl. Pharmacol. 102, 300-315.

Cairns, T. (1980): The ED_{01} study: Introduction, objectives and experimental design. J. Environ. Pathol. Toxicol. 3, 1-7.

Cohn, M. S. (1987): Sensitivity analysis in pharmacokinetic modeling. In Pharmacokinetics in Risk Assessment, Vol. 8, pp. 265-272. National Academy Press, Washington, D.C.

Crump K.S. and Howe R.B. (1984): The multistage model with a time dependent dose pattern: application to carcinogenic risk assessment, Risk Analysis, 4, 163-176.

Cukier, R. I., Fortuin, C. M., and Shuler, K. E. (1973): Study of the sensitivity of coupled reaction systems to uncertainties in rate coefficients. I theory. The Journal of Chemical Physics 59, 3873-3878.

Drescher, K., Timm, J., Wosniok, W. (1983): Risikoabschätzungen für N-Nitroso-Diethanolamin (NDEIA). In: Beurteilung des Risikos kleiner Dosen von krebserzeugenden Stoffen für den Menschen (Berichte des Umweltbundesamtes 2/83), Erich Schmidt Verlag, Berlin 45-63.

Ford, I., Kitsos, C.P., and Titterington, D.M. (1989): Recent advances in nonlinear experimental design. Technometrics 31, 49-60.

Gart, J.J., Krewski, D., Lee, P.N., Tarone, R.E., and Wahrendorf, J. (1986): Statistical methods in cancer research, vol III: The design and analysis of long-term animal experiments. International Agency for Research on Cancer, Lyon.

Gearhart, J. M., Mahle, D. A., Greene, R. J., Seckel, C. S., Flemming, C. D., Fisher, J. W., and Clewell III, H. J. (1993): Variability of physiologically based pharmacokinetic (PBPK) model parameters and their effects on PBPK model predictions in a risk assessment for perchloroethylene (PCE). Toxicol. Lett. 68, 131-144.

Godfrey, K. R., and DiStefano, J. J. (1987): Identifiability of model parameters. In Identifiability of Parametric Models (E. Walter, Eds.), pp. 1-20. Pergamon Press, Oxford.

Hartley, H.O. and Sielken, R.L. (1977): Estimation of "safe doses" in carcinogenic experiments. Biometrics 33, 1-30.

Hetrick, D. M., Jarabek, A. M., and Travis, C. C. (1991): Sensitivity analysis for physiologically based pharmacokinetic models. J. Pharmacok. Biopharm. 19, 1-20.

Iman, R. L., and Helton, J. C. (1988): An investigation of uncertainty and sensitivity analysis techniques for computer models. Risk Anal. 8, 71-90.

Kennedy, W.J. and Gentle, J.E. (1980): Statistical Computing. Marcel Dekker, New York.

Kitsos, C.P, Titterington, D.M., and Torsney, B. (1988): An optimal design problem in rhythmometry. Biometrics 44, 657-671.

Kitsos, C.P. (1992): Adopting sequential Procedures for biological experiments. In: Müller, W., Wynn, Zhigljavsky (eds.): Model oriented data analysis. Physica-Verlag, 3-9.

Kitsos, C.P., and Müller, C.H. (1995): Robust estimation of non-linear aspects. In: Kitsos, C.P. and Müller, W. (eds.): Model oriented data analysis. Physica-Verlag, 223-233.

Koda, M., McRae, G. J., and Seinfeld, J. H. (1979): Automatic sensitivity analysis of kinetic mechanisms. International Journal of Chemical Kinetics 11, 427-444.

Kopp-Schneider, A., and Portier, J. (1991): Distinguishing between models of carcinogenesis: The role of clonal expansion. Fundamental and Applied Toxicology 17, 601-613.

Krewski, D., Gaylor, D.W. and Lutz, W.K. (1995): Additivity to background and linear extrapolation. In: Olin, S., Farland, W., Park, C., Rhomberg, L., Scheuplein, R., Starr, T and Wilson, J (eds.): Low-dose extrapolation of cancer risks: issues and perspectives. ILSI Press, Washington D.C.

Liepmann, D. (1983): A closed ecosystem model: development and global sensitivity analysis via the Fourier Amplitude Sensitivity Test, M.S. thesis, California Institute of Technology.

Liepmann, D., and Stephanopoulos, G. (1985). Development and global sensitivity analysis of a closed ecosystem model. Ecological Modelling 30, 13-47.

Littlefield, N.A., Farmer, J.H. and Gaylor, D.W. (1980): Effects of dose and time in a long-term, low-dose carcinogenic study. J. Environ. Pathol. Toxicol. 3, 17-34.

McRae, G. J., Tilden, J. W., and Seinfeld, J. H. (1982): Global sensitivity analysis – a computational implementation of the Fourier Amplitude Sensitivity Test (FAST). Computers and Chemical Engineering 6, 15-25.

Moolgavkar, S.H. and Venzon, D.J. (1979): Two-event models for carcinogenesis: Incidence curves for childhood and adult tumors. Math. Biosci. 47, 55-77.

Moolgavkar, S.H. and Knudson, A.G. (1981): Mutation and Cancer: A model for human carcinogenesis. JNCI 66, 1037-1052.

Portier, C. and Hoel, D. (1993): Low-dose-rate extrapolation using the multistage model. Biometrics 39, 897-906.

Portier, C. and Hoel, D. (1984): Design of animal carcinogenicity studies for goodness-of-fit of multistage models. Fundam. Appl. Toxicol. 4, 949-959.

Pukelsheim, F. (1993): Optimal design of experiments. John Wiley and Sons, New York.

Saltelli, A., and Marivoet, J. (1990): Non-parametric statistics in sensitivity analysis for model output: A comparison of selected techniques. Reliability Engineering and System Safety 28, 229-253.

Silvey, S.D. (1980): Optimal Design. Chapman and Hall, London.

Spear, R. C., Bois, F. Y., Woodruff, T., Auslander, D., Parker, J., and Selvin, S. (1991): Modeling benzene pharmacokinetics across three sets of animal data: parametric sensitivity and risk implications. Risk Anal. 11, 641-654.

Tan, W.Y. (1991): Stochastic models of carcinogenesis. Marcel Dekker, New York.

Chapter 8

INFORMATIVE CASE STUDIES

E. G. Luebeck[1], C. Travis[2], and K. Watanabe[2]

[1]Fred Hutchinson Cancer Research Center, Seattle, USA
[2]Tulane University Medical Center, New Orleans, USA

8.1. RADON, CIGARETTE SMOKE, AND LUNG CANCER: THE COLORADO PLATEAU URANIUM MINERS' COHORT

Much of what we know about the interaction of radon and tobacco smoke in the etiology of human lung cancer derives from studies of uranium miners. The Colorado Plateau uranium miners' cohort is one of the oldest and most thoroughly studied cohorts showing the effect of radon exposures on lung cancer incidence in miners. It has also served as one of the first epidemiological data sets where the exact solution of the two-mutation clonal expansion model was employed for the analysis (Moolgavkar et al., 1993). See Chapter 6 for a description of this model and for definitions of the central quantities used in the likelihood analysis of time-to-tumor data. The analysis described here presents an example of the recursive scheme for the computation of tumor probabilities when exposure patterns are piecewise constant (see section 6.5).

The Colorado Plateau miners' cohort consists of 3,346 miners who worked in the mines from 1950-1964. There is detailed information on the pattern of radon and cigarette exposure for each individual in the cohort. This includes the ages at which exposure to radon and cigarette smoke began, the ages at which these exposures stopped, the cumulative exposure to radon in Working Level Months (WLM) and the number of cigarettes smoked per day. In addition, the age at last observation or death was given and whether or not the individual died of lung cancer. A lag period of 3.5 years was assumed between malignant transformation of lung tissue and death from lung cancer. Thus, exposure is only relevant for times up to 3.5 years before death from tumor. With contiguous periods of smoking and/or radon exposure there are up to 5 time intervals for the integration of the cumulative hazard (see section 6.5 and 6.6 for mathematical

Perspectives on Biologically Based Cancer Risk Assessment, edited by Cogliano *et al.*
Kluwer Academic/Plenum Publishers, New York, 1999.

details). A summary of this analysis that also shows the various patterns of exposure is shown in Fig. 8.1.

Because there are very few unexposed (non-smoking) miners in the cohort a simultaneous analysis of the miners cohort together with the British doctors' cohort was conducted. Two distinct dose-response scenarios (referred to as model A and model B) were investigated. Let d_s denote the rate of cigarette exposure in cigarettes per day and d_r the rate of radon exposure on working level months (WLM) per month, then we assume that

$$\nu(d_s, d_r) = a_0 + a_s d_s + a_r d_r,$$

$$\mu(d_s, d_r) = b_0 + b_s d_s + b_r d_r$$

i.e. linear dose-response relationships for the first and second mutation rates, and for the net cell proliferation parameter, $\alpha - \beta$ we assume

$$(\alpha - \beta)(d_s, d_r) = c_0 + c_{s1}(1 - \exp[-c_{s2} d_s]) + c_{r1}(1 - \exp[-c_{r2} d_r])$$

for the Colorado miners' data, and

$$(\alpha - \beta)(d_s) = e_0 + e_{s1}(1 - \exp[-e_{s2} d_s])$$

for the British doctors' data. For both data sets we choose

$$X = 10^7 \quad \text{and} \quad \beta/\alpha = constant,$$

i.e. the number of normal target cells, X, and the ratio of cell death rates and cell birth rates are assumed to be independent of the level of exposure to radon or tobacco smoke. Preliminary analyses showed that $a_0 = b_0$, i.e. the mutation background rates could be assumed to be equal, and $b_s = b_r \simeq 0$, namely the second mutation rate did not show a dose-response to either radon or cigarette smoke. Further, a non-sigmoid saturation in the intermediate cell kinetics was found to give better fits to the data, motivating our choice for $\alpha - \beta$. Model A was then defined by the separate treatment of the cell proliferation in the two cohorts (British doctors and Colorado uranium miners), while Model B assumed that $c_0 = e_0, c_{s1(2)} = e_{s1(2)}$, equating the dose-response to tobacco smoke for the cell proliferation in the two cohorts. The observed and expected number of tumors for the various exposure patterns are shown in Fig. 8.1 for the miners cohort.

In conclusion we find no indication that radon and tobacco smoke interact on the level of the cell, i.e. additional terms proportional to $d_s \times d_r$ in the above parameter functions did not improve the fits significantly. Despite this, the relative risk of joint exposure is somewhere between additive and multiplicative. We also find no indication that radon or tobacco smoke affect the second mutation rate, consistent with our earlier findings in rats exposed to radon (Moolgavkar et al. 1990b) and, for cigarette smoke, in the British doctors' cohort (Moolgavkar et al. 1989). Tar in tobacco smoke contains mutagens that may require metabolic activation. If intermediate cells lose the capacity for metabolic activation, then tobacco smoke is not expected to increase the second mutation rate.

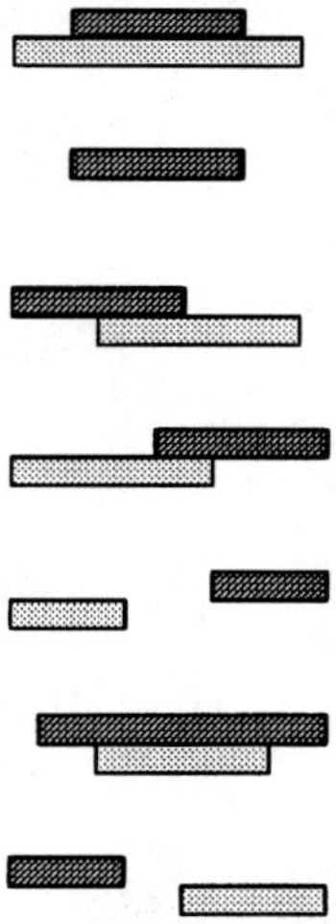

Group	Exposure profile	No. of miners	No. of lung cancer deaths		
			observed	Model A	Model B
I. no exposure		8	0	.0084	.0046
II. Radon Tobacco smoke		2224	235	237.1	234.4
III. Radon Tobacco smoke		477	13	16.04	12.03
IV. Radon Tobacco smoke		116	15	15.25	16.02
V. Radon Tobacco smoke		118	20	14.18	12.72
VI. Radon Tobacco smoke		159	8	8.17	6.10
VII. Radon Tobacco smoke		19	3	0.71	0.68
VIII. Radon Tobacco smoke		11	0	0.53	0.40
Total		3132	294	292.0	282.4

Figure 8.1: *Schematic representation of patterns of exposure. Length of bars does not represent actual duration of exposure. In each category the number of miners, the observed number of lung cancer deaths and the expected numbers generated by models A and B are shown. See text for more details*

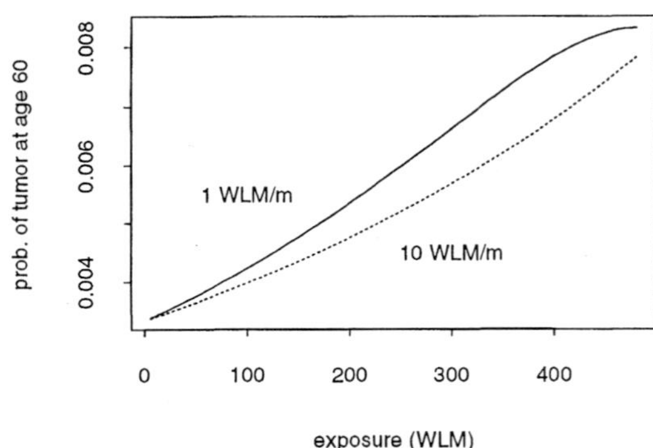

Figure 8.2: *The inverse dose-rate effect with radon. The probability of tumor at a specific age is plotted against total exposure for two exposure rate regimen.*

Intriguing is the prediction of an inverse dose-rate effect, i.e. fractionation of a given total dose of radon increases the life time risk of tumor (see Fig. 8.2). In the two-mutation clonal expansion model this effect can be attributed to the difference in weight between duration of exposure and exposure rate. For a given total exposure the duration of exposure is more important for the probability of tumor than equivalent increases in the rate of exposure.

8.2. MODELING COLON CANCER

Recent laboratory work suggests that a number of specific genetic changes are associated with colon carcinogenesis (for a comprehensive overview, see Cavanee and White (1995)). Here we will demonstrate that either two or three rate-limiting steps are sufficient to explain the incidence of colon cancer in the general population and among polyposis cases. However, based upon the particular estimates of the transformation parameters a three stage model seems to agree better with the experimental evidence. Moreover, the comparison of the incidence curves from sporadic and polyposis cases suggests that a mutation at the Familial Adenomatous Polyposis (FAP) locus may not be one of the rate-limiting steps on the pathway to colon cancer. In other words, the occurrence of colon cancer in FAP subjects does not appear to follow the retinoblastoma paradigm as postulated by Knudson (Knudson, 1971) for the embryonal cancer retinoblastoma.

In order to test the assumptions of biological models for colon cancer, we analyzed two distinct data sets: Colon cancer incidence rates among the general population of Birmingham, England from 1968-1972, and data on patients with FAP, who were diagnosed with colon cancer at Saint Mark's Hospital in London, England, between 1925 and 1965. The latter data were taken from a publication by Ashley (1969). Fig.8.3

shows the observed colon cancer incidence as a function of age for the Birmingham data together with fitted curves from the Armitage-Doll model and the 2-(or 3-) mutation model. Details of the analyses presented here are covered in depth in Moolgavkar and Luebeck (1992).

8.2.1. How Many Rate-limiting Events for Colon Cancer?

The Armitage-Doll model (see Chapter 5 for a description) can be used to obtain an upper bound on the number of rate-limiting steps involved since it does not consider the clonal expansion of intermediate cells. By fitting the formula $I(t) = ct^k$ to the age-specific incidence rates of colon cancer per year per 10^5 males in Birmingham, England, we obtain the parameter estimates $\hat{c} = 4 \times 10^{-2}$ and $\hat{k} = 4.54$. Since in the Armitage-Doll model k equals one less than the number of rate-limiting steps required for malignant transformation, the estimate of k suggests that maximally 5 or 6 steps are required for malignancy. Further, the estimate of $\hat{c}$ allows us to compute the individual mutation rates λ (in the notation used earlier: $c = 10^5 N\lambda_0 \cdots \lambda_{n-1}$, where N is the number of stem cells in the colon). They are 2 to 3 orders of magnitude higher than measured mutation rates in specific loci, which are typically around $10^{-7} - 10^{-8}$ per cell division. We conclude that incidence data alone (without further biological information) are not sufficient to estimate the number of rate-limiting genetic events that are necessary for tumor formation. What, however, are the consequences of assuming a smaller number of rate-limiting steps (2 or 3) together with the capacity of intermediate cells to proliferate? For simplicity, as was done for the analysis with the Armitage-Doll model, we will assume that mutation rates are the same for all compartments. Let us denote the mutation rates into the *ith* compartment by μ_i, then our assumption translates into $\mu_1 = \mu_2$ for the two-mutation model and $\mu_1 = \mu_2 = \mu_3$ for the three-mutation model.

The two- and three-mutation models provide excellent fits to the general incidence data displayed in Fig.8.3. However, the two-mutation model predicts a mutation rate that is around 3×10^{-10} *per cell division*, a rate that seems too low for a specific locus mutation ($\sim 10^{-7} - 10^{-8}$), unless a mutation at a particular subsite (for instance at the codon level) is required. The estimates of the mutation rates ($\mu_1 = \mu_2 = \mu_3$) are approximately 2 orders of magnitude higher than the ones found for the two-mutation model, therefore are more in line with experimental values. Interestingly, we did not find an increase in the net cell proliferation rate of the first stage, i.e. $\alpha_1 - \beta_1 \simeq 0$, while $\alpha_2 - \beta_2 \simeq 0.1$ per cell per year for the second (penultimate) stage. The parameter estimates of fitting the two- and three-mutation model to the Birmingham data are summarized in Table 8.1.

Thus, a three-mutation model gives a consistent description of the colon cancer data and is more in tune with biological facts than a two-mutation model. Yet, it is not clear which gene loci should be identified with the postulated rate-limiting events. Consistently, $p53$ mutations are found in colon carcinoma, and this gene seems clearly involved. However, the DCC (Deleted in Colon Cancer) gene is also frequently mutated in colon cancer, but is believed to play a role only later during tumor progression.

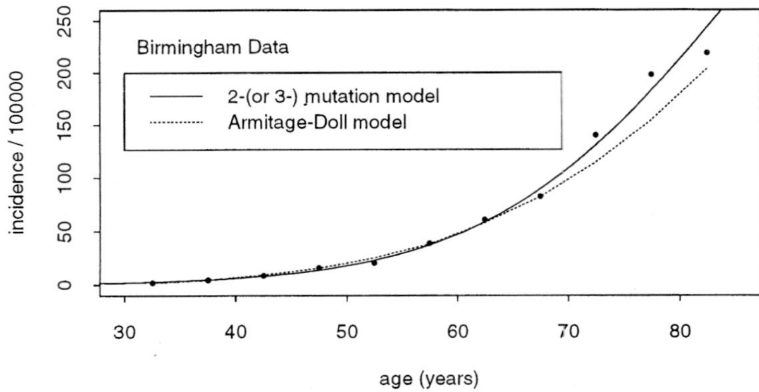

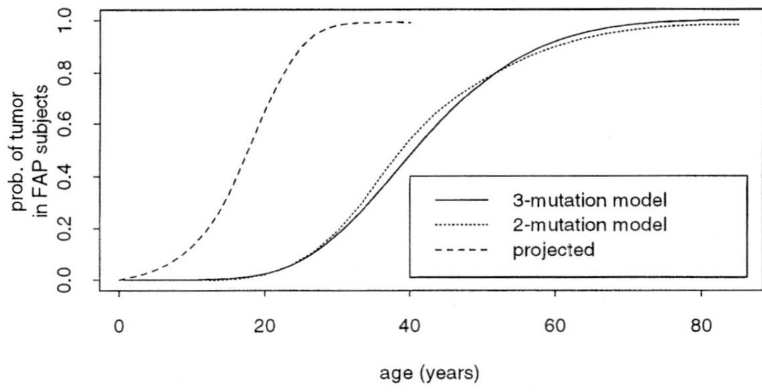

Figure 8.3: *Upper panel: Annual age-specific incidence rates of colon cancer among males in Birmingham, England (shown by bullets) together with the annual age-specific incidence curves generated by the Armitage-Doll model (dashed line) and by the two- and three-mutation models (solid line). The curves generated by the latter two models are indistinguishable. Lower panel: The probability of developing colon cancer by a given age, as predicted by the two- and three-mutation models plotted against age. Solid line to the lower right represents the predicted probability in the male population of Birmingham. For this population, the predictions made by the two models are virtually identical. Solid line and dashed line in the middle represent the probabilities of colon cancer in the FAP patients that are predicted by the three- and two-mutation models, respectively. They are very similar. The curve labeled P denotes the conjectured probability of developing colon cancer in polyposis subjects patients if inheritance of the polyposis gene were equivalent to inheriting one of the rate-limiting mutations in a three-mutation model.*

Two-mutation model				
estimates	$\mu_1 = \mu_2$	$\alpha - \beta$	β/α	
males	3×10^{-8}	0.107	0.999	
females	3.1×10^{-8}	0.108	0.999	
Three-mutation model				
estimates	$\mu_1 = \mu_2 = \mu_3$	$\alpha_1 - \beta_1$	$\alpha_2 - \beta_2$	$\beta_1/\alpha_1 = \beta_2/\alpha_2$
males	4.8×10^{-6}	~ 0	0.106	0.929
females	4.6×10^{-6}	~ 0	0.112	0.963

Table 8.1: *Estimates of parameters for the two- and three-mutation models fitted to incidence rates of colon cancer in the general population of Birmingham, England.*

Two-mutation model				
estimates	$\mu_1 = \mu_2$	$\alpha - \beta$	β/α	
	4.5×10^{-7}	0.207	0.998	
Three-mutation model				
estimates	$\mu_1 = \mu_2 = \mu_3$	$\alpha_1 - \beta_1$	$\alpha_2 - \beta_2$	$\beta_1/\alpha_1 = \beta_2/\alpha_2$
	2.6×10^{-5}	~ 0	0.307	0.954

Table 8.2: *Results of fitting the two- and three-mutation models to incidence rates of colon cancer in polyposis patients. Data were taken from the table in Ashley [ref]*

Certain $p53$-mutations are known to lead to transdominant loss of the wild-type allele and, hence, a three-mutation model would be sufficient to explain the loss of function in both, the DCC gene, and the $p53$ tumor suppressor gene. These considerations are speculative, but are based on hypotheses generated from the model.

8.2.2. Analysis of Colon Cancer Data in Patients with FAP

FAP is a dominantly inherited condition, the locus of which has been mapped to chromosome 5q. The gene isolated that appears to cause FAP is commonly referred to as the APC gene. People who inherit the mutated APC gene develop hundreds of adenomatous polyps in their colon and rectum. These polyps are quite generally thought of as benign precursor lesions that enormously increase the risk for developing colon carcinoma. Our analysis suggests that by age 45 years, a person with FAP is approximately 700 times more likely to get colon cancer than a person in the general population (see Fig.8.3).

The role of the APC gene can be modeled in two ways. First, if a mutation in the APC gene represents a necessary step toward malignancy, then it should be possible to fit the FAP incidence data with one stage less than the number of stages employed for fitting the Birmingham data. It should be possible to do this without much change in the parameters that describe the common somatic events that lead to colon cancer. However, this approach does not give a satisfactory fit to the FAP data as can be seen from Fig.8.3. The curve labeled P represents the conjectured age-specific probability of tumor if the inheritance of the FAP gene were equivalent to inheriting one of the rate-limiting steps in the three-mutation model. It predicts that 80% of the FAP subjects would develop colon cancer by age 20, a percentage that is considered much too high.

An alternative explanation for the role of the APC gene is to think of the APC gene as a promoter gene, that is, to assume that it increases cell proliferation of intermediate cells (especially of cells in compartment 2 of the three-mutation model). This effectively may lead to the increase of the mutation rates as seen by the estimates of μ presented in Table 8.1 and 8.2.

In summary, our analyses suggest a common pathway to colon cancer in the general population and in patients with polyposis coli. This pathway would involve the same three mutations in both, the difference being increased cell proliferation due to a mutation in the polyposis gene. The increase in symmetric stem cell divisions would also explain the concomitant increase in the mutation rates as estimated from the data.

8.3. QUANTITATIVE ANALYSIS OF ENZYME ALTERED FOCI (EAF)

8.3.1. Effects of PCBs on the Initiation and Promotion of EAF

The first example here is the analysis of an initiation and promotion experiment with DEN as initiator and a number of PCB congeners as promoters (Luebeck et al., 1991). The protocol is shown schematically in Fig. 8.4. There were two sacrifice points, the first 1 week after stop of promotion, the second 8 weeks later. From the data we were able to estimate the net cell proliferation parameter $\alpha - \beta$ during promotion and after promotion together with the corresponding ratios β/α, measuring the extinction of initiated cells. Focal transections were stained for 2 distinct marker enzymes (ATPase and GGT) on two adjacent sections. Three distinct phenotypes were defined according to whether foci were predominantly ATPase negative (class 1), predominantly GGT positive (class 2) or showed both changes concomitantly (class 3). Table 8.3 lists the estimated parameters together with their standard errors for class 1. All the investigated PCB congeners were found to be strong promoters. Class 3 lesions (results not shown here), showing both enzyme alterations, were found to proliferate significantly faster under promotion compared to class 1 or class 2 lesions. Furthermore, the probability of extinction, as measured by the ratio β/α, was strongly reduced for foci in class 3. No promoter induced spontaneous initiation by the examined congeners was detected.

8.3.2. Effects of Chronic Administration of N-nitrosomorpholine on Liver EAF and Hepatocellular Carcinoma (HCC)

When one group of animals is monitored for premalignant lesions and another, independent, group for malignant lesions, the joint analysis is rather straightforward. We illustrate by means of an example.

The data in this example are from an experiment in which a group of female Lewis rats were administered NNM in their drinking water in different concentrations (0, 0.1, 1, 5, 10, 20, 40, 80 parts per million (ppm)). The animals receiving the highest dose (80 ppm) were not considered further because of toxicity. Animals from each dose

Estimates of Promotion Parameters				
	ATPase dominant			
compound	$\alpha_1 - \beta_1$	$\alpha_2 - \beta_2$	β_1/α_1	β_2/α_2
corn oil	$.0286 \pm .0030$	-	$.968 \pm .011$	-
4-MCBP	$.0433 \pm .0066$	$-.0021 \pm .0037$	$.965 \pm .013$	$1.300 \pm .150$
2,2',4,5'-TCBP	$.0592 \pm .0061$	$.0024 \pm .0026$	$.829 \pm .061$	$.998 \pm .002$
3,3',4,4'-TCBP	$.0587 \pm .0056$	$.0214 \pm .0019$	$.769 \pm .077$	$.898 \pm .045$
3-MC	$.0552 \pm .0061$	$.0090 \pm .0027$	$.872 \pm .044$	$.995 \pm .003$
Estimates of Initiation Parameters				
all	ATPase dominant		$\nu_o X$	$\nu_1 X$
			5963 ± 1800	6.8 ± 1.8

Table 8.3: *Maximum likelihood estimates (m.l.e.) and standard errors (s.e.) for the listed PCB compounds for ATPase dominant foci (class 1). On each of the time intervals, $I_1 = (0, t_1)$ during the treatment and $I_2 = (t_1, t_2)$ after the treatment ended until sacrifice the likelihood can be expressed in terms of the net proliferation parameters $\alpha_i - \beta_i$ and the ratios of cell death to cell division rates: β_i/α_i, $i = 1, 2$ (see Fig. 8.4). The parameter $\nu_o X$ represents the number of cells altered by the DEN treatment per ml of liver and $\nu_1 X$ the number of spontaneously altered cells per ml per day during the experiment.*

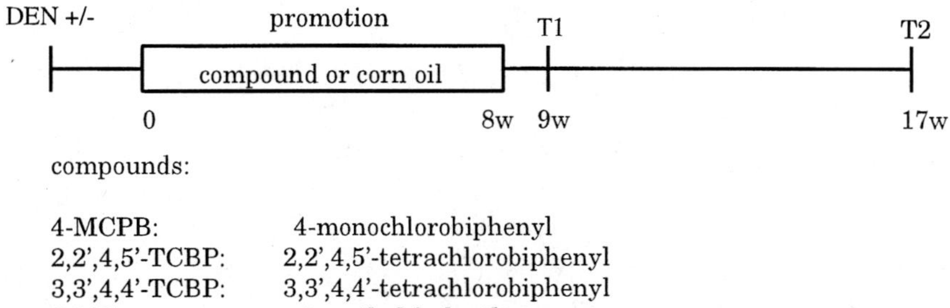

Figure 8.4: *Experimental protocol for the PCB experiment by Buchmann et al. (1991). DEN was administered for 10 consecutive days. Animals were killed at 9 or 17 weeks after the start of promoter treatment. See Luebeck et al. (1991) for more details.*

group were periodically killed, and their livers examined for ATPase deficient foci. The number of observed transections per section area and the size (area) of each transection were recorded. From each dose group some animals were followed until death, and their livers examined for the presence or absence of HCC. For the statistical analysis of the data, the malignant tumors were considered to be fatal. Among 107 animals followed in this way, there were 38 malignant tumors.

The analysis of the foci data follows section 6.7 and was first reported in Moolgavkar et al. (1990a). For the joint analysis discussed here, we assume a linear dose-response in the net cell proliferation rate and the first mutation rate, i.e. $\alpha-\beta = a+b\times d$ and $\nu X = \nu_o X + \nu_1 X \times d$. The second mutation rate $\mu = \mu_o + \mu_1 d$, but μ_1 is estimated in this analysis to be zero. We assume that only surface cells undergo cell division while interior cells are resting. This assumption needs elaboration: In the original foci analysis, all the cells in an ATPase deficient focus were assumed to have the same probability of division (volume growth model: m, the number of cells in a particular clone is given by the ratio of clone volume to cell volume, i.e. $m = (r/r_c)^3$). In fact, there is probably a great deal of heterogeneity among the cells of a focus, and there is evidence that, at least in large foci, cells close to the surface are more likely to divide (Buchmann et al., 1994). We have made an attempt to incorporate heterogeneity by assuming that only cells on the surface of foci undergo division (i.e. we assume $m = \pi(r/r_c)^2$). This is undoubtedly an oversimplification, but it fits the data better than the assumption of homogeneity within foci. Each animal whose liver was examined for altered foci contributes to the likelihood as described in section 6.7. Each animal that was followed until death makes one of two contributions to the total likelihood. If the animal had a malignant liver tumor, then the contribution is the density function for the time-to-tumor distribution derived from the two-mutation clonal expansion model, $P'(t)$. If the animal died without malignant tumor, then the contribution is the probability of no malignant tumor by the time of death derived from the same model, $1-P(t)$. The total likelihood is the product of likelihood contributions from all animals, and is a function of all the parameters of the model. These parameters were estimated by maximizing the likelihood.

The results of the analysis are summarized in Table 8.4. They show that NNM affects the first mutation rate, i.e., increases the rate at which normal hepatocytes acquire the ATPase deficient phenotype, and also increases the net proliferation rate of altered foci. However, no effect of NNM on the second mutation rate was observed. The asymptotic probability of extinction, β/α, is high, 98.6%.

In a previous publication (Moolgavkar et al., 1990a) we had concluded that NNM was a strong initiator and a weak promoter. The joint analysis shown here (using the surface growth model) yields the same conclusion. Both, the rate of initiation and the net rate of proliferation of initiated cells, are consistent with a linear increase with dose of NNM. As noted earlier, the second mutation rate appears to be independent of dose of NNM. Moreover, the background rate of the second mutation is estimated to be about 8×10^{-10} per cell per day. This appears to be far too low a number. One interpretation within the framework of the model is that only a small subset of ATPase deficient foci is made up of truly initiated cells. Our estimate of the second mutation

Parameter	Estimate	95% C.I.
a	.00543	(.0048, .0062)
b	.00018	(.00016, .0002)
β/α	.986	(.982, .990)
$\nu_o X$	4.18	(3.08, 5.66)
$\nu_1 X$	8.06	(6.74, 9.65)
$\mu_o \times 10^{10}$	8.0	(5.70, 11.2)

Table 8.4: *Parameter estimates and their confidence intervals (C.I.) for the N-nitrosomorpholine (NNM) example using the surface growth model. Net cell proliferation rate defined as $\alpha - \beta = a + bd$, and first transformation rate per ml liver defined as $\nu = \nu_o + \nu_1 d$, where d is the dose in ppm. Unit of time is days.*

rate is based on the assumption that all ATPase deficient cells are equally likely to go on to malignancy. Another explanation of this finding is that malignant cells too have a large probability of extinction so that our estimate of the second mutation rate represents a lower bound only.

Based upon the assumed linearity of the dose-response a simple definition of initiation and promotion potencies can be given readily by the ratio of the slope and the corresponding intercept. This ratio is given per unit dose. For our NNM example we get (per *ml* liver)

$$\nu X(d) = 4.18 + 8.06\, d$$

$$\Rightarrow \text{initiation potency} \quad = 1.93\ /ppm$$

and similarly for the net cell proliferation parameter $(\alpha - \beta)$

$$(\alpha - \beta)(d) = .00543 + .00018\, d$$

$$\Rightarrow \text{promotion potency} \quad = 0.033\ /ppm$$

This result may lead to the conclusion that NNM is a strong initiator but only a weak promoter. However, the promotional effect of NNM may still be important since intermediate cell clones grow exponentially under the model while newly initiated cells accrue only linearly over time. Thus, sooner or later, the promotional effects will dominate the tumor risk.

8.4. THE ROLE OF CELL PROLIFERATION IN URINARY BLADDER CARCINOGENESIS

Cohen and colleagues (Cohen et al., 1991; Cohen and Ellwein, 1993) have thoroughly studied the tumor promoting effects of Sodium Saccharin, Sodium Ascorbate and related acids in rat bladder. These compounds have been shown to be non-genotoxic, but administered after initiation with N-[4-(5-nitro-2-furyl)-2-thiazolyl]formamide (FANFT), nitrosamines or MNU show increased tumor response.

Another interesting finding is the synergy between genotoxicity and non-genotoxic effects of FANFT, as demonstrated by Cohen and colleagues in the male rat bladder. FANFT is a classical genotoxic bladder carcinogen in a variety of animals. It is metabolically activated to an intermediate that binds directly to DNA leading to DNA damage. At higher doses, however, FANFT also stimulates urothelial cell proliferation, causing bladder tumors to appear within one year, while at lower dose (less than 0.01% in the diet) no tumors were produced within 2 years. No evidence for a threshold in the genotoxicity of FANFT was apparent since the its metabolites continued to be present in the urine of the animals even at low doses. This observation is readily explained in the framework of the two-mutation clonal expansion model. While at higher doses FANFT is both initiating and promoting, at the lower doses it ceases to promote. Indeed, labeling index data in the rat bladder indicate a threshold in the cell proliferation response to FANFT. The observed effects on bladder tumor prevalence in male F344 rats was modeled explicitly and described quantitatively by Cohen and Ellwein. Their model is briefly described in Chapter 6. According to these authors, it would be erroneous to describe the no-effect level of FANFT exposure as a true threshold since tumors would eventually be picked up if the animals were followed up long enough. This fact is of importance for species extrapolation. Scaling time to human life spans could possibly result in an increased lifetime tumor probability.

The absence of promoting activity at low doses of FANFT can be substituted by a non-genotoxic promoter. When 5% Sodium Saccharin is given together with 0.005% FANFT in the diet, a carcinogenic effect is seen in the rat bladder, whereas no effect is observed when these compounds are given separately.

In contrast to the mechanism of action described for FANFT, it has been shown that certain non-genotoxic agents that cause calculus formation in the bladder, such as uracil, melamine and calcium oxalate, cause bladder tumors when given at high enough doses. At lower doses, however, no calculus production is observed in the urine and no tumors are scored. Since these substances are non-genotoxic, the no-effect threshold constitutes a true threshold phenomenon in contrast to the 'pseudo-threshold' observed for FANFT.

These examples show the importance of a distinction between genotoxic (initiating, transforming) and non-genotoxic (promoting) agents. While genotoxic agents are thought of leading necessarily to increased tumor rates, the concomitant or subsequent action of a promoting agent may lead to a drastic acceleration of the tumor rates, giving rise to a pseudo-threshold. However, promoting agents alone may be sufficient to increase the probability of tumor, if they cause an increase in cell division rates. Cell proliferation that works through an inhibition of apoptosis should not show such an increase. Thus, compounds that are mitogenic at higher doses and lead to an accumulation of DNA replication errors may be safe at lower levels where cell proliferation mechanisms are inactive.

8.5. N-NITROSOMORPHOLINE: COMPARISON OF MULTISTAGE MODEL AND TWO-EVENT CLONAL EXPANSION MODEL

It is of interest to see the differences in risk or potency estimates that arise from the use of different risk models. Of particular interest is the question of how simultaneous information on premalignant lesions, such as EAF, alter the conclusions drawn from classical risk assessment procedures using, for example, the linearized multistage model. For the purpose of low-dose extrapolation, within a given animal species, the inclusion of precursor lesions on the pathway to cancer is of great importance. Precursors may act as a magnifying glass for the low dose region of an experiment, showing dose related effects long before malignant tumors can be detected.

Potency estimates (in terms of ED10s) for exposure to NNM have been derived (U.S. EPA) using the studies by Ketkar et al. (1983) and Lijinski et al. (1988). The Ketkar study showed that NNM induced a statistically significant increase in respiratory and digestive tumors in male in female Syrian golden hamsters, while the Lijinski study showed that NNM increases the incidence in liver tumors in female F344 rats. However no measurements on EAF were taken in the study of Lijinski et al. (1988) that could be incorporated into a risk assessment of NNM. The NNM study of Schwarz et al. (1989), while much smaller in terms of animals per dose group, and using a different strain of rat (female Lewis rats), also gathered information on EAF in select animals. Other animals (in all dose groups combined, 107) were kept alive until they died of malignant liver tumor (38 of them), or from other causes. Even though the number of animals used in Schwarz's NNM study is much smaller than in Lijinski's study, an internal comparison of risk estimates obtained from different models may give important insights.

The dose at 10% excess risk (ED10) is derived from maximum likelihood estimates of parameters associated with specific cancer models. Usually, no estimate of an upper confidence bound for the computed risk is used for ED10. However, the uncertainty of such estimates should be dealt with even when risk levels are only moderately low, since the size of the experiment, in terms of number of animals and dose groups used, and other factors of heterogeneity, can have a strong impact on these estimates.

Several approaches can be taken to construct the likelihood. If the information on the times of death from tumor is ignored, as is often the case, then the tumors are grouped together and analyzed using a binomial likelihood with mean $nP(d)$, if there are n animals in the group given dose d. This, however, would only approximate the true likelihood provided the animals developed incidental (non-fatal) tumors. If the tumors are fatal, the probability density of tumor (see section 6.3), must be used instead. Even when tumors are considered incidental, the survival times provide important information that should be included in the analysis.

Let us compute ED10 for the NNM data by Schwarz et al. (1989) using (a) the multistage model, assuming that the probability of tumor is given by

$$P(t, d) = 1 - \exp[(a_o + a_1 d + a_2 d^2) t^n],$$

and (b) using $P(t, d)$ derived from the two-mutation clonal expansion model (section 6.3) with and without foci information. The excess risk, $R(t, d)$ is defined as

nominal dose	no. of animals	no. of HCC observed	multi stage model Armitage-Doll	2-mutation model without foci	2-mutation model with foci
0. ppm	24	1	.35	.39	.48
.1 ppm	28	0	.51	.67	.76
1. ppm	12	0	.30	.36	.66
5. ppm	11	7	5.7	4.8	3.5
10. ppm	13	11	17.1	13.5	8.7
20. ppm	9	9	9.9	8.6	9.7
40. ppm	10	10	4.1	9.7	14.1

Table 8.5: *NNM experiment (Schwarz et al., 1989), excluding animals sacrificed for EAF. The group given 80 ppm is excluded from this analysis because of strong toxicity. Expected values are computed using the cumulative hazard function.*

$$R(t,d) = \frac{P(t,d) - P(t,0)}{1 - P(t,0)}.$$

A short summary of the frequency (observed and expected) of hepatocellular carcinoma (HCC) in the different dose groups of this experiment is shown in Table 8.5. As in the previous section, we assume that the liver tumors of interest (in this case hepatocellular carcinomas) are fatal. In addition, we study the behavior of the tumor probability when information on time of death is ignored in the likelihood construct (binomial analysis). Results of this comparison are shown in Fig. 8.5 for the lifetime excess risk. Lifetime of the animals is assumed to be 2 years.

The shapes of the curves shown in Fig. 8.5 vary widely. While the two-mutation model yields approximately linear slopes at low doses the multistage model shows quadratic behavior. It is perhaps surprising that the two-mutation model still gives a linear dose-response, even when the foci are not included in the analysis. It should be noted, however, that the uncertainty in the risk estimate is much greater in this case.

ED10s, expressed in nominal dose of NNM concentration, vary from 0.3 to somewhat over 2 ppm, depending on model and analysis used. The curve for the excess risk for HCC in the 100 week exposure group used in the study by Lijinski et al. (1988) coincides with the corresponding curve for the Schwarz study. The ED10 values for both studies, based upon a grouped data analysis, lie near 2 ppm. As mentioned above, this type of analysis ignores the individual survival times of the animals. If the survival times are taken into account, the risk curve changes dramatically (multistage model, based on incidence versus grouped data analysis). Still there is very little agreement between these curves and the one obtained by using the two-mutation model, with foci included, except that they cross each other near the ED10 dose. At very low risk ($< 10^{-3}$), the discrepancy between multistage model and the biologically motivated two-mutation model becomes more pronounced because the estimate of the linear term in the excess risk for the multistage model is very small. Thus, the two-mutation model would give a more conservative 'safe dose' estimate in this case.

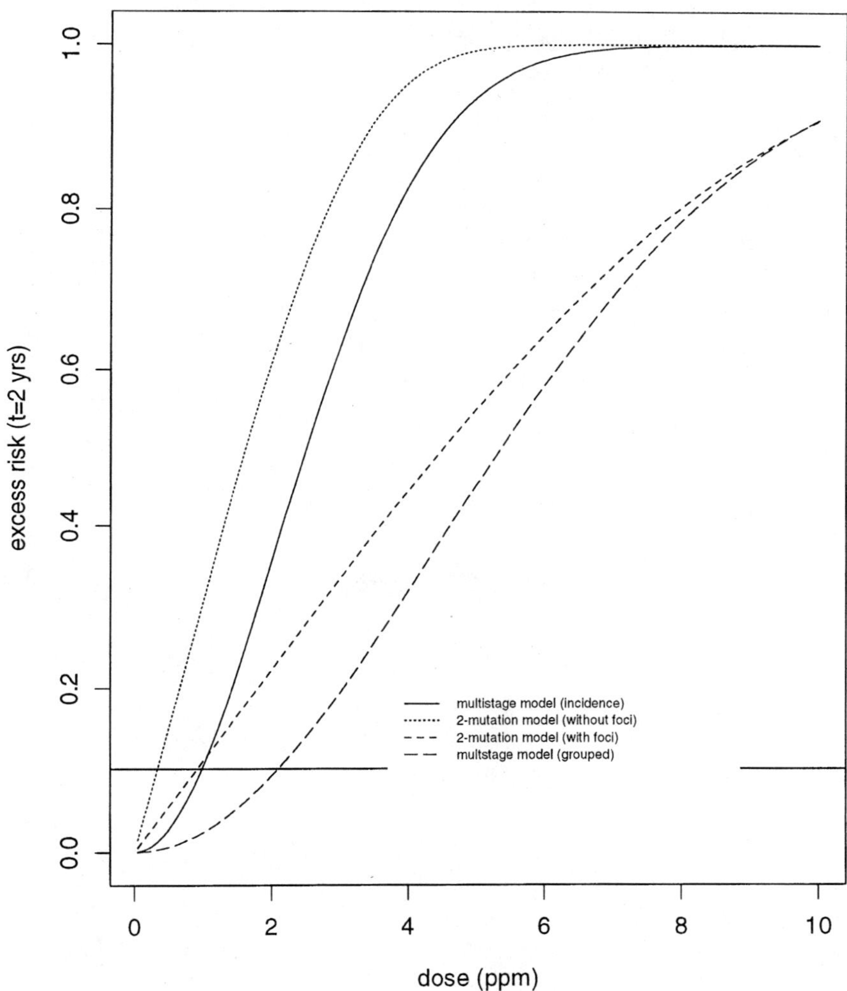

Figure 8.5: *Comparison of excess risks from multistage model and two-mutation model. Data are from the NNM experiment by Schwarz et al. (1989). See text for details.*

8.6. CALCULATION OF TETRACHLOROETHYLENE RISK ESTIMATES

In this section we calculate human unit risks from the exposure of mice to tetrachloroethylene (PCE). Three approaches are taken with the first two utilizing the multistage model and the third incorporating the two-stage model. In the first example, we use the administered dose. Next, we calculate risks based on the target tissue dose predicted by a physiologically based toxicokinetic model. Finally, in a biologically-based risk assessment we use the PBTK model and the two-stage model to predict human risks.

8.6.1. Classical Risk Assessment Methodology

8.6.1.1. Interspecies Extrapolation The first step in the classical risk assessment approach is the choice of an appropriate measure of equivalent carcinogenic dose in mice and humans. Equivalent dose can be expressed in terms of a concentration per medium or quantity per animal body weight. In this example, we use equivalent doses in terms of mg/kg body weight and mg/m^2 surface area.

8.6.1.2. Dose-Response Relation in Animals In its Guidelines for Carcinogen Risk Assessment (Federal Register, 1986) , the United States Environmental Protection Agency (EPA) suggests that the cancer incidence at the most statistically sensitive tumor site in the most sensitive animal species and strain should be used as the basis for estimations of human risk. Thus, for tetrachloroethylene, the EPA indicates that risk estimates should be based on dose-response data for hepatocellular carcinomas in female B6C3F1 mice resulting from inhalation exposure.

In accordance with the assumption that there is no threshold of carcinogenic response and that dose-response is linear in the low-dose range, we used a linearized, multistage model, GLOBAL83 (Howe, 1983), to compute the dose response curve. GLOBAL83 calculates the dose-response relation for carcinogens by the formula

$$P(d) = 1 - \exp(-q_0 - q_1 d - q_2 d^2). \tag{8.1}$$

Thus, incremental cancer risk can be defined as

$$F(d) = \frac{P(d) - P(0)}{1 - P(0)} = 1 - \exp(-q_1 d - q_2 d^2). \tag{8.2}$$

From this, the model derives q_u, the 95% upper bound for the linear slope, q_1. At low doses, the upper bound risk, R, can be predicted by $q_u d$, where d is the measure of dose. The first step in the process is to estimate the administered doses in the inhalation study of B6C3F1 mice (National Toxicology Program, 1986).

Mice in the NTP study were exposed to 100 and 200 ppm, 6 h/day, 5 days/week, for 104 weeks. A 100 ppm exposure concentration can be converted to administered dose according to equation (8.3).

$$\frac{100\text{mol PCE}}{10^6\text{mol air}} \times \frac{165.8\text{g/mol PCE}}{24.45/\text{mol air}} \times \frac{1000\text{mg}}{1\text{g}} \times 0.0315\frac{\text{L}}{\text{min}} \times 360\frac{\text{min}}{\text{day}} \times \frac{1}{0.032\text{kg}} \tag{8.3}$$

	Administered Dose (ppm)[a]	Number of Animals[a]	Tumor Bearing Animals[a]	Administered Dose LAE (mg/kg/day)	Body Weight Extrapolation		Surface Area Extrapolation	
					q_u	Human Risk	q_u	Human Risk
Males	0	49	7	0				
	100	49	25	152.4	3.3×10^{-3}	6.3×10^{-7}	4.1×10^{-2}	7.8×10^{-6}
	200	50	26	304.8				
Females	0	48	1	0				
	100	50	13	159.4	2.7×10^{-3}	5.1×10^{-7}	3.6×10^{-2}	6.8×10^{-6}
	200	50	36	318.8				

[a] Source: National Toxicology Program (1986)

Table 8.6: *Overall tumor incidence data, potency estimates for B6C3F1 mice exposed to PCE by inhalation, and human risk estimates for exposure to 1 $\mu g/m^3$ PCE.*

$$= 240.3 \text{mg/kg/day}$$

Here we are assuming a ventilation rate of 0.0315 L/min for a mouse weighing 0.032 kg. When experimental exposure conditions are not continuous over the lifetime of the animal, the EPA risk estimates are based on a lifetime average exposure (LAE). Assuming a lifespan of 112 weeks, the following conversion applies (U.S. Environmental Protection Agency, 1985):

$$240.3 \frac{\text{mg}}{\text{kg} \cdot \text{day}} \times \frac{5\text{days}}{7\text{days}} \times \frac{104\text{weeks}}{112\text{weeks}} = 159.4 \frac{\text{mg}}{\text{kg} \cdot \text{day}} \text{LAE}. \tag{8.4}$$

Table 8.6 presents the potency, q_u, for the LAE doses administered to male and female mice. The q_u values in column 5 are calculated assuming mg/kg body weight provides the best measure of equivalent dose, and the values in column 7 are based on surface area as the measure of equivalent dose.

8.6.1.3. Calculation of Administered Dose in Humans In assessing the risk to humans exposed to a particular compound, United States regulators calculate the human risk that results from exposure to a standard unit of concentration, $1\mu g$ of compound inhaled per m^3 of air breathed in. Use of this standard unit of exposure concentration allows comparison of risk from one compound with the risks produced by exposure to other compounds. The risk due to human exposure to $1\mu g$ of a compound per m^3 of air is known as the *unit risk.*

In order to calculate the unit risk of PCE, we must begin by calculating the administered dose to humans (in units of mg/kg/day) that results from exposure to the unit concentration of $1\mu g/m^3$. We estimate it as the product of the exposure concentration and daily air intake divided by human body weight. Since not all inhaled air is available for gas exchange in the lungs, the alveolar ventilation rate is used instead of the total ventilation rate. The estimated administered dose associated with human exposure to

$1\mu g/m^3$ of PCE in air is

$$D = (1\mu g/m^3)(13.4m^3/day)(1/70kg)(1 \times 10^{-3}mg/\mu g)$$

$$= 1.9 \times 10^{-4}mg/kg/day$$

where 13.4 m^3/day is the daily alveolar ventilation rate of a 70 kg person based on a daily air intake of 20 m^3/day. This calculation also assumes 100% absorption of the compound. In actual situations, the percentage of compound absorbed would decrease with length of exposure due to saturation of the blood's ability to take up additional chemical (Bolanowska and Golacka, 1972). As a result, this method of dose calculation overestimates actual human exposure. PBTK models can account for this phenomena in a more realistic fashion.

8.6.1.4. Classical Calculation of Human Risk This estimation of administered dose can now be used with the potencies (q_u) to compute the human risk due to exposure to 1 $\mu g/m^3$ of PCE in air (see Table 8.6). At low doses the upper bound risk, R, equals the product of the potency (q_u) and dose (d).

$$R = q_u d \tag{8.5}$$

Based on q_u derived from the female mouse data and mg/kg body weight as the equivalent dose metric, the risk to humans associated with $1\mu g/m^3$ of PCE in air is

$$R = (2.7 \times 10^{-3})(1.9 \times 10^{-4}) = 5.1 \times 10^{-7}.$$

Table 8.6 contains additional risk estimates based on male mice and surface area extrapolations.

8.6.2. Toxicokinetic Risk Assessment Methodology

The cancer process can be separated into a toxicokinetic phase and a toxicodynamic phase. The former relates applied dose to effective dose at target tissue, while the latter relates effective dose with biological effect.

8.6.2.1. Interspecies Extrapolation In the classical (administered dose) approach to risk assessment, it is assumed that when administered dose is expressed in the proper units (body weight basis or surface area basis), cancer incidence will be the same in all species. Thus, the equivalent dose metric is assumed to account for interspecies differences in both the toxicokinetic and toxicodynamic phases for the cancer process. In the toxicokinetic approach to risk assessment, the PBTK model accounts for interspecies differences in toxicokinetics. The PBTK model is assumed to provide the proper species-specific relation between exposure and effective dose to target tissue. However, it is still not known if a unit of toxin per unit of mouse tissue results in the same response as an equal unit of toxin per unit of human tissue. That is, the question arises as to the proper measure of effective dose to target tissue so that toxicodynamic response is the same in all species. Again, possible choices are mg metabolite/kg weight of target tissue

	Administered Dose (ppm)	Effective Dose LAE (mg/kg/day)	Body Weight Extrapolation		Surface Area Extrapolation	
			q_u	Human Risk	q_u	Human Risk
Males	0	0				
	100	42	1.7×10^{-2}	5.3×10^{-7}	2.2×10^{-1}	6.8×10^{-6}
	200	51				
Females	0	0				
	100	42	1.0×10^{-2}	3.1×10^{-7}	1.3×10^{-1}	4.0×10^{-6}
	200	53				

Table 8.7: *Physiologically based toxicokinetic model effective doses, potency estimates for B6C3F1 mice exposed to PCE by inhalation, and human risk estimates for exposure to 1 $\mu g/m^3$ PCE*

per day or mg metabolite/m^2 surface area target tissue per day. Since organ sizes scale approximately with body weight across species, equivalent metabolized dose in target tissue can be expressed in units of mg/kg body weight per day or mg/m^2 surface area per day.

8.6.2.2. Dose-Response Relation in Mice The classical method of estimating risk assumes that the biological effects of a particular compound are directly related to the administered dose. Toxicokinetic estimation of risk assumes that biological effect is related to the quantity of parent chemical that actually reaches the target tissue, the liver. In the case of PCE, the dose of concern appears to be the amount of metabolite produced along the nonlinear mixed function oxidase pathway since this metabolite correlates best with hepatocellular carcinoma incidence in the female mice. Thus, in order to determine the dose-response curve for the nonlinear metabolite, a PBTK model for PCE (Ward et al., 1988) was used to determine the amount of nonlinear metabolite in the liver which results from a known administered dose.

By using equation (8.4), the nonlinear metabolized doses calculated by the PBTK model at 100 and 200 ppm are converted to lifetime average doses for the females of 42.4 and 52.9 mg/kg/day, respectively. The potency of PCE in mice, q_u, can now be determined by applying the multistage model to the lifetime average metabolized dose in the liver and the incidence of hepatocellular carcinomas. At low doses the upper bound risk, R, equals the product of potency, q_u, and effective dose d_{eff}. This formula is equivalent to assuming that the toxicodynamic relation is linear at low effective doses to the liver.

As with exposure of administered dose, the appropriate measure of equivalent metabolized dose in mice and humans must be determined. Table 8.7 presents q_u based on the effective dose of PCE (nonlinear metabolite in the liver) in male and female mice. The q_u values in columns 3 and 5 are computed on the basis of body weight extrapolation and surface area extrapolation, respectively.

8.6.2.3. Calculation of Effective Dose in Humans We use the potencies presented in Table 8.7 with toxicokinetically derived metabolized dose to estimate the human risk resulting from continuous exposure to 1 $\mu g/m^3$ of PCE in air. In the toxicokinetic approach to risk assessment, the dose to humans is based on the PBTK model estimate of the amount of PCE nonlinear metabolite that reaches the liver. PBTK model simulation of PCE transport in humans estimates that a continuous exposure to 1 $\mu g/m^3$ of PCE in air results in an effective dose to the liver of 3.1×10^{-5} mg/kg/day.

Furthermore, the PBTK model predicts that metabolized dose to the liver does not increase linearly with exposure dose absorbed through the lungs, but rather reaches a maximum level and remains constant. Exposure to 1 ppm of PCE produces 3.3 mg of PCE metabolite, which increases to 22.8 mg metabolite at 10 ppm and 63.3 mg metabolite at 100 ppm. However, because of saturation of the nonlinear pathway, at 1000 ppm only 81.1 mg metabolite are produced. Thus, unlike the classical method, which assumes that effective dose increases linearly with exposure dose, use of the PBTK model assumes that at higher dose levels, the amount of active compound reaching the liver does not increase. This phenomenon is a direct result of saturation of the nonlinear metabolic pathway and implies that carcinogenic risk to humans does not continue to increase with administered dose of PCE.

8.6.2.4. Toxicokinetic Calculation of Human Risk The potencies based on the effective dose and the PBTK model estimation of metabolized dose to the liver may be used to calculate a toxicokinetically derived estimate of human risk due to continuous exposure of 1 $\mu g/m^3$ of PCE in air (see Table 8.7). Using equation (8.5) when mg/kg body weight is considered to be the appropriate measure of equivalent dose, potency is computed for female mice, the risk to humans associated with 1 $\mu g/m^3$ of PCE in air is

$$R = (1.0 \times 10^{-2})(3.1 \times 10^{-5}) = 3.1 \times 10^{-7}.$$

8.6.3. Biologically Based Risk Assessment Methodology

In this example, we use the effective doses predicted by the PBTK model as the basis for the relationship between PCE and its cellular effects (initiation, cell division and cell death) in the two-stage model. The cell division rate (α) and the first mutation rate (ν) are assumed to be linear over effective dose, the ratio of cell death to cell division (β/α) is assumed to be constant and the second mutation rate (μ) is assumed to be equal to the first. The number of normal hepatocytes in mouse liver, X, is assumed to be 10^8. Thus,

$$\begin{aligned}
\alpha &= a_0 + a_1 d_{eff}, \\
\nu &= c_0 + c_1 d_{eff}, \\
\beta/\alpha &= \text{constant}, \\
\mu &= \nu, \text{ and } X = 10^8.
\end{aligned}$$

8.6.3.1. Dose-Response Relation in Mice Only the terminal rates for hepatocellular carcinoma reported in the NTP bioassay (see Table 8.8) were used to estimate

	Administered Dose (ppm)[a]	Effective Dose LAE (mg/kg/day)	Number of Animals[a]	Tumor Bearing Animals[a]	Estimate of a_1 $(0.1 g/kg/day)^{-1}$	Estimate of c_0 $(0.1 g/kg/day)^{-1}$	Human Risk
Males	0	0	46	6			
	100	42	25	8	2.8×10^{-1}	6.9×10^{-8}	1.2×10^{-7}
	200	51	32	14			
Females	0	0	36	1			
	100	42	31	8	7.5×10^{-1}	1.8×10^{-8}	1.3×10^{-7}
	200	53	19	16			

[a] Source: National Toxicology Program (1986)

Table 8.8: *Terminal tumor incidence for B6C3F1 mice, two-mutation model parameter estimates, and 95% upper bound human risk estimates for exposure to 1 $\mu g/m^3$ PCE*

the two-mutation model parameters, since individual failure times are not compiled in the NTP report. Thus a clear distinction should be made between these data and the overall tumor rates used in the first two examples where the failure times were not considered at all.

Preliminary analysis of the male and female mouse data together yielded estimates of $\beta/\alpha = 0.97$, a_0 and c_1 equal to 0. Because estimation of β/α caused convergence problems in estimating the 95% upper confidence bound of the human risk as derived from the mouse data, β/α was set at 0.97. The value of a_0 equal to 0 indicates that the mutation rates are sufficient to explain the occurrence of the control group tumors. In other words, increasing the initiated cell population by clonal expansion thereby enlarging the number of cells at risk for malignancy, is not necessary to explain the background tumor incidence. However, we know that there is some cell division among initiated cells. Hence, we assume a small background level of cell division (i.e. a_0) of 0.01 day^{-1}. Finally, a value of c_1 equal to zero implies that tetrachloroethylene has no genotoxic effect. Thus, the mutation rates, ν and μ, are simply the background or spontaneous rates of mutation.

Further analysis of the male and female mouse data separately with the estimated model parameters described above allowed us to estimate values of a_1 and c_0 from these data sets. Table 8.8 contains the estimates for these parameters.

8.6.3.2. Calculation of Human Risk Human risk of exposure to 1 $\mu g/m^3$ PCE (PBTK effective dose of 3.1×10^{-5} mg/kg/day) was predicted by the two-mutation model using the parameters estimated from the dose-response data obtained in mice. The delta method (Bishop et al., 1975) was used to calculate the 95% upper confidence bound on the incremental risk (see Table 8.8).

8.6.4. Comparison of Human Risk Estimates

We can compare directly the human liver cancer risk estimates (female mouse results in Tables 8.6 and 8.7) calculated with the multistage model based on administered dose and the multistage model based on effective dose. The biologically-based risk estimate given here (Table 8.8) relies on a subset of the mouse liver tumor incidence data and should not be considered final. Thus a direct comparison is questionable. However, inclusion of the tumor incidence prior to the termination point of the experiment and information on the pathology of the tumors would strengthen the biologically-based risk assessment. Since this information is not published in the NTP report, we confine our analysis to the terminal rates of hepatocellular carcinoma, knowing that the animals were sacrificed at 104 weeks. Furthermore, we can assume that the tumors observed at this time were incidental.

We provide this calculation to demonstrate the method, not to advocate a reduction in human risk by using the two-stage model as presented here.

Multistage model potencies were extrapolated between species using both mg/kg/day (body weight extrapolation) and mg/kg$^{0.67}$/day (surface area extrapolation). Our calculations assumed that a female mouse weighs 0.032 kg and inhales 0.067 m^3 of air per day and that a person weighs 70 kg and inhales 20 m^3 of air per day. Regardless of the method of extrapolation, at low exposures, incorporation of toxicokinetics into the risk assessment for PCE exposure lowered the risk estimates by a factor of at least 1.6.

As the nonlinear pathway saturates and the amount of metabolite reaching the liver stabilizes, however, incorporation of toxicokinetics into the risk assessment greatly reduces the estimation of human risk. At small administered doses (1 μg/m^3 to 1 ppm) the reduction in risk gained from use of the effective doses in the multistage model remains constant at a factor of 1.6. As administered dose increases, the resulting reduction in risk also increases linearly with dose. At an exposure concentration of 100 ppm, for example, use of the PBTK model reduces the risk estimate by about a factor of 24. At an exposure concentration of 500 ppm, use of toxicokinetics reduces the risk estimate by about 118 times.

Based on the terminal incidence data, the 95% upper bound on the human risk from exposure to 1 μg/m^3 PCE is 1.3×10^{-7}. This prediction depends on the model assumptions, e.g., that the first and second mutation rates are equal or that the cell division rate is linearly dependent on effective dose. Moreover, our choice of model assumptions impacts the parameters that are estimated and subsequently, the uncertainty in the risk estimate. As such, it becomes important to have data on the model inputs to reduce uncertainty and gain a better understanding of the carcinogenic process.

The biologically-based risk approach demonstrated here combines a toxicokinetic model with the two-stage model in the calculation of human risk. We can improve upon the risk estimate by incorporating the time to tumor and the pathology of the hepatocellular carcinomas. In addition, cellular kinetic data need to be obtained in order to achieve a better understanding of the cancer process and to reduce the uncertainty in biologically-based risk assessment.

Study	C_{inh}[a] (mg/L)	Duration (min)	Postexposure Period (min)	Measurements
1. Teisinger and Fiserova-Bergerova (1955)	0.08	480	2040	Amount of total urinary phenol
2. Srbova et al. (1950)	0.313	90	390	Expired air and venous blood concentrations
3. Sato et al. (1974)	0.08	120	300	End-tidal air and venous blood concentrations
4. Sato et al. (1975): males	0.08	120	300	End-tidal air and venous blood concentrations
5. Sato et al. (1975): females	0.08	120	300	End-tidal air and venous blood concentrations

[a] C_{inh} = inhalation exposure concentration. To convert to ppm, divide by 0.003207 assuming T=25° C and P=1 atmosphere.

Table 8.9: *Summary of the human data used in parameterizing the PBTK model. Single exposures were used in all experiments.*

8.7. CONSIDERATIONS FOR BENZENE TOXICOKINETIC EXTRAPOLATION

Extrapolation of physiologically based toxicokinetic models raises the question of how well the extrapolated models predict the human target tissue dose. In most cases, this question cannot be answered because human data are difficult to acquire. However, human and animal toxicokinetic data for benzene are available. In the following, we allometrically extrapolate ten rat PBTK model parameter vectors to represent humans. The PBTK model is also fitted to human data independently to provide ten human model parameterizations. Comparison of the predictions made by both sets of models shows that the outcome depends largely on the quantity of interest. Furthermore, the rat may not provide a good kinetic model of benzene distribution in humans.

8.7.1. Methods

8.7.1.1. Experimental Data The experimental protocol of the four human studies used to parameterize the PBTK model are summarized in Table 8.9. In the rest of this section, the experiments are coded as "T" for Teisinger and Fiserova-Bergerova (1955), "Sr" for Srbova et al. (1950), "Sa74" for Sato et al. (1974), and "Sa75" for Sato et al. (1975). Table 8.10 describes the animal data we used and the experimental conditions under which the information was obtained.

8.7.1.2. Model A PBTK model (Woodruff et al., 1992), shown in Fig. 8.6 to consist of a lung, fat, bone marrow, and central (comprised of liver, well-perfused, and poorly-perfused tissues) compartment, was used to simulate benzene distribution in the body

Experiment	Animal	C_{inh}[(a)] or Dose	Exposure Type and Duration	Postexposure Period (min)	Quantities Measured
Rickert (1979)	male F344 rats	1.28 mg/L	chamber inhalation; 6 hours	540	Benzene in expired air, blood, liver, adipose tissue, and bone marrow
	male F344 rats	1.28 mg/L	chamber inhalation; 8 hours	0	Benzene in blood, bone marrow, and adipose tissue
Sabourin (1987)	male F344/N rats	0.5 - 300 mg/kg	gavage	2880	Benzene in expired air and metabolites excreted in urine and feces
	male F344/N rats	0.33-2.26 mg/L	nose cone inhalation; 6 hours	3360	Benzene in expired air and metabolites excreted in urine and feces
Sabourin (1988)	male F344/N rats	0.12 mg/L	nose cone inhalation; 6 hours	480	Benzene in blood and liver

[a] C_{inh} = inhalation exposure concentration.

Table 8.10: *Summary of the rat data. Single exposures were used in all of the experiments.*

(see Appendix A for definitions and the calculation of derived values). This structure was shown to adequately represent benzene disposition in rats (Woodruff et al., 1992) and humans (Watanabe, 1993; Watanabe et al., 1994).

The overall structure of the model is the same for rats and humans, but three differences exist. 1) In the rat model, a *Stress* parameter is used to account for differences in benzene inhalation. For example, a rat exposed to benzene in a chamber may breathe more deeply than one exposed through a nose cone apparatus. This parameter is allowed to vary between 0.5 and 1.5 in the rat model, but it is set to 1.0 in the human model. 2) The human model has a parameter defining the fraction of metabolites eliminated as phenol or phenol conjugates which is not present in the rat model because only total metabolites were measured in rats. 3) An intestinal absorption coefficient is present in the rat model, but not in the human model since oral administration data were not available in humans.

Monte Carlo simulations were used to parameterize the PBTK model. In one iteration, the model parameters were selected randomly, the system equations solved numerically to predict the measured values, and the quality of fit assessed by the sum of squared deviates in logarithmic space (SS log). This procedure was used to obtain values for the scaling coefficients which were uniformly or log-uniformly sampled from the biologically acceptable ranges described in Table 8.11.

The initial bounds of each parameter range were determined from the literature. For humans, if no information on the parameter was available, measurements made in animals were used and extrapolated allometrically. This scaling was used only to define the ranges and did not impact the final human parameters since the Monte Carlo procedure further defines the parameter values providing good fits to the data. The parameters were sampled either uniformly or log-uniformly depending on their range.

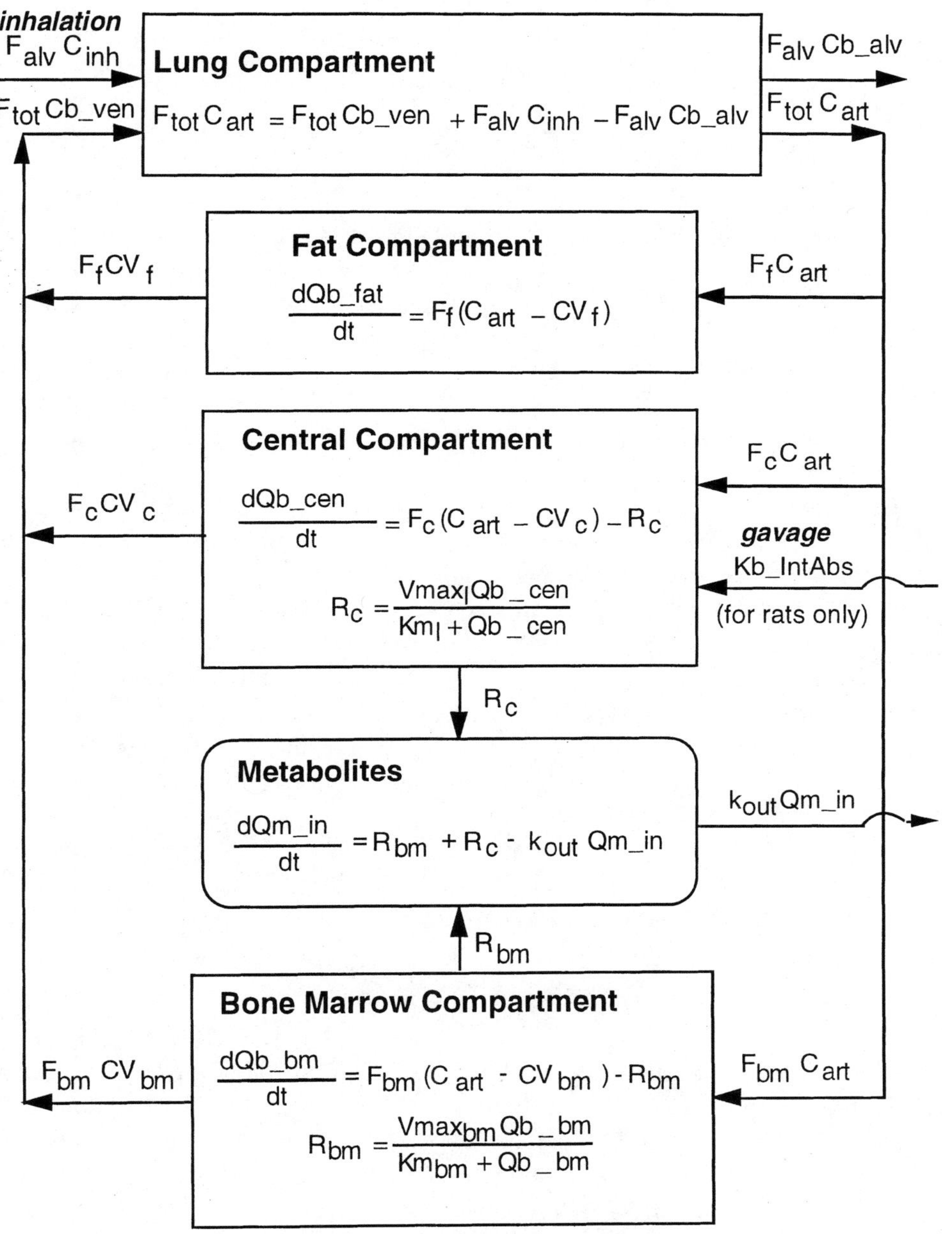

Figure 8.6: *Diagram of the physiologically based pharmacokinetic model.*

If the ratio of the upper to lower bound was greater than a factor of 50, the log uniform distribution was used.

The sum of squared deviates in logarithmic space, equation (8.6), was used as the objective function.

$$SS\ \log = \sum_{i=1}^{n}[ln(Obs_i/Pred_i)]^2 \tag{8.6}$$

where, Obs_i and $Pred_i$ are the observed and predicted values, and n is the number of data points. This measure is based on the assumption of a log normal distribution of measurement error.

Each Monte Carlo series contained N Monte Carlo simulations and was started with a different number as the input into a pseudo-random number generator. In order to test the robustness of the parameterization procedure, a total of 10 series of Monte Carlo simulations were performed for each of the data sets (human and rat). Three series of 100,000 simulations and seven series of 50,000 simulations were performed. In this study, the best rat data-fitted parameter vector from each series (total of ten vectors) was extrapolated and the extrapolated model predictions were compared to those from the ten best parameterizations of the model fitted to human data.

The relative difference between the SS log after N simulations and 50,000 simulations was used to determine the best rat parameter vector from each series. The termination condition was set at a relative difference of 2% or less which corresponded to extrapolating the ten best rat parameter vectors obtained after 30,000 simulations. In other words, each rat parameter vector produced a fit within 2% of the best fit after 50,000 simulations.

Fitting the model parameters to rat data required more computational time (measured in central processing unit, cpu, time) than fitting the model parameters to human data. This occurred partly because 100 rat data points were used to fit the model compared to 36 human data points. For this reason an equivalent number of "human" simulations to "rat" simulations was calculated as 47,000 to 30,000 respectively. This ratio is the number of "human" simulations that can be performed in the amount of cpu time per data point that it takes to perform 30,000 rat simulations. Thus, the best human model parameter vectors were recorded after 47,000 simulations.

8.7.1.3. Extrapolation The best rat parameter vector after 30,000 simulations from each series was extrapolated allometrically. The exponents used in the allometric scaling (see Table 8.11) were 0.75 for the cardiac output, alveolar ventilation, blood flows, and Michaelis-Menten maximum rates of metabolism (V_{max}) and an exponent of 1.0 for the compartment volumes (Fiserova-Bergerova and Hughes, 1983; Mordenti, 1986; Travis et al., 1990b) . Two parameters in the rat model, Stress and Kb_IntAbs, were not scaled because they are specific to the rat model only.

In the remaining text, a *model* is one parameterization of the PBTK model structure described earlier. Thus, there are ten extrapolated models (parameters vectors allometrically extrapolated from the model fitted to rat data) and ten human models (parameter vectors obtained from the model fitted to human data).

Physiologic Parameter	SC	Multiplier	Human SC Lower Bound	Human SC Upper Bound	Rat SC Lower Bound	Rat SC Upper Bound
Cardiac output, F_{tot}	Sc_Flow_tot	$BW^{0.75}$ * Stress	0.188	0.543	0.25	0.4
Alveolar ventilation, F_{alv}	VPerf_Rat	F_{tot}	0.500	1.50	0.6	1.25
Blood flows[c]						
Bone marrow, F_{bm}	Flow_bm	F_{tot}	0.00821	0.0665	0.01	0.06
Fat, F_f	Flow_fat	F_{tot}	0.0203	0.0784	0.04	0.1
Volumes[d]						
Bone marrow, V_{bm}	V_bm	BW	0.010	0.060	0.01	0.06
Fat, V_f	V_fat	BW	0.109	0.337	0.08	0.2
Blood/air partition coefficient	PCb_art	1	1.66	17.9	8.00	18.0
Tissue/blood partition coefficients						
Bone marrow	PCb_bm	1	3.03	29.3	3.00	12.0
Fat	PCb_fat	1	23.0	70.5	23.0	39.0
Central compartment	PCb_cen	1	2.02	20.1	2.00	5.00
Maximum rates of metabolism						
Central compartment, $Vmax_l$	Vab_cen	$BW^{0.75}$	0.00104	0.170	0.05	0.17
Bone marrow, $Vmax_{bm}$	Vab_bm	$Vmax_l$	0.020	0.300	0.02	0.30
Vmax/Km ratios						
Central compartment[e]	Kab_cen	1	0.00533	0.362	0.01	0.3
Bone marrow[e]	Kab_bm	1	0.000358	0.495	0.002	0.5
Elimination rate constant	k_{out}	1	0.000211	0.0028	0.001	0.00135
Fraction of metabolites excreted as phenol or phenol conjugates	PhFraction	1	0.600	1.00	– [f]	– [f]
Effect of external conditions on blood flow and alveolar ventilation	Stress	1	1	1	0.5	1.5
Gastrointestinal absorption coefficient	Kb_IntAbs	1	– [f]	– [f]	0.002	0.05

[a] Physiologic parameter = scaling coefficient × multiplier. Units: BW = body weight in kg, flows in L/min, volumes in L, Vmax in mg/min, Vmax/Km in 1/min.

[b] Initial lower bounds and upper bounds were obtained from the literature or scaled from animals. All scaling coefficients were sampled from uniform prior distributions except where otherwise noted.

[c] The central compartment blood flow, F_C, was computed at each run so that the sum of the flows equaled 100% of the total flow.

[d] The central compartment volume, V_C, was computed at each run so that the sum of the volumes was equal to 90% of the body volume. Bones constitute the remaining 10%.

[e] The variable was sampled using a log uniform distribution (i.e., uniformly sampled after log transformation).

[f] Parameter not defined in this model.

Table 8.11: *Physiologic parameters and their scaling coefficients (SC) for benzene toxicokinetics in humans and rats, with the corresponding Monte Carlo sampling ranges.*[a,b]

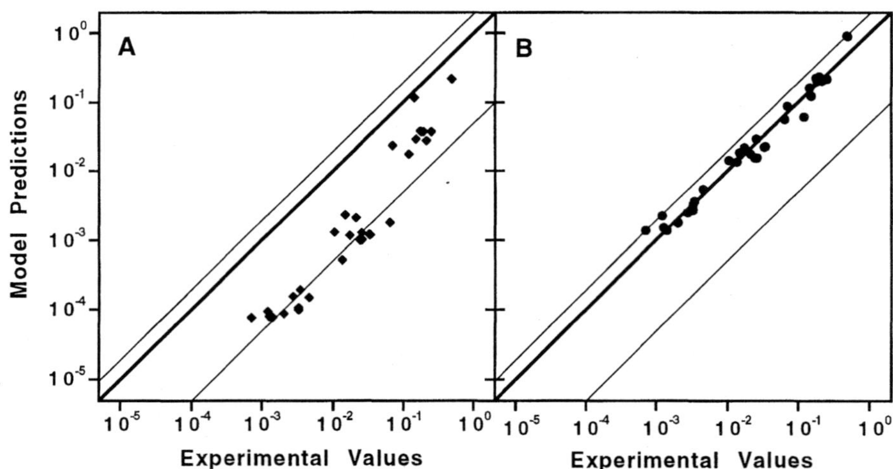

Figure 8.7: *Predicted values versus experimental human values for: (A) the best of ten models extrapolated allometrically; and (B) the best of ten models fitted to the human data. The thin lines represent the largest deviation of the human model predictions from the experimental values (±95%).*

8.7.1.4. Extrapolated Model Predictions The *SS* logs for predictions of the human data were calculated for the extrapolated models and compared to the *SS* logs for the human model predictions. Only Sr, Sa74, and Sa75 human data were predicted since the rat model is unable to generate quantities of urinary phenol (no PhFraction in the model).

The extrapolated rat models and the independently fitted human models were then used to predict the total exposure of bone marrow to benzene (AUCb_bm) and the cumulative quantity of metabolite produced in bone marrow (Qmet_bm) in humans. Predictions were made at 4320 minutes (three days) after a single inhalation exposure at time zero of either 32 ppm for 15 minutes (E1) or 1 ppm for 480 minutes (E2).

8.7.2. Results and Discussion

Fig. 8.7 plots human data predictions made by the best allometrically extrapolated rat model and the best human model. In general, the extrapolations underpredict the experimental human values. The *SS* log corresponding to the allometrically scaled model (Fig. 8.7A) is 207.9 and the human model *SS* log (Fig. 8.7B) is 3.4. In general, the sums of squares in log space for the predictions made by the ten extrapolated rat models are about 50 times those of the human models.

8.7.2.1. Extrapolated Model Predictions Predictions of AUCb_bm and Qmet_bm are shown in Figures 8.8 and 8.9. The extrapolations predict a much lower mean for AUCb_bm compared to the human model predictions. Slight dose rate effects are present in the ten, human model, AUC predictions whose values obtained from exposure 1 are larger than exposure 2 by 0.5-1.9%. In contrast, the predictions of Qmet_bm

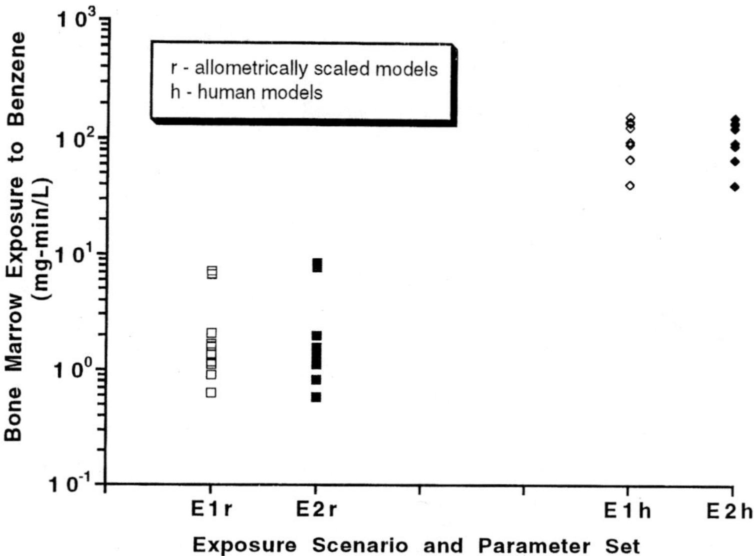

Figure 8.8: *E1: 32 ppm benzene exposure for 15 min. E2: 1 ppm benzene exposure for 480 min. Predictions of the total exposure of bone marrow to benzene (AUCb_bm).*

are similar for the extrapolations and the human models. Again, the human model values of Qmet_bm from exposure 1 are greater than exposure 2 by 0.5-1.9%.

The predictions of AUCb_bm made by the extrapolations are much lower than those generated by the fitted human model parameter vectors because the rate of benzene metabolism in the central and bone marrow compartments is higher, thereby reducing the benzene blood concentration throughout the body. Furthermore, the bone marrow tissue to blood partition coefficient is lower in the extrapolated models than in the human models, which results in less benzene entering the bone marrow tissue. Yet, the Qmet_bm predictions are in the same general range although the rate of metabolism is higher for the extrapolated models. This occurs because initially the formation of metabolite predicted by the extrapolations is higher than the human model, but decreases rapidly as benzene is depleted. In contrast, the metabolite formation predicted by the human models decreases more slowly over time, resulting in final cumulative metabolite quantities similar to the extrapolated model predictions.

Assuming the structure of the PBTK model to be correct, the model can be used to determine the efficacy of rats as a kinetic model for humans. The allometrically scaled rat parameter vectors do not yield predictions of the human data comparable to the fitted human model predictions. In fact, they are considerably worse, despite utilizing tissue data in rats which we expect to provide a better description of the system dynamics than the non-tissue specific data in humans. This result could be a limitation of the allometric extrapolation method although it may also mean that the rat does not provide a good kinetic model of benzene distribution in humans.

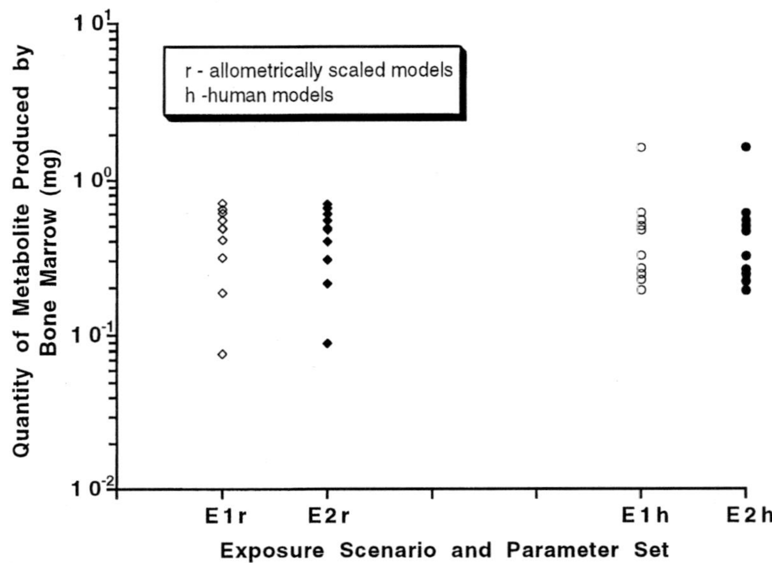

Figure 8.9: *E1: 32 ppm benzene exposure for 15 min. E2: 1 ppm benzene exposure for 480 min. Predictions of the cumulative quantity of metabolite produced in the bone marrow (Qmet_bm).*

This study has shown that the prediction performance depends greatly on the quantity of interest (i.e., a dose surrogate). For the total exposure of bone marrow to benzene, the extrapolations predict lower values than the human models. Yet, the extrapolations and the human models predict similar values for the cumulative quantity of metabolite produced by bone marrow. Validation with target tissue data would be enlightening to get some measure of the accuracy of extrapolated PBTK model predictions and how they affect risk assessment.

8.8. REFERENCES

Ashley, D.J.B. (1969): Colonic cancer arising in polyposis coli. J. Med. Gen. 6, 376-378.

Bishop, Y.M.M., Fienberg, S., and Holland, P. (1975). Discrete Multivariate Analysis. MIT Press, Cambridge.

Bolanowska, W., and Golacka, J. (1972). Absorption and elimination of tetrachloroethylene in humans under experimental conditions. Medical Pr 23, 109-119.

Buchmann, A., Ziegler, S., Wolf, A., Robertson, L.W., Durham, S.K. and Schwarz, M. (1991): Effects of polychlorinated biphenyls in rat liver: Correlation between primary subcellular effects and promoting activity. Toxicol. Appl. Pharmacol. 111, 454-468.

Buchmann, A., Stinchcombe, S., Kürner, W., Hagenmaier, H.P. and Bock, K.W. (1994): Effects of 2,3,7,8-tetrachloro- and 1,2,3,4,6,7,8-heptachlorodibenzo-p-dioxin on the proliferation of preneoplastic liver cells in the rat. Carcinogenesis 15, 1143-1150.

Cavanee, W.K. and White, R.L. (1995): The genetic basis of cancer. Sci-Am. 272, 3, 72-9.

Cohen, S.M., Ellwein, L.B., Okamura, T., Masui, T., Johansson, S.L., Smith, R.A., Wehner, J.M., Khachab, M., Chappel, C.I., Schoenig, G.P., Emerson, J.L. and Garland, E.M. (1991): Comparitive Bladder Tumor Promoting Activity of Sodium Saccharin, Sodium Ascorbate, Related Acids, and Calcium Salts in Rats. Cancer Research 51, 1766-1777.

Cohen, S.M. and Ellwein, L.B. (1993): Use of Cell Proliferation Data in Modeling Urinary Bladder Carcinogenesis. Environ. Health Persp. 101, 111-114.

Federal Register (1986). Guidelines for carcinogen risk assessment. Fed. Regist. 51, 33992-34003.

Fiserova-Bergerova, V., and Hughes, H. C. (1983). Species differences on bioavailability of inhaled vapors and gases. In Modeling of Inhalation Exposure to Vapors: Uptake, Distribution, and Elimination, Vol. II (V. Fiserova-Bergerova, Ed.), pp. 97-106. CRC Press, Boca Raton.

Howe, R. B. (1983). GLOBAL83: An Experimental Program Developed for the U.S. Environmental Protection Agency as an Update to GLOBAL82: A Computer to Extrapolate Quantal Animal Toxicity Data to Low Doses. Ruston, LA: K.S. Crump and Co., Inc. (unpublished).

Mordenti, J. (1986). Man versus beast: pharmacokinetic scaling in mammals. J. Pharm. Sci. 75, 1028-1040.

Ketkar, M.B., Holste, J., Preussmann, R. and Althoff, J. (1983): Carcinogenic Effect of Nitrosomorpholine administered in the Drinking Water to Syrian Golden Hamsters. Cancer Lett. 17(3), 333-338.

Knudson, A.G. (1971): Mutation and Cancer: Statistical study of retinoblastoma. Proc. Nat. Acad. Sci., USA, 68, 820-823.

Lijinsky, W., Kovatch, R.M., Riggs, C.W. and Walters, P.T. (1988): Dose Response Study with N-Nitrosomorpholine in Drinking Water of F-344 Rats. Cancer Research 48, 2089-2095.

Luebeck, E.G., Moolgavkar, S.H., Buchmann, A., and Schwarz, M. (1991): Effects of polychlorinated biphenyls in rat liver: Quantitative analysis of enzyme-altered foci. Toxicol. Appl. Pharmacol. 111, 469-484.

Moolgavkar, S.H., Dewanji, A., and Luebeck, G. (1989): Cigarette smoking and lung cancer: reanalysis of the British doctors' data. J Natl Cancer Inst 81, 415-420.

Moolgavkar, S.H., Luebeck, E.G., de Gunst, M., Port, R.E., and Schwarz, M. (1990a): Quantitative analysis of enzyme-altered foci in rat hepatocarcinogenesis experiments I: Single agent regimen. Carcinogenesis 11, 8, 1271-1278.

Moolgavkar, S.H, Cross, F.T., Luebeck, E.G., and Dagle, G.E. (1990b): A two-mutation model for radon-induced lung tumors in rats. Radiation Research 121, 28-37.

Moolgavkar, S.H. and Luebeck, E.G. (1992): Multistage carcinogenesis': Population-based model for colon cancer. J. Natl. Cancer Inst. 84, 610-618.

Moolgavkar, S.H., Luebeck, E.G., Krewski, D., and Zielinski, J.M. (1993): Radon, Cigarette Smoke, and Lung Cancer: A Reanalysis of the Colorado Plateau Uranium Miners' Data. American Journal of Epidemiology, Vol. 4, no.3, 204-217.

National Toxicology Program (1986). NTP Technical Report on the Toxicology and Carcinogenesis of Tetrachloroethylene (Perchloroethylene), CAS 127-18-4, in F344/N Rats and B6C3F1 Mice (Inhalation Studies). (Report #NTP TR 311, NIH Publ. No. 86-2567). U.S. Department of Health and Human Services, Public Health Service, National Institutes of Health, NTP, Washington, D.C.

Rickert, D. E., Baker, T. S., Bus, J. S., Barrow, C. S., and Irons, R. D. (1979). Benzene disposition in the rat after exposure by inhalation. Toxicol. Appl. Pharmacol. 49, 417-423.

Sabourin, P. J., Bechtold, W. E., Birnbaum, L. S., Lucier, G., and Henderson, R. F. (1988). Differences in the metabolism and disposition of inhaled [^{3}H]benzene by F344/N rats and B6C3F1 mice. Toxicol. Appl. Pharmacol. 94, 128-140.

Sabourin, P. J., Chen, B. T., Lucier, G., Birnbaum, L. S., Fisher, E., and Henderson, R. F. (1987).

Effect of dose on the absorption and excretion of [^{14}C]benzene administered orally or by inhalation in rats and mice. Toxicol. Appl. Pharmacol. 87, 325-336.

Sato, A., Nakajima, T., Fujiwara, Y., and Hirosawa, K. (1974). Pharmacokinetics of benzene and toluene. Int. Arch. Arbeitsmed. 33, 169-182.

Sato, A., Nakajima, T., Fujiwara, Y., and Murayama, N. (1975). Kinetic studies on sex difference in susceptibility to chronic benzene intoxication - with special reference to body fat content. Brit. J. Ind. Med. 32, 321-328.

Schwarz, M., Pearson, D., Buchmann A. and Kunz, W. (1989): The use of enzyme-altered foci for risk assessment in hepatocarcinogenesis. In: Biologically Based Methods for Cancer Risk Assessment, edited by C.C. Travis, NATO ASI Series A: Life Sciences Vol 159, Plenum Press, New York, 31-39.

Srbova, J., Teisinger, J., and Skramovsky, S. (1950). Absorption and elimination of inhaled benzene in man. Arch. Ind. Hyg. Occup. Med. 2, 1-8.

Teisinger, J., and Fiserova-Bergorova, V. (1955). Valeur comparée de la détermination des sulfates et du phénol contenus dans l'urine pour l'évaluation de la concentration du benzène dans l'air. Arch. Mal. Prof. Med. Trav. 16, 221-232.

Travis, C. C., White, R. K., and Ward, R. C. (1990b). Interspecies extrapolation of pharmacokinetics. J. Theor. Biol. 142, 285-304.

U.S. Environmental Protection Agency (1985). Health Assessment Document for Tetrachloroethylene (Perchloroethylene). (Report #EPA/600/8-82/005F). Office of Research and Development, Office of Health and Environmental Assessment, Environmental Criteria and Assessment Office, USEPA.

Ward, R. C., Travis, C. C., Hetrick, D. M., Andersen, M. E., and Gargas, M. L. (1988). Pharmacokinetics of tetrachloroethylene. Toxicol. Appl. Pharmacol. 93, 108-117.

Watanabe, K. H. (1993). Mathematical Modeling of Benzene Disposition: A Population Perspective, Ph.D. dissertation, University of California, Berkeley.

Watanabe, K. H., Bois, F. Y., Daisey, J. M., Auslander, D. M., and Spear, R. C. (1994). Benzene toxicokinetics in humans - bone marrow exposure to metabolites. Occupational and Environmental Medicine 51, 414-420.

Woodruff, T. J., Bois, F. Y., Auslander, D., and Spear, R. (1992). Structure and parametrization of pharmacokinetic models: Their impact on model predictions. Risk Anal. 12, 189-201.

8.9. APPENDIX A

MODEL PARAMETERS AND VARIABLES

C_{art} = benzene concentration in the arterial blood (mg/L)
Cb_ven = benzene concentration in the venous blood (mg/L)
C_{inh} = benzene concentration in the inhaled air (mg/L)
Cb_exp = benzene concentration in the expired air (mg/L)
Cb_alv = benzene concentration in the alveolar air (mg/L)
CV_{bm} = bone marrow compartment venous blood benzene concentration (mg/L)
CV_c = central compartment venous blood benzene concentration (mg/L)
CV_f = fat compartment venous blood benzene concentration (mg/L)
F_{tot} = cardiac output (L/min)
F_{alv} = alveolar ventilation rate (L/min)
F_{bm} = blood flow rate to the bone marrow compartment (L/min)
F_c = blood flow to the central compartment (L/min)
F_f = blood flow to the fat compartment (L/min)
Kb_IntAbs = gastro-intestinal absorption coefficient (1/min)
Km_{bm} = Michaelis-Menten quantity (mg) at half the maximum reaction velocity for bone marrow
Km_l = Michaelis-Menten quantity (mg) at half the maximum reaction velocity for the central compartment
k_{out} = rate constant for the urinary excretion of metabolites (1/min)
PCb_art = equilibrium concentration ratio of benzene in blood to air
PCb_bm = equilibrium concentration ratio of benzene in bone marrow tissue to blood
PCb_cen = equilibrium concentration ratio of benzene in central compartment tissues to blood.
PCb_fat = equilibrium concentration ratio of benzene in adipose tissue to blood
Qb_bm = quantity of benzene in the bone marrow (mg)
Qb_cen = quantity of benzene in the central compartment (mg)
Qb_fat = quantity of benzene in the fat compartment (mg)
Qm_in = quantity of benzene metabolites in the body (mg)
Qm_out = cumulative quantity of benzene metabolites excreted in urine (mg)
Qph = cumulative quantity of metabolites excreted as phenol or phenol conjugates (mg)
Stress = the effect of external conditions on cardiac output and alveolar ventilation
$Vmax_{bm}$ = bone marrow compartment Michaelis-Menten maximum reaction velocity
$Vmax_l$ = central compartment Michaelis-Menten maximum reaction velocity
V_{bm} = volume of the bone marrow compartment (L)
V_c = volume of the central compartment (L)
V_f = volume of the fat compartment (L)

DERIVED VALUES

Cb_alv = Cart/*PCb_art*

Cb_exp = 0.3 * Cb_inh + 0.7 * Cb_alv
CV_{bm} = Qb_bm / (V_{bm} * *PCb_bm*)
CV_c = Qb_cen / (V_c * *PCb_cen*)
CV_f = Qb_fat / (V_f * *PCb_fat*)
F_{tot} = *Sc_Flow_tot* *(body weight)$^{0.75}$ * *Stress*
F_{alv} = *VPerf_Ratio* * F_{tot}
F_{bm} = *Flow_bm* * F_{tot}
F_c = 1.0 - *Flow_bm* – *Flow_fat*
F_f = *Flow_fat* * F_{tot}
Km_{bm} = $Vmax_{bm}$/*Kab_bm*
Km_l = $Vmax_l$/*Kab_cen*
Qm_out = $\int$ k_{out} Qm_indt
Qph = *PhFraction* * Qm_out
$Vmax_{bm}$ = *Vab_bm* * $Vmax_l$
$Vmax_l$ = *Vab_cen* * (body weight)$^{0.75}$
V_{bm} = *V_bm* * body weight
V_c = 0.9 - *V_bm* – *V_fat* (assumes that bone volume is 10%)
V_f = *V_fat* * body weight

Notes: Italicized quantities represent the sampled model parameters.

Chapter 9

CONCLUSIONS AND RECOMMENDATIONS

J. J. Amaral-Mendes[1], J. V. Cogliano[2], A. Kappas[3], C. Kitsos[4], E. D. Kroese[5], E. G. Luebeck[6], E. Pluygers[7], C. Travis[8], K. Watanabe[8], W. Wosniok[9], and G. A. Zapponi[10]

[1]University of Evora, Evora, Portugal
[2]U.S. Environmental Protection Agency, Washington DC, USA
[3]National Centre for Scientific Research "Demokritus", Athens, Greece
[4]Department of Statistics, Athens University of Economics and Business, Athens, Greece
[5]Rijksinstituut voor Volksgezondheid en Milieuhygiene, Bilthoven, The Netherlands
[6]Fred Hutchinson Cancer Research Center, Seattle, USA
[7]Oncology Department, Jolimont Hospital (honorary), La Louvière, Belgium
[8]Tulane University Medical Center, New Orleans, USA
[9]Institute of Statistics, University of Bremen, Bremen, Germany
[10]National Institute of Health, Rome, Italy

9.1. INTRODUCTION

The present report addresses several key issues in quantitative cancer risk assessment pertaining to the dose- response analysis of initiator and promoter carcinogens. Most problems addressed in this report fall into one of the following categories of questions:

1. What does each source of experimental data contribute to our knowledge and ability to model?

2. What kinds of information are needed to develop a biologically based model?

[2]The views expressed in this chapter are those of the authors and do not necessarily reflect the views or policies of the U.S. Environmental Protection Agency.

Perspectives on Biologically Based Cancer Risk Assessment, edited by Cogliano *et al.*
Kluwer Academic/Plenum Publishers, New York, 1999.

3. How does linearity enter into empirical models and biologically based models?

4. How does a biologically based model help us understand intraspecies variability?

5. How does a biologically based model help us understand interspecies variability?

6. What are the uncertainties associated with a biologically based model?

9.2. WHAT DOES EACH SOURCE OF EXPERIMENTAL DATA CONTRIBUTE TO OUR KNOWLEDGE AND ABILITY TO MODEL?

Epidemiologic information is often unavailable; when it does exist, it can be sparse or confounded by exposures to other potential carcinogens, lifestyle factors, and variations with geographic location and culture. Thus, experimental information has played an important role in identifying potential carcinogens and understanding their effects.

For many years the long-term animal bioassay, most often using rats and mice, has been the principal source of information used to test chemical substances for carcinogenicity in humans. Advantages are obvious: the studies are performed under highly controlled conditions, often restricted to specific strains and study durations where spontaneous tumor rates are known, and experimental protocols often closely monitor carcinogen uptake. On the other hand, the use of rodent bioassays to make inferences about human carcinogenicity has been, and will likely remain, highly problematic. Aside from the formidable problem of translating results from one species to another, experiments are also performed with relatively high doses (often near the maximal tolerated dose), mostly for economic reasons. Thus, an extrapolation of risk estimates (hazards, relative risks, or excess risks) to doses many orders of magnitude lower than those used in typical bioassays is necessary in order to quantify cancer risk to human populations.

Credibility of an assessment is higher when extrapolation is based on a model that uses information indicating that effects observed at high doses in animals are relevant to lower doses in humans. The sources of information discussed in chapters 3 and 4 can each contribute something to a biologically based model. We know that a cell has to mutate and grow uncontrollably in order to result in cancer. In vitro studies and short term tests provide mechanistic information about the mode of action, including identification of loci (in addition to their historical use in screening to identify putative carcinogens for further testing in long-term bioassays). Cell proliferation studies elucidate the relationship of cell proliferation as a function of dose, which then can be input into the cancer model. Toxicokinetic studies are specifically designed to investigate the distribution (absorption, metabolism, elimination) of a toxicant in the body; this source of data is fundamental to being able to extrapolate risks across species. In long-term animal bioassays, serial sacrifices can be performed in order to monitor intermediate endpoints and to study their relationship to cancer. Thus, in vitro studies, biomarkers, and animal experiments provide indispensible data sources for studying carcinogenic effects under highly controlled conditions. Bioassays remain important in their ability to provide an in vivo indication of carcinogenicity.

Physiologically based toxicokinetic (PBTK) models have been utilized to improve the estimate of effective dose in dose-response analyses for cancer risk assessment. They are useful in cases where the applied dose is not directly proportional to the effective dose due to absorption, metabolism, or excretion of the toxicant. These models incorporate the mechanisms affecting the distribution of toxicants in the body, and with appropriate development they can be useful tools in extrapolating from high to low doses and across species. As demonstrated in section 8.7, however, extrapolated model predictions of a dose surrogate can vary greatly from predictions made by the model fitted to human data. The incorporation of PBTK models in biologically based risk assessment is considered to improve the extrapolation process, however, additional research can be performed in this area. Tissue-specific data are needed in humans to validate these models and provide some assurance that an extrapolated animal model, in fact, represents the disposition of the toxicant in humans. Human biomarkers may be able to provide data for this purpose.

The paradigm presented here for a more comprehensive and quantitative cancer risk assessment has emerged over the last 5 to 10 years. It is based upon a better understanding of carcinogenesis in terms of the underlying genetic processes, in particular the role of oncogene activation and anti-oncogene (tumor suppressor gene) inactivation in the cell. Further, the ability to quantify molecular changes due to carcinogenic exposures, and to identify metabolic pathways and interactions of metabolites with DNA and other cellular components, has led to new data sources that need to be incorporated into the risk assessment process.

9.3. WHAT KINDS OF INFORMATION ARE NEEDED TO DEVELOP A BIOLOGICALLY BASED MODEL?

With a steady stream of new information on the genetics, biology, and biochemistry of cancer, we are challenged to develop better and more realistic cancer models that can be descriptive as well as predictive. Thus, whenever sufficient information about the tumor response is available, a biologically based model should be used in the analysis of the data. To this extent, time-to-tumor and censoring information needs to be recorded and made available. In many cases this information has been recorded during the study, but due to the large volume and intermediate nature of these data they are not published or easily accessible. We recommend that this information be made available in electronic form so it can be used by modelers and other investigators.

The question arises whether risk estimates obtained with biologically based models using tumor incidence alone should be used for risk prediction without further confirmation of the cellular responses postulated by the model. When using the model to predict cancer risk, additional sources of information should be included to strengthen the credibility of the risk estimates. As a class of models, the biologically based model provides a natural interface for the inclusion of laboratory data into risk analysis. For example, measurements of mitotic rates in premalignant lesions at different doses can be compared to estimates of these parameters generated by the model. We note that these cellular kinetic studies are starting to be routinely included in bioassay protocols. We encourage use of this information to confirm biologically based modeling results.

Biologically based models need not assume homogeneity of processes across species (for example, a compound may cause liver cancer in one species but bladder cancer in another). Because of the richness of the parameters in a biologically based model, these models have the ability to explain heterogeneity across species; for example, the dose might increase the mitotic rate in mouse liver cells and rat bladder cells. The incorporation of cross-species toxicokinetic information can indicate how target tissues and dose levels differ across species. Rates measuring cellular processes can indicate differences in response to equivalent doses of the toxicant in different species.

Hypothesized mechanisms and model predictions should be scrutinized on the basis of data that provide direct measurements of these mechanisms. For instance, if an agent is found to be a promoter (in the analysis of tumor data alone with the model), we expect to find increased levels of mitotic activity or decreased levels of apoptosis or necrosis. As an example, in the case study of tetrachloroethylene risk estimation (see chapter 8), the compound was found to promote the growth of premalignant tumors, but was not found to be an initiator. This hypothesis could be confirmed with biological data on the growth kinetics of intermediate lesions. Obviously, the use of curve-fitting models precludes this feedback for developing more comprehensive models, since their parameters bear no physical or biological significance. Thus, biologically based models stand the best chance to be useful guides for experimental work and better risk prediction.

9.4. HOW DOES LINEARITY ENTER INTO EMPIRICAL MODELS AND BIOLOGICALLY BASED MODELS?

The notion of a linear relationship between dose and cancer response is used in different ways. In empirical models, the relationship between dose and risk is defined to be linear. The justification to use a linear description may be an approximation argument, if a situation near to a dose of zero is investigated. Besides the assumption of linearity, the starting and ending point of the linear curve must be specified, which means in particular an assumption about a baseline risk (at a dose of zero). If linearity is assumed over a large dose range, and not only in the vicinity of zero, then if the true relation has a sigmoid form, the low-dose risk may be highly overestimated in some cases and underestimated in others.

In biologically based models (including biologically based multistage models, such as the Armitage-Doll model) the relationship between risk and dose is a consequence of all the model assumptions made before. From these it follows whether the relationship is linear or not; in most cases it is not. (Of course, any model may, within a limited domain and level of accuracy, be approximated by a linear function, for example, using a Taylor expansion. This is a general mathematical property of every continuous function, not a model assumption like it is for the empirical models.) There is, however, a place in biologically based models where linear functions may enter by assumption. It is common to assume that the cell transition rates (ν and μ in the two-stage model) and the cell kinetic rates (α and/or β in the two-stage model) are linear functions of dose. This is an assumption which must, as every other one, be discussed for each particular case. Support for a chosen dose-rate function may possibly be derived from the approach of physiologically based modelling, previous experience, or specific experiments devoted to this problem. It should be noted that errors in the specification of these dose-rate functions may propagate to the final risk estimate.

In many practical cases strong arguments can be made in favor of low-dose linearity. This, however, should not be confused with the problem that arises when risks are extrapolated linearly to low doses. If risk assessment is based on purely statistical models, absolutely no guarantees can be given that the model will extrapolate risk correctly to lower doses. Many animal experiments are designed with exposures that induce tumors in a relatively high fraction of animals. A priori, there is no reason to believe that the modeled dose-response relationship actually continues to hold at very low doses. It is our fundamental belief that a model should properly reflect real physical processes, possibly too complex to be described in every detail, but that capture essential biological mechanisms that can be observed (in related experiments at the cellular level) at doses much lower than the doses used in the typical animal experiment. It is clear that questions with regard to modifications of the low-dose behavior due to the presence of threshold or saturation phenomena and such are more easily addressed in models that contain parameters having a biological interpretation, that is, which can be measured in principle.

9.5. HOW DOES A BIOLOGICALLY BASED MODEL HELP US UNDERSTAND INTRASPECIES VARIABILITY?

Differences among susceptibilities of human individuals and subpopulations to cancer risk factors may involve metabolism, halflife in the body, mutagenicity, and other relevant parameters. A number of biomarkers provide indications of these differences. They include levels of enzymes that may transform inactive carcinogens into active ones, levels of detoxifying enzymes, levels of DNA binding, and indicators of DNA repair capacity. Variability in individual susceptibilities detected by biomarkers may be accounted for by biologically based models. As an example, instead of single values or average values of model parameters, suitable parameter distributions or statistical indicators of variability may be used.

9.6. HOW DOES A BIOLOGICALLY BASED MODEL HELP US UNDERSTAND INTERSPECIES VARIABILITY?

A "biologically based" interspecies extrapolation of toxicological parameters should ideally consider both the toxicokinetics and toxicodynamics of the process under study. In other words, a reference is needed to the relationships existing in the involved species between the exposures (or external doses) and the corresponding active doses at the target, as well as the relationships between the doses at the target and the biological effects at the target. Biological monitoring and biomarkers of both exposure and effect are extremely relevant in providing information for this purpose.

As an example, differences may exist in the examined species in the distribution of a chemical in different target organs or tissues, as well as in the possible metabolic processes leading to the formation of active metabolites. Moreover, as in the case of forestomach tumors in the mouse, relevant differences may also exist in the physiology of experimental animals and humans. Lastly, differences may exist in the mechanisms leading to cancer induction (as, for example, differences in DNA repair efficiency) in experimental animals and humans. These aspects need to be considered in the assessment.

9.7. WHAT ARE THE UNCERTAINTIES ASSOCIATED WITH A BIOLOGICALLY BASED MODEL?

A distinction has to be made between uncertainty in its genuine sense and uncertainty in the form of variability. While the first term refers to nonexistent knowledge about the appropriateness of assumptions, the latter denotes the uncertainty which is essentially caused by random effects. These carry over to a certain extent to the statements that are finally made, thus endowing them with a certain imprecision. This kind of uncertainty will be dealt with under the name of variability.

The main source of uncertainty in risk assessment is model misspecification. This may have the form of choosing an inadequate mathematical formulation to describe the relation between dose, time, and risk, or by unknowingly omitting important factors. Misspecification may be indicated by a poor model fit, particularly if the error was to exclude a relevant variable. However, model fit is not a good indicator of appropriateness. It is possible that in the range of observed dose values there is a perfect model fit, while outside this range the model prediction might be drastically wrong because different biological laws exist outside the observed range.

Measurement error is another source of uncertainty in biologically based risk assessment. One cannot eliminate this source of uncertainty, but a modeling methodology that incorporates a reasonable estimate of this error can be applied in a biologically based risk assessment.

Distributional approaches, such as Monte Carlo analysis, can be used to address uncertainty and variability in the model. Toward this end, all averaged data from cancer bioassays, toxicokinetic studies, and biomarker studies should be reported with standard deviations, and the raw, individual data should be made available in electronic form. When the sample size is large enough, empirical distributions can be used for the input model parameters.

Today's models are increasingly able to handle more information of different types. All input data need to be made available so that models can provide realistic estimates of the uncertainty and variability in the model outputs.

Contributors

José J. Amaral-Mendes, University of Evora, Evora, Portugal

Leonello Attias, National Institute of Health, Rome, Italy

V. James Cogliano, U.S. Environmental Protection Agency, Washington DC, USA

Andreas Kappas, National Centre for Scientific Research "Demokritus", Athens, Greece

Christos Kitsos, Department of Statistics, Athens University of Economics and Business, Greece

E. Dinant Kroese, Rijksinstituut voor Volksgezondheid en Milieuhygiene, Bilthoven, The Netherlands

E. Georg Luebeck, Fred Hutchinson Cancer Research Center, Seattle, USA

Ida Marcello, National Institute of Health, Rome, Italy

Eric Pluygers, Oncology Department, Jolimont Hospital (honorary), La Louvière, Belgium

Curtis Travis, Oak Ridge National Laboratories, Oak Ridge, USA

Gerasimos Voutsinas, National Centre for Scientific Research "Demokritus", Athens, Greece

Karen Watanabe, Tulane University Medical Center, New Orleans, USA

Werner Wosniok, Institute of Statistics, University of Bremen, Bremen, Germany

Giovanni A. Zapponi, National Institute of Health, Rome, Italy

Index